SEXUAL ENERGY ECSTASY

A Practical Guide to Lovemaking Secrets
of the East and West

David and Ellen Ramsdale

Illustrated by Allan Parker

BANTAM BOOKS
NEW YORK • TORONTO • LONDON • SYDNEY • AUCKLAND

This book has been written to provide information in regard to the subject matter covered. It is sold with the understanding that the publisher and authors are not engaged in rendering medical, psychological or other professional services. Therefore, if medical or other expert assistance is required, the services of a competent professional should be sought.

SEXUAL ENERGY ECSTASY
A Bantam Book / published by arrangement with the authors

PUBLISHING HISTORY
Peak Skill Publishing edition published 1985, 1991
Bantam edition / August 1993

Library of Congress Cataloging-in-Publication Data
Ramsdale, David Alan
Sexual energy ecstasy : a practical guide to lovemaking secrets of the East and West / David and Ellen Ramsdale ; illustrated by Allan Parker.
p. cm.
Includes bibliographical references and index.
ISBN 0-553-37231-9
1. Sex instruction. 2. Sexual intercourse. 3. Sensuality.
4. Tantrism. I. Ramsdale, Ellen. II. Parker, Allan.
III. Title.
[HQ31.R197 1993]
613.9′6—dc20   93-10329
CIP

Published simultaneously in the United States and Canada

Bantam Books are published by Bantam Books, a division of Bantam Doubleday Dell Publishing Group, Inc. Its trademark, consisting of the words "Bantam Books" and the portrayal of a rooster, is Registered in U.S. Patent and Trademark Office and in other countries. Marca Registrada. Bantam Books, 1540 Broadway, New York, New York 10036.

PRINTED IN THE UNITED STATES OF AMERICA
RRH   20 19 18 17 16 15 14 13 12

SEXUAL ENERGY ECSTASY

A Practical Guide to Lovemaking Secrets
of the East and West

David and Ellen Ramsdale

Illustrated by Allan Parker

BANTAM BOOKS

NEW YORK • TORONTO • LONDON • SYDNEY • AUCKLAND

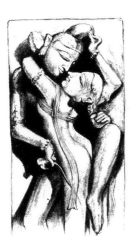

This book is dedicated to Divine Mother, whose beautiful embodiment is this Earth.

"By practice, even without understanding, it will be made plain; your body will understand it long before your mind puts words to it. No amount of understanding without practice will work. It is not necessary that knowledge precede experience. Performance will produce knowledge."
— Shiva, the Father of Tantra

CONTENTS

OPENING TO BLISS 11

Baby's Mind 13
The New Sexual Revolution 14
Sexual Energy Ecstasy 15
Supreme Ultimate (T'ai Chi) 18
Consort 21
Tantra 23
Honesty 25
Holistic Loving 26
Intimacy 27
Life Energy 28
Relax–Release 29
Tantric Orgasm 31
Sex 33
Sexual Freedom 35
Love Spot 36
Open The Door 38

READY FOR LOVE 39

Lifestyle 40
Sexy Bodymind 41
Attract Your Ideal Consort 41
Complete Breath 42
Deep Relaxation 46
Diet For Sexual Well-Being 54
Drugs And Sexual Performance 62
Energy Centers 63
Exercise For Sexual Well-Being 67
Hara 68
Herbs For Lovers 70
Meditation And Tantra 74
Orgasm And Energy 78
Pelvic Expression 84
Pleasure, Health And
The Anus 88
Pompoir Power 91
Safer Sex 94
Selfloving 95
Sexercises 101
Sexual Energy Recycling 118
Taoist Circle Of Gold 122
Technology For Lovers 126
Ultra-Intimacy 127

FOR PLAY 129

Harmony Signs 130
It's The Thought That Counters 132
Making Love Is A Touching
Experience 134
For Play 135
Aculoving 135
Aural Sex 142
Boudoir Basics 146
Charge Up 150
Do It Rite 152
Dream Lover 156
Educe Each Other 159
Energize Your Hands 163
Erotic Massage 163
Extended For Play 165
Good Times 167
Oriental Arousal 169
Pair Bonding And Tuning 171
Pleasuring The Lingam 177
Pleasuring The Yoni 184
Spreading 193

SWEPT AWAY 197

Conscious Conflict 198
The Art Of Erotic Awakening 199
Co-Inspiration 200
Complete Circuits 203
Elevate Energy 207
Focus 213
Full Stop 214
God And Goddess 216
Ground And Store Energy 219
Inspire Yourself 221
Love Tap 227
Make Love With Your Mind 228
Peaceful Positions 234
Soaking 236
Sound Sex 240
Stairway To Heaven 245
Stay Together 246
Tension Positions 248

CLIMAX 251

Where Do You Go? 252
Creative Sex 253
Peace Of Ass 255
Voluntary Creative Climax 256
Anger And Orgasm 256
Creative Orgasm 257
Grand Orgasm 264
Metasexual Orgasm 264
Peak Experience 265
Total Orgasm 266
Voluntary Orgasm For Men 268
Voluntary Orgasm For Women 282

NIGHTS OF TANTRA 293

Making Love Is A Model
For Living 294
Nights Of Tantra 295
Sleeping Together 299
Extrasensory Sex 302
Bio-Electric Sex 304
War And Peace 307
Magnetic Sex 311
Karezza 313
OTV–On The Verge 320
Tao Of Sex 324
Ragamaya Tantra 333
Slow Motion 339
Imsak 340
Fusion Breath Sex 346
Tantric Ritual Sex 354
Kabbazah Sex 358
Third Eye Sex 363

WAVE OF BLISS 365

Happiness Is Knowing You
Are Single 366
Endless Orgasm 366
Wave Of Bliss 369

APPENDIX 371

BIBLIOGRAPHY 373

INDEX 377

FOREWORD This book is a lovemaking guide of enormous practical value, and it properly belongs in the how-to sex manual genre. But you will not find quick relief recipes or tables of survey statistics, as useful as such information is. *Sexual Energy Ecstasy* not only offers sexual knowledge, it offers sexual wisdom as well.

The authors assume that Westerners are ready to learn from Tantric and Taoist traditions and other holistic sources. The skill with which they weave a tapestry of the old and new, of ancient Chinese Deer exercises and 1990s verbal affirmation techniques, may just make their assumption a reality. This unique sex therapist–massage therapist team, who are also husband and wife, has developed a pragmatic yet provocative holistic approach to enhancing the sexual experience for a culture that puts a higher premium on instant gratification than on well-earned satisfaction.

While many of the lovemaking styles and skills described herein will ask you to stop rushing after your "solitary crescendos," the authors are not purist advocates of deceleration per se. They would have us embrace the historical perspective embodied in the holistic lovemaking concept. They have presented us with a gracious gestalt of the sexual legacies of the world, including the little-known American sacred sexuality legacy, that we can understand and use and benefit from immediately.

Edmund Chein, M.D., J.D.

ACKNOWLEDGMENTS The authors would like to thank the following persons for their comments and suggestions: Alex Comfort, M.D., D. Sc., Arnold Cinman, M.D., Fred Kuyt, M.D., Andrew Lewin, M.D., Edmund Chein, M.D., J.D., Richard Moss, M.D., Lewis Durham, Ed.D., M.Th., William Hartman, Ph.D., Wayne Dyer, Ph.D., William Schutz, Ph.D., Jack Rosenberg, Ph.D., Paul Bindrim, Ph.D., Jack Kornfield, Ph.D., Kenneth Ray Stubbs, Ph.D., Steven Koenigsberg, Ph.D., Sage King, Ph.D., Brenda Morgan, Ph.D., Dr. Jonn Mumford, Randy Martin, Ph.D., O.M.D., C.A., Whitfield Reeves, C.A., Jonathan Robinson, M.A., M.F.C.C., Marty Klein, M.A., Joseph Giovannoni, M.A., M.S., Paulette Rochelle-Levy, M.A., M.F.C.C., Joani Blank, M.P.H., Barbara Roberts, L.C.S.W., Stephanie Wadel, M.A., Bryce Britton, M.S., Sedonia Cahill, M.A., Al Manning, C.P.A., D.D., Ven. Shinzen Young, Dio Urmilla Neff, Joe Vitale, Bill Hamilton, Dan Poynter, Dolores Winton, Irwin Zucker, Jack Frost, Jeff Labno, our parents and other friends, students and associates too numerous to mention. We would also like to thank Dr. Stephen Chang for permission to quote him, Charles Neighbors, Inc. for permission to quote Robert K. Moffett on the dedication verso page and pages 66 and 295, Steven Halpern Ph.D. and Terry Patten for contributing original material, Lee Perry for editorial services, Mike Jablonski for computer consultation and Cathy Riggs for design expertise.

Opening
To
Bliss

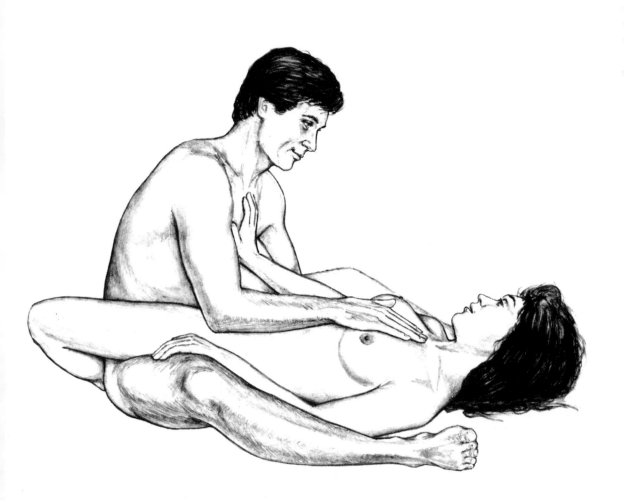

TO OUR READERS

This book is divided into more than one hundred highly concentrated sections full of valuable, practical information. While you can start here and read straight through, we also encourage you to skip to the sections that interest you most and immediately apply what you read. Do read *Opening To Bliss* first, though.

In order to help you find information in other parts of this book related to the topic you are reading, we have italicized the names of the relevant sections. Usually, we will say it like this: (see *Sexercises*). Of course, the titles of books (and a few other special words) are italicized, too.

Please enjoy this book. Use it often. It is our gift to you.

BABY'S MIND   *here is the secret:*

*forget everything
you ever learned about sex*

*from mom and dad
to Masters and Johnson
and everybody else
for
sexual maps are not the sexual territory*

*enjoy again
the baby's mind
not knowledgeable about sex
yet the body whole
one ecstatic organ*

*baby's mind
quiet and calm
yet full of life
like the meeting place
of
sand and sea
body and mind*

*set aside please
the familiar past
as much as you can*

*enjoy this adventure
of
baby's mind
in adult body*

Sexual Energy Ecstasy

THE NEW SEXUAL REVOLUTION

there is a new "sexual revolution"
authentic
spontaneous
natural
free to all

not in conflict with morality
immorality
itself

unanticipated
by those
in favor of
sex without love
or
love without sex

this
new sexual revolution
is
happening now

this evolutionary revolution
simply helps make
making love
a statement of fact

enjoy now
the new intimacy
"sexualove"

a vibrant blending of sexual energy
and love
in a marriage of happy intelligence

SEXUAL
ENERGY
ECSTASY

making love is all about
people
becoming naked

the nakedness
begins with the body
but
it doesn't have to
end with the body
only

we can enjoy
emotional nakedness
mental nakedness
nakedness of
our innermost essence

some people rush
their lovemaking

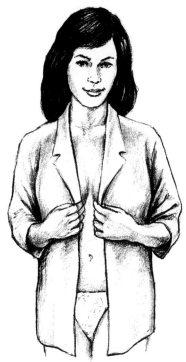

they prefer just
physical nakedness
with maybe
a few flashes
of naked feeling
here and there

some people
feel burdened
by the flesh

they long to soar
as souls
through the sky

listen

our bodies
are not the baggage . . .
our bodies are the ticket

for example
men and women report that
while making love
their bodies seem to
contract

expand
liquefy
shake
burn
glow
melt
merge

they say
they feel like they are flying
they feel two people become one
they see brilliant colors
they feel like king and queen, noble and royal
they feel really "high"—naturally
some even say
they disappear for awhile

in other words
they experience that
making love
expands
their consciousness

these people were not on drugs
they were on sex

Sexual Energy Ecstasy
is a very safe
fantastic
natural high

sexual energy
is not a special or unique energy
in fact
sexual energy
is the energy of life
expressing itself
in sex

that is all

while you make love
you experience
this energy of life
quite intensely

while you make love
you feel more alive
while you make love
you ARE more alive

though we claim
our society is "sexually liberated"
sex and love
are still divorced

people feel a great sadness in their hearts

the revolutionary union
of sex and love
starts in your bedroom

it will be so beautiful

peace will smile
in the eyes of all of us

heaven and earth
will be in accord

MAKE LOVE, NOT WAR

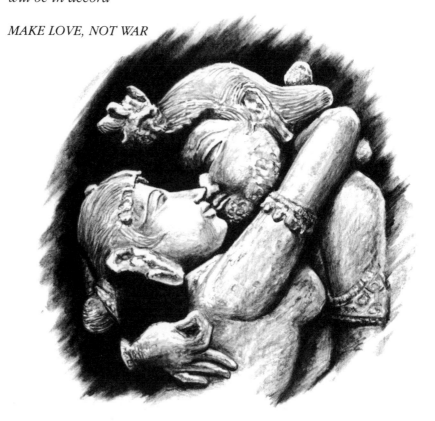

MAITHUNA *right*
Khajuraho, 11th century.
His right hand is in the
energy recycling gesture
Gyana Mudra ("OK" sign).

SUPREME ULTIMATE (T'AI CHI)

here is the sexual secret of the T'ai Chi symbol:

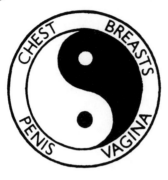

*man juts out
or projects
from the bottom*

*woman juts out
or projects
from the top*

*a man's projection
is called
penis*

*a woman's projection
is called
breasts*

*a man draws in
or introjects
from the top*

*a woman draws in
or introjects
from the bottom*

T'AI CHI *above*
Each contains the seed of the other. Symbol of dynamic change within wholeness, it holds the secrets of life and love.

*a man's introjection
has no official name
in our society
a woman's introjection
is called
vagina*

T'ai Chi
reveals the complete secret
of ultimate sexual intimacy:

penis penetrates vagina
and
breasts penetrate chest

this is the mystery
of the second penetration

projection and introjection
must fuse
at both points of contact

two keys will enter
two locks
and open them

the first lock
is well known:
vagina

the second lock
is not well known

the second lock
is the mysterious place
located
in the treasure chests
of both sexes

here is the palace of joy
the heart
the feeling center
the psychic core
the soul
the inner radiance
the essence of
the person
this precious place
we call
the Love Spot

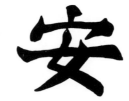

the key to the first lock
is well known: penis

what is the key to the second lock?

when the connections
above and below
are fused
a completed circuit
is created which takes the shape
of a luminous circle (or sphere)

we have felt and seen
this radiant circle (sphere)
and so have friends of ours

you may see and feel it too
there are many possible signs
such as an all-consuming joy

this great circle is T'ai Chi
the sexual super battery

the experience of
ultra-intimacy

relax
become the depth
you will be filled

you will be
T'ai Chi

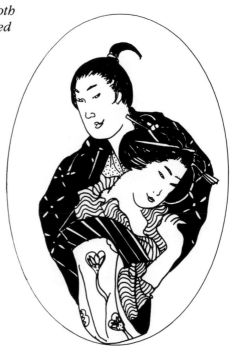

CONSORT   *god and goddess*
play, or consort, together
in a realm made heavenly
by the harmony of their interpersonal relations

in English translations of many Eastern texts
the sexual partner lover wife husband
the intimate associate of a god or goddess
is called a consort

to consort is to unite

the dreariness of daytime duties is dissolved
by the ten thousand bodies and faces seen
in the twilight theater of uninhibited loving

your most loving gift to each other
is to forget who you are
names faces ages beliefs histories
leave your driver's license identities
in your purse and wallet

husband and wife are often the worst offenders
love and ecstasy do not spring
from knowing another well
but from not knowing each other at all
from consorting
without constricting
from revealing nakedness
not from insulating
the soft feeling touching secret skin
in short-sighted certainties

sustain the enchantment
be forever mystified

slyly merge the thrill of meeting
the mysterious stranger
with depth of trust
developed over time

this is real sex magic

in the faces of the gods and goddesses
united beyond sadness
in the statues and pictures you will see

they are blissful with wise innocence

when you look into the eyes of your sexualover
your consort
on some wonderful day
just after making love
or just before
say these or similar words
out loud or silently
with feeling in your heart

my sexualover
my consort
you are the mystery
you are the secrets
you are
the beginning and the end
and most important of all
you are me

even if our bodyminds
never touch again
I have touched eternity
through you

by making use
of the friendly valuable gift
of your bodymind
I have understood
that eternity is my only companion
my one true consort

so I insist
we are consorts
we are god and goddess
and nothing less

CLOUDS AND RAIN *right*
After a woodblock print
by Shunchosai. Japan,
18th cent ury A.D.

TANTRA   *Tantra is about love*

not "souped-up nookie"

it is not techniques of
breathing
visualizing
positioning

Tantra says
deep inside you are already free
you are already unblocked
you are already radiant
you are the beginning and ending
you are the source
you are the earth
you are the sun and the moon
you are the universe

so relax

do whatever you want

only do not knowingly
harm another

there is no god or goddess
other than your true Self

Tantra says
what is not here
is not anywhere

Tantra says
enjoy
what is here

below the superficial self
lies an inner darkness
the negative self-image
we avoid yet protect

there in hidden chambers
we judge ourselves
just as
we have judged others

Tantra says
get to know
this image

Tantra says
let go
of this image

it is not
what it seems

it is not
worth the trouble

it is not
you

Tantra says
love and forgive
all your images
of self and other

be free of imagery

be free
to be

enjoy the feeling
of just being

Tantra
is the art of
unblocked feeling
the natural way of
radiance

Tantra is about you
the real you
the you
you already are
that cannot be added to
or diminished
or changed
or improved
Tantra is about
your true shining Self:

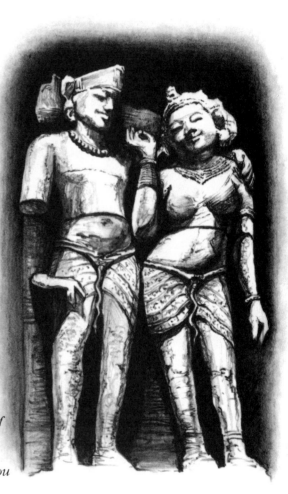

TANTRIC LOVERS *right*
Raja Rani Temple, 11th
century, Bhuvanesvar,
Orissa, India.

always happy
forever free
completely content

relax
be aware
you are
already there

HONESTY *when our bodies make love*
emotions and minds
and innermost we
make love too

ideally
all of me is naked
with my consort

emotions and mind
innermost me
as well as
this precious flesh

honesty in thought, word and action
apart from lovemaking
is lovemaking, too

during sexualove
doing Tantra
emotional garbage will appear

it is a by-product of opening
the door
to the heart

my pain and anger and fear and doubt
will confront me
in my quest for the heart of gold

good
better sooner than later . . .
better now than then . . .
better from making love

HOLISTIC LOVING

holistic, wholistic:
whole

the whole of lovemaking
includes both
hard and soft
yang and yin
ways
to make love

hard style lovemaking
is more familiar to most of us

it makes excellent use of abilities
like setting and achieving goals

soft style lovemaking
is new to many of us

it makes excellent use of abilities
like feeling and intuiting

information about hard style
is easy to get
in our time and place
(Masters and Johnson)

information about soft style
is not so easy to get

soft does not mean weak
soft is simply
the complement to
balance for
and opposite of
hard

this book is about soft, yin style lovemaking
including Tantric lovemaking
and
hard, yang style lovemaking
with a soft touch

INTIMACY   *Our word intimacy*
has its roots
in a Latin word
that meant
"innermost"

people make love in order to

reproduce
relieve sexual tensions
experience pleasure
strengthen interpersonal bonds
enjoy a different state
of consciousness
(such as orgasm)
and so on

why do you make love?

what would the
ultimate experience
of sexual intimacy
be like for you?

this book describes
some great ways
to experience
intimacy
while making love

new ways
(soft ways)
to reach the
innermost place
the heart or core
of your consort
and
of yourself

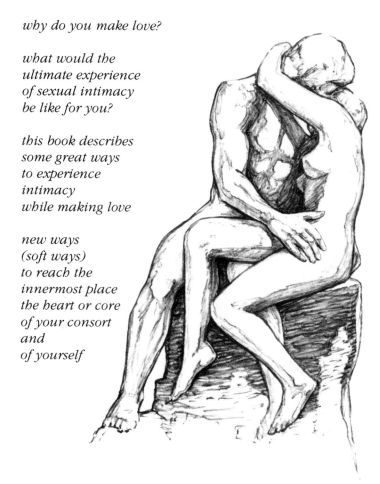

LIFE ENERGY

*life energy is simply that energy which, though invisible to
the ordinary eye, makes the difference between a corpse
and a living, breathing, animated person*

*life energy is that which vitalizes or gives life
life energy is not yet a fact of conventional science*

*as artists of sexualove, we don't have to wait for the
scientific proof*

*as compassionate life-giving lovers, we can make love
AS IF life energy were a fact of love (if not of life), and give
and receive and share and otherwise fully feast upon a
banquet of life energy over and over again with our
consorts*

*this concept of a life energy dimension to lovemaking
opens the door to a wonderful new world*

*life energy is a concept
that stimulates imagination, creativity, sensitivity
it is not necessary to believe in it*

*if life energy becomes a part of your direct experience,
fine*

if not, fine

to act or play AS IF is plenty good enough

*change nothing
simply allow for the possibility of something flowing to and
through and around and within and between you and
your consort as you make love, something which has the
essence of magic in it*

make room for miracles

RELAX–RELEASE   *relief is different from release*

when I relieve myself
I am dumping
discarding
discharging
what I choose
not to contain

during lovemaking
a charge
is built up

it is not easy for me
to hold a lot of charge
when I'm very tense
because the increase in charge
increases the feeling of tension

release
on the other hand
is the letting go
of tension
without a loss of charge

I can choose to make love
in a relaxed way
or in a tense way

what I do when I make love
whether it's soft or hard
yin or yang
is not nearly as important
as how
I do what I do

there's a lot of emphasis nowadays
on building up sexual tension

just to get the rush of relief
that may follow

take the peak
quickly
then jump off
it's a fast ride down

*today's hard styles
encourage this response*

*soft styles
on the other hand
encourage relaxation
and release
I can choose to*

*stay at the peak or in the valley
stay where I am and be filled by that*

*soft styles
are especially handy
for learning
to relax during lovemaking
and hold more charge*

*even so
one's not better
than the other*

*we find that
a balance is beautiful*

*we like
both hard and soft
tension and relaxation
relief and release*

*frankly
what we like
most of all
is having the choice*

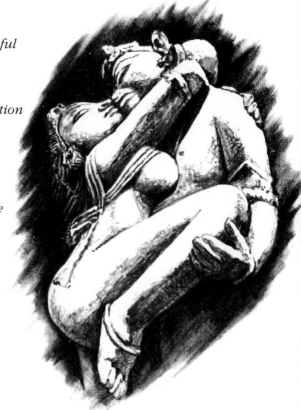

MAITHUNA *right*
Devi Jagadamba
Temple, Khajuraho,
India, 11th century.

TANTRIC ORGASM

*when somebody asked you
"Did you orgasm?"
after making love
how did you answer it?*

you are an individual

*orgasm
refers to quite a few
possible experiences
even for one person . . . you*

*for example
it is well known that
some men and women
who do not experience scientifically verifiable
physical orgasmic release
may still experience an exquisite release
of a different kind
an emotional climax*

*just as there are so many different ways
that people have the familiar kinds of orgasms
there are lots of wonderful things
that can happen during lovemaking
for which there are no names
in the English language*

*there is an enchanting uncharted world
in there (out there?)*

*where you go
what you see and feel
is unique to you
though you will share experiences in common
with others*

*here's the plan: relax totally
during lovemaking
(and we mean totally)
body and mind
and see where that takes you*

*moving or motionless
relaxation is total
you are the river*

*of clear light
that flows
to the endless shining sea*

*effortless release
the way of royalty*

*when you really relax
while making love
and don't make the usual orgasm your goal
you become available
to a grand new brand of
sexual peak experiences*

*experiences like these may happen
without making any special efforts to relax
there are many, many ways
but relaxation is a very reliable approach*

*the relaxation strategy enables you
to have these experiences
again and again*

perhaps you have experienced such climaxes

*if you have
you know
how elegant and beautiful
this whole new range of sexual opportunities is*

*in other words
there are other kinds of orgasms or climaxes
not yet the subject of scientific investigation*

*they are not just a head trip
or somebody's fantasy*

*they are as substantial and real as
the orgasms studied in laboratories today
only different, of course*

*their main features are the feeling of unity
between you and your lover
that lasts and lasts
the rushes of powerful energies and wonderful feelings
the expansion and elevation of awareness*

some people describe it as "holy" or "sacred"
however
oneness can take many forms
and be of different degrees and qualities and duration

energy can flow in all directions
in many ways
with multiple effects

the good feelings can be of various kinds
and intensities and tones

the change in awareness will be drawn from the limitless
array of possiblities

these are the orgasms or climaxes of complete relaxation
(they may occur with conventional orgasms, too)

known in Tantra as Tantric Orgasm

SEX   *the emphasis on sex*
in our society
whether sex is put
in a negative light
or a positive light
is an attempt to fill a vast emptiness

in their heart of hearts
what people really want
is
unconditional love

the ultimate interpersonal gift

sex is a gift too
but the wrapping
makes all the difference

when the gift of sex
is wrapped in love
where is this problem of sex?

what can sex solve then?
the healing power of sex
is love in action

sex is
neither question nor answer
but magnificent gift
akin to the great gift of life itself

the emphasis on sex is by default
when the door to the heart is rusted shut
from lack of use
people are stuck in the basement

in spite of what people say
giving and receiving and being
unconditional love
is it

people look and look and look and look and
when they find themselves
they find unconditional love also
everywhere they look

the image of sex
which before was furtively molded
to meet their needs
they will now see
with clarity
is their own face

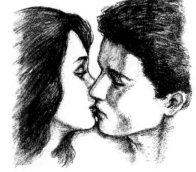

sex is beautiful
but its beauty is drawn
from the same source
as sunrise and sunset
flowers and fire
ocean and mountain
birth and death

sex can take me to that source
but I must forget to use sex
and let sex use me

I must forget to think sex
and let sex embody me

I must forget to hold onto sex
and let sex embrace me

for sex is none other than life itself

"good sex" is one thing

leaving the raft of thought
and diving into a pure ocean of sensation
swimming in a sea of self-loss
is quite another

many centuries ago
Western civilization took a wrong turn

sex was such a convenient scapegoat
it is considered so difficult to feel love
so easy to feel sex
now is the time to get back on the road
that leads to happiness

the fate of our Mother
is in our hands

by suppressing the sex urge
and denying its power to express love
violence is created

anti-sex is anti-life and anti-Earth

let us be sex-positive
and love unconditionally
the miraculous process
that gave us our birth
on this beautiful blue
planet of love

peace will prevail
once again

SEXUAL   *one person's sexual freedom*
FREEDOM *is another person's*
         sexual prison

one person's sexual truth
is another person's
lie

puritan organizations sell "No On Sex!"
pornographer businesses sell "Yes On Sex!"

they would both like us to think
that we will discover our sexual integrity
by listening to them and buying their products
neither is right
only love is right

SEXSEXSEXSEXSEXSEX
is
the primary creative urge at play

it cannot be legislated
it cannot be controlled
it cannot be sold

what is for sale
is only sadness

do not be fooled
true sexual freedom is not for sale anywhere
yet honest vulnerable consorts enjoy it for free

THE LOVE SPOT   *In this society the focus is so great upon the genitals that a balancing focus is needed, the Love Spot or heart center.*

The specific gland that corresponds to the Love Spot is the thymus, which is located a little higher than the Love Spot location at the center of the breastbone. This gland can be activated by thumping it with the fist (see Love Tap*). The thymus plays a vital role in our bodymind's self-defense system. It helps maintain and distribute physical energy. It is the glandular equivalent of "I love myself."*

The Love Spot corresponds to the danchu acupuncture point. It also corresponds to the anahata heart chakra of yoga (see Energy Centers*).*

The Love Spot is simply a door into a much larger room. This heart door swings open easily. Only a gentle push is needed. The Love Spot is connected to the spine. Have a friend place the palm of one hand over your Love Spot and the palm of the other hand over the spine directly behind it. You may be able to feel the flow between these two special points.

This much larger room into which the Love Spot opens is sometimes referred to as the heart space. Mystics who explored it thoroughly found it was so vast that they described it as being limitless. According to their reports, a brilliant light fills this vastness with warmth and joy.

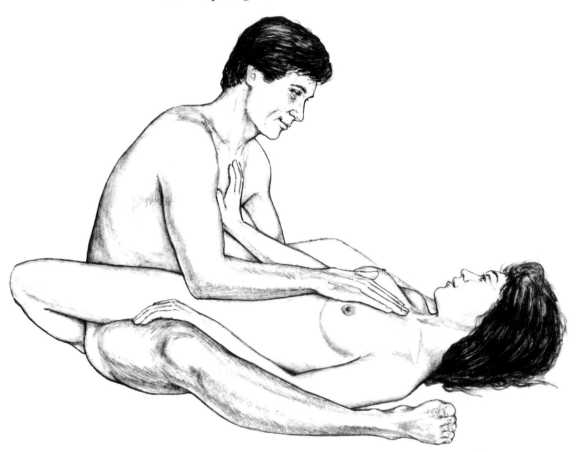

THE LOVE SPOT *above*
Keep the pressure gentle.
Speak through your hand
without moving it.

*Visualized, the Love Spot is really more like a Love Cave.
Here is the core of our ability to deeply feel. On the surface
are felt the more inconsequential emotions, whether they are
positive, negative or neutral in content. Deep within the
chest are somehow felt the soul emotions, the deep personal
and interpersonal feelings that shake and move and bind
sincere consorts.*

*Not everyone feels this place or core to this extent. Evi-
dently, some people hardly feel it at all. You may be able to
feel it extending back to the spine or, starting from the other
end of the Love Cave, from the spine to the chest.*

*The renowned Hindu sage Ramana Maharshi noted that
when a person wants to identify themselves, they point to
their chest. Try this as an experiment or just observe yourself
in a social situation. During profound energy intimacy
unusually sweet, noble, inspiring emotions may rise inward
and upward from the chest. Tears may appear.*

*These are signs that your Love Spot has been activated
through your lovemaking. There are many such signs. Posi-*

tive changes in your life are the surest sign of Love Spot activation.

It helps to have a specific area of the bodymind to refer to when talking about feelings of love. We talk about thinking from the head and desiring from the genitals. It seems equally sensible to talk about love from the heart and to give this love activity an equally specific location.

The ancient experts taught that to bring feeling and energy up to the Love Spot and open the heart, or deep feeling center, is the big challenge. Once this is learned, energy can be directed throughout the bodymind, including the glands and the psychic centers in and above the head.

What is the difference between making love and having sex? If your Love Spot is stimulated, you are making love. If your Love Spot is not stimulated, if your energy, feelings and attention stay below the belt, you are having sex.

You can send love energy from your Love Spot to your consort at will. Try it. The more relaxed you are, the easier it will be. This skill is especially rewarding shared as a prelude to making love (see Pair Bonding And Tuning*).*

To feel, to breathe and to be in the present is enough to fully activate the Love Spot. Yet to do just this may prove more difficult than any other style or skill presented in this book. By working with these styles and skills, though, you will find it much easier to just simply make love.

Free of distracting thoughts or disturbing emotions, you enjoy a fusion of ecstasy and light as you become the primal god/goddess and face the original mind. Developing this ability to just be is a major act of power that will so clearly benefit your life in every area you will be amazed.

OPEN THE DOOR   *Sex is not what you think. In fact, you do not know what sex is. We don't know either. Sex is beyond the mind.*

When sex is good, you say "I lost my mind!"

Losing your mind in this way is wonderful. Don't you agree? But soon it is over.

Good sex shows you that you are happy and free when you let go of your mind. But good sex is not enough. Even great sex with deep love is not enough. Even that is not the ultimate, intimate sexual experience.

In sex is hidden a door to infinity. Open it.

Ready
For
Love

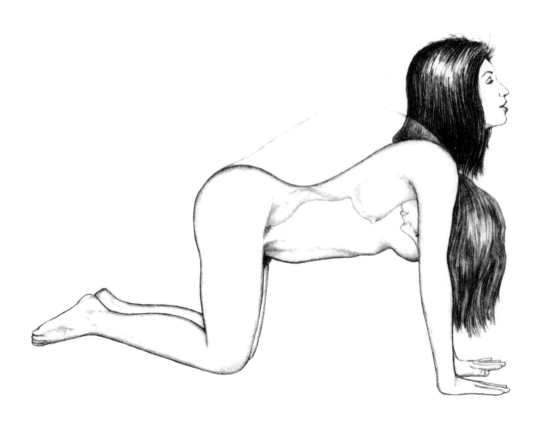

LIFESTYLE *lifestyle, lovestyle, mindstyle*
are the same apple
viewed from different angles

slice the apple
you destroy the apple

an apple is a unity
you are a unity

eat wholesome food
exercise
take time to relax
and clear the mind

be aware of the possible side effects
of any drugs you are taking
prescription drugs included

if your personal energy
is not strong and clear
your sex life won't be
strong and clear either

if you're under lots of stress
this too may negatively affect
your sexual functioning

you can learn tricks
to attract a consort

take the time instead
to learn to love

a true consort
will fall at your feet

you will be a natural sex magnet
of the finest kind

SEXY BODYMIND

What is a sexy bodymind? A whole bodymind is a sexy bodymind. A bodymind that is bursting with life and emotional warmth has an automatic sex appeal, a wholesome sex magnetism. Such a bodymind is not just a sex magnet. It is a life, love and happiness magnet, too.

Attitude is the mysterious catalyst that will bring it all together for you. How you feel about yourself in your heart of hearts, more than anything else, makes you a sexual dud or a sexy body that turns heads or, ideally, a fully magnetic bodymind that attracts life's blessings, including the sweetness of sexual contentment.

Sexual fulfillment is a synergy, a complex combination of many factors. A healthy, relaxed bodymind, a surplus of personal energy and a positive mental attitude are the most important ingredients.

ATTRACT YOUR IDEAL CONSORT

What is the secret to attracting the ideal consort? How can you find that person who is just right for you physically, emotionally, mentally and spiritually? Does this person even exist?

Every relationship is a mirror and, if you are very sincere, a door as well. The best way to attract your ideal consort is to grow as a person and deepen your relationship with yourself. Find new ways to give to and be with other people. Like attracts like.

If you begin to take an assertive role in your community by doing work that reduces the suffering of others, your being is suffused with the highest sort of magnetism. Beautiful people will be drawn into your life and the chances of finding an ideal consort for practicing High Romance or Tantra (sexual mysticism) is greatly increased.

Here is our plan for attracting your ideal consort. This plan will increase your personal magnetism in the most positive way.

○ Begin to do some kind of growth work on yourself every day, i.e., yoga, meditation, journal writing, bodywork, men's or women's groups. There are many options. The key is to begin working through your emotional blocks. Explore forgiveness and unconditional love (for yourself as well as others) as a realistic choice in your life.

○ Do this to grow as a human being as well as a way to meet people. In fact, your motivation determines the outcome. If you're doing this just to have sex, others will detect this and be turned off. If you do it to grow, it will show.

○ Do exercises to energize your genitals and pelvic region.

○ Begin to get involved in actively helping to reduce the suffering in the world. Volunteer at least two hours a week to some group or organization or individual that is doing something you really believe in. If you cannot find time to reach out to others in some way, how can you expect others to reach out to you?

○ At some point, be willing to become extremely visible as a representative of something positive and beneficial. For example, we met while David was giving a lecture on astrology at the Sivananda Yoga Center in Los Angeles. Of course, you don't have to go into public speaking. The idea is that you are now making the step of communicating to others the value of service.

The inevitable outcome of these noble activities is that you will become a dynamic, happy, magnetic human being. In order to attract and keep in your life a dynamic, happy, magnetic consort, you must be such a person yourself.

Don't worry about how long this process takes. If you take on this plan in earnest, your life will soon have so much richness in it that you will no longer be concerned about finding the right person. You will be content in knowing that you are becoming the right person. The person that was missing from your life all along was you.

COMPLETE BREATH

Human beings have a natural way to breathe that is complete, beautiful and instinctive. To see this natural breath in action, watch a healthy naked baby.

People seem to fall into two categories: chest-breathers and belly-breathers. Chest-breathers are more self-assertive but less grounded. Belly-breathers are more grounded but need to assert self more. The balance, obviously, is found in breathing completely from both chest and belly. In the complete breath and other breath training methods, the upper lobes and the back of the lungs are also accessed.

Both men and women tend to hold their breath during lovemaking. When this is intentional, such as during semen stopping or in *Tension Positions,* it is rewarding. Holding the breath before or during orgasm can also be done on purpose, intensifying or otherwise altering your orgasm experience.

Unintentional holding of the breath is very frequently an unwelcome expression of tension. The basic remedy is simply to remember to breathe completely and deeply. This may prove surprisingly difficult to do as the old habits are often very set.

The complete breath consists of four natural stages: inhalation, retention, exhalation and pause. The art of working with these stages is highly developed in the Taoist and hatha yoga schools. Still, it all begins with learning the complete breath which, though it may seem strange at first, quickly feels much more natural than the old way.

Whole schools of psychotherapy and self-improvement have developed around the power of complete breathing and its many variations. For example, negative emotional states, such as anxiety or depression, are often symptoms of low energy. You do not, in effect, have enough octane in your fuel mix. If, at such a time, you make the effort to do some dedicated deep complete breathing, you may find that your symptoms diminish or even vanish.

It is a classic observation in psychotherapy that people withhold the breath in order to avoid feeling pain. They are then literally using shallow breathing as an anesthetic. This is maladaptive, however, as you quickly discover when you set out to enjoy a potentially ecstatic situation like lovemaking and find that pleasure and deep satisfaction evade you. Even so, we prefer the natural, easy way of discovering the breath as it is rather than trying to change it.

Easy Complete
Breath

sit erect
but comfortable

hands on your hips or in your lap

close your eyes
breathe through your nose
relax

now consciously draw the breath
deeply
so that it scrapes the back of your throat
and flows down against your spine

let it go all the way down
till it can't go any further
and it naturally flows upward
into your lower belly and navel

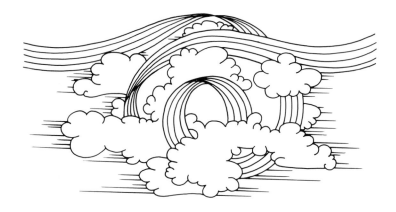

when your belly is comfortably full
let the air rise
and expand your ribs
and let the chest rise
if your shoulders rise a little
that's OK . . . but only a little
you are now
full of air

you filled yourself
from bottom to top
from belly to chest
now empty yourself
from top to bottom
from chest to belly

compress the chest firmly
as if an invisible hand
pressed upon its center
(use your own hand at first if it helps)

you may have been holding
the shoulders up
let them down if you were
exhale very slowly, very gently
no need to rush
you breathe 21,600 times a day

WINDS *above*
The life force is like
the wind. The breath
is the easiest way to
work with its energy.

your belly deflates
automatically

you have just completed one complete breath

You can do the complete breath lying on your back, too. Practice this process just a few minutes a day. The above instructions can be read aloud to you by a friend. Or you can record them on tape.

The best time for breath training is early morning. You will avoid the bulk of the air pollution. Do complete breathing as soon as you get out of bed or even in bed before getting up if you prefer. If you become dizzy while doing this or any other breathing process, stop.

Exhalation is more important than inhalation. If exhalation is complete and deep, inhalation will take place automatically. Exhalation, which helps remove toxins and stale air from the lungs, tends to be neglected. When instructed to breathe more deeply, many people just inhale deeper. A major secret of breath development is to emphasize the length and strength of the exhalation.

A concern of some people about the complete breath is that they will develop a pot belly. This is easily avoided. The following refinement of the complete breath should be practiced after you are beyond the early beginning stage: when you are retaining the breath, pull the lower part of the belly (at the *Hara* point below the navel) in and hold. Done properly, you will feel a strong sense of power and control. This added step is said to benefit the adrenal glands.

By practicing the complete breath just a few minutes a day for a few weeks, you will become aware of your current breathing habits. It would be useful for you to know, for example, that you tend to prevent the breath from being full and complete by tightening your belly during the inhalation.

Many people have this habit. A new awareness like this can enrich your lovemaking in unexpected ways.

Alternate nostril breathing *(nadi shodhana pranayama)* from yoga is a good preparation for lovemaking. Swami Vivekananda of the Bihar School of Yoga in India states that five minutes of alternate nostril breathing balances the hemispheres of the brain, calming the emotions as well as improving mental functioning.

Breathing through just the left nostril for five minutes or less creates a right brain dominant condition ideal for sensitive lovemaking. He reports that this has been verified by brain wave tests.

Alternate nostril breathing is easy. Place the middle and index fingers of your right hand on the forehead. Close off the right nostril with the thumb.

Inhale easily through the left nostril. Close both nostrils using the thumb and the fourth finger. Now lift the thumb but keep the left nostril closed with the fourth finger and exhale gently through the right nostril.

Inhale serenely through the right nostril. Close off both nostrils. Now lift the fourth finger but keep the right nostril closed with the thumb and exhale calmly through the left nostril.

You have completed one cycle. To breathe through the left nostril continuously keep the right nostril closed off with the thumb.

Repeat for up to but no longer than five minutes. If you feel dizzy, discontinue immediately. Alternate nostril and left nostril only breathing are powerful. Start off with just a minute or two and gradually build up to five minutes.

Yogis teach that this process purifies the nervous system. If you wish to go more deeply into these techniques, please get individualized instruction from a certified yoga teacher with experience teaching breath techniques *(pranayama)*.

DEEP RELAXATION

The delights of deep relaxation just before, during or after lovemaking are so incredible that it is like entering another world. The combination of deep relaxation and lovemaking not only makes sex better, it liberates the hidden potential in lovemaking that consorts often sense but rarely tap.

It may be hard to believe that such a new wonder world is only twenty minutes away, the time it takes to go through a basic deep relaxation routine. But it is. How can such a simple act as a few minutes of strategic relaxation make such a difference?

There is an inner compulsive drive in most people that rushes them past the present in a whir of nearsighted concerns. They run through life's precious moments as if the reward for existence could only be found at the end of the race. Like a vacuum cleaner gone berserk, they swallow whatever is in their path without tasting it. Is it any wonder that the modern adult is referred to as a consumer?

The popularity of fast food restaurants testifies to this stampede for instant gratification. Food and sex habits are intimately linked. Contemporary bedroom strategies reflect this connection. Modern lovers leap into bed and grab for the gusto as if their bedroom was a fast sex restaurant and their lover an instant orgasm burger in a plain white sack.

When you take the time to deeply relax, you effectively short-circuit this compulsive drive to rush through your experiences. As you do so again and again, the stranglehold on your senses loosens up more and more. Blind compulsion is replaced by wide-eyed appreciation. Your life, your love life included, is changed for the better forever.

There are many, many deep relaxation methods. These include yoga, the relaxation response, meditation, prayer, massage, self-hypnosis, breath work, biofeedback, progressive relaxation, autogenic training, floating in tanks and the Copper BioCircuit™ (see *Technology For Lovers*).

Many people find audio cassette programs helpful. *Experience Yoga Nidra* is a guided deep relaxation and meditation experience combining an ancient Tantra yoga method taught by Swami Janakananda with music by Roop Verma. This highly effective technique is a very powerful induction into altered states of consciousness that is also an excellent preparation for Tantric lovemaking.

Find an approach that works for you and stick with it. Do it every day. In this way you establish a relaxation baseline that will help you significantly with stress reduction. Excess stress, of course, can greatly inhibit relationships as well as sexual performance and enjoyment.

Resting inside a flotation tank, for example, effortlessly results in a state of deep physical relaxation and mental clarity that you may find ideal for lovemaking. Research at the Medical College of Ohio reveals that endorphins, the organic opiates in the brain, are released during floating to create an euphoric effect. As no special training is required, you can make use of this holistic technology breakthrough right now. While flotation tanks can be purchased, there are centers in major cities where tank time can be rented. In our experience, flotation tanks really do work. A practical hint— see your consort immediately after floating. That is when your natural high will be at its peak.

Relaxation And Meditation

Deep relaxation and deep meditation are not the same thing. Deep relaxation develops calmness, a prerequisite for deep meditation. This calmness makes it possible to see things more clearly.

In deep meditation, this clarity aspect is encouraged to develop as well. As the waves of the mind ocean become still, we are able to see clear to the bottom and retrieve the treasures hidden there.

This combination of calmness and clarity releases deep personal resources in a useful way. People who meditate regularly can experience an enormous acceleration in their personal growth, effectiveness and sense of well-being. Just as there are many ways of achieving deep relaxation, there are many ways to meditate (see *Appendix*). The key is to find something that works for you and stick with it.

Our favorite basic ways to relax and meditate are as follows. Allow about twenty minutes per process.

Simple Deep   *lie on your back on a rug or blanket*
Relaxation   *with your eyes closed*

your arms comfortably away from your body
your hands palms up

your legs spread comfortably apart
your feet angle outwards from the heels

if you can do so comfortably
keep the small of your back against the floor
if not
that's OK
(you can try placing some padding underneath
to see if you like the feeling of support there)

breathe through your nose
slowly and gently
do this for a few minutes

simply be aware of the passing of air
in and out of the nostrils
nothing more

if thoughts distract you
allow them to be
and return to the breath

they will leave when they see
you are not interested in them

now
feel the weight of your body
feel the pull of gravity
surrender to it
give in to gravity

take plenty of time to do this
to surrender to gravity

it is a beautiful experience

it reconnects you with the earth

now
feel your contact with the ground
become aware of this contact exactly
between the ground and you

from the edge of your heels
to the back of your head
and every place in between
slowly discover

take plenty of time to do this

you may never have felt how the ground
supports you
feel the heaviness of your body
again

you are sinking
sinking
sinking
into the ground
it is a wonderful feeling

the ground
the earth
is caring for you

the Great Mother
holds you in the palm
of her loving hand

let go of your concerns
you have nothing to do
but lie here
nestled in her palm
let go
enjoy this feeling of being
totally and effortlessly supported

though your body is heavy
you may feel as if you are floating

this is normal
this is natural

now that you have let go
of your concerns
you are light

this ends
the simple deep relaxation

Another way to achieve deep relaxation is to tense the muscles of the body to a count of three and then relax them. Muscle groups can be tensed separately, starting with the muscles of the feet and going up to the neck. Or they can be tensed simultaneously. If you have time, do both and end by tensing the whole body at once.

Hold the breath while tensing. Exhale while releasing and relaxing.

Take in a comfortable amount of breath, such as half your usual capacity. Avoid straining. This is not a contest.

After releasing the tension in each muscle group, reinforce the relaxation by affirming it. For example, after tensing and releasing your left foot, say "My left foot is relaxed, my left foot is relaxed, my left foot is relaxed. My left foot is now completely relaxed."

You can perform this total tension technique as soon as you lie down and then proceed with simple deep relaxation for maximum results. Whole body tensing by itself is a quick and convenient substitute. It can be very handy on those occasions when you need to relax and energize, but are unable to lie down or take the time to do the longer versions.

Simple Meditation   *sit with your spine straight*
in any way that is comfortable for you

if you sit in a chair
place your feet flat on the floor
do not cross them

place your hands on your thighs or knees
in a comfortable way

palms up
palms down
in a little cup
clasped together
interlaced
whatever is comfortable
will be right

the chin tends to float up
so tuck it down and in slightly
but only slightly

now begin to breathe through your nose
slowly and gently

simply be aware of the passing
of air
in and out of the nostrils

nothing more

if thoughts distract you
allow them to be
and return to the breath

they will leave when they see
you are not interested in them

simply be aware of the sensation
of air passing
in and out of the nostrils
nothing more

return gently
to this physical sensation
again

there is no need to change
the way you breathe

to be aware of the breath
as it is
is enough

there is nothing
to interpret
or figure out

nothing is happening
except the breath
and it happens by itself
there is only
this physical sensation
of the air

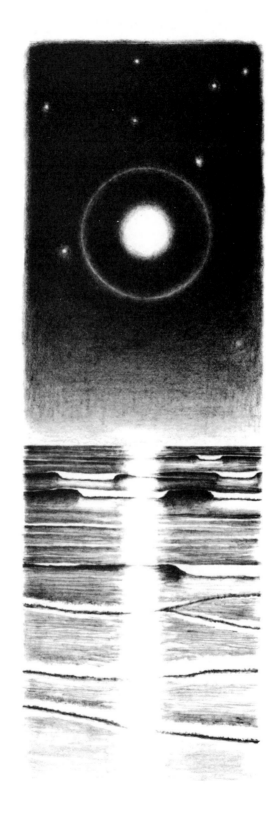

passing in and out
of your nostrils

in this moment
and this moment
and this moment

gently return
to this physical sensation
as often as needed

be kind
to yourself
when you stray
from the breath

the breath
doesn't mind

just return
come home
to the breath
you will be welcome

simply be aware
of the sensation
of air passing
in and out of the nostrils
nothing more

return gently
to this physical sensation again

there is no need to change
the way you breathe

to be aware of the breath
as it is
is enough

this ends
the simple meditation
on the breath

MOON OVER WATER
opposite
When the mind is quiet,
it is like a reflection of
the moon in still water,
there and yet not there.

Come back to the everyday world slowly. Your senses will
be wide open. Enjoy the priceless, private luxury of relaxation.

If you find it difficult to keep your attention focused on the breath, try this technique a friend of ours used on a meditation retreat. She visualized a giant arrow with the words "You are here!" inscribed on it, not unlike an eye-catching billboard. The arrow pointed right at her nostrils.

These processes can be read out loud slowly by a friend as you do them. You can put them on tape yourself. Or just absorb the gist of the instructions, referring to them before or after a relaxation or meditation session.

DIET FOR SEXUAL WELL-BEING

No holistic approach to the art of making love would be complete that did not take diet into account. Since we are each biochemically unique, there is no one set plan of diet and supplementation for everybody. Each must work out his or her own optimum nutritional program for personal and sexual well-being.

Be sure to consult with your physician—nutritionally-oriented, if at all possible—regarding any and all changes in sexual activities, diet and supplementation that you may want to make. There is evidence that many sexual difficulties respond to improved nutrition (see *Appendix*).

Garbage In— Garbage Out

Eat fresh wholesome foods. Eat to live. Don't live to eat. Sugar, salt, saturated fat and chemical food additives in the quantities found in the average American diet can impair your sexual performance and enjoyment. Minimize your red meat, preserved meat and smoked meat consumption, as these are known to contain toxins, stress the liver and contribute to high blood pressure, reducing sexual well-being.

Chronic sugar overindulgence can lead to hypoglycemia or diabetes, both of which can interfere with sexual functioning. A person with hypoglycemia (low blood sugar), for instance, may get headaches, experience mental confusion, feel depressed, lack energy or be subject to extreme mood swings. Due to a side effect of kidney dialysis, many diabetic men must take supplementary zinc in order to function normally sexually.

Regular indulgence in alcohol, tobacco or coffee has a price tag. For example, if you smoke you may need fifteen times as much vitamin C as someone who doesn't in order to maintain your resistance to disease. These substances leech vitamins and minerals vital to your sexual well-being from your bodymind, making extra supplementation essential. Smoking can also cause circulatory problems.

Ingredients in alcohol, tobacco and coffee irritate the prostate of the male and there is some evidence that sugar and salt in the large amounts consumed today do as well. This irritation of the prostate increases the need to ejaculate. If a man wants to try ejaculating less and recycling sexual energy, he should use these substances sparingly. Uric acid, found in red meat, may need to be avoided for the same reason.

Some women who were subject to severe premenstrual stress symptoms found relief by going on a low-salt diet for ten days prior to the onset of menstruation. Eating lightly may reduce unpleasant menstrual symptoms.

Ellen has found that with her vegetarian diet, she rarely experiences menstrual cramps. However, since the uterus is swollen, she may feel discomfort due to the passage of food through her body. This problem is alleviated when she fasts on vegetable juice for one or two days just prior to the beginning of her cycle. Eating lightly—mostly vegetables and fruits—has also proved helpful.

Some holistic physicians are convinced that most sexual problems are the result of vicarious elimination of toxic substances in the diet via the sexual organs. Problems such as frigidity, lack of sensitivity in the breasts and vagina, non-orgasm and even the feeling of being only mechanically involved during sex may all be much more nutritionally based than most of us realize. Likewise, problems such as impotence, early ejaculation and low libido may also be, in many cases, fundamentally nutritional.

One well-known fact lends support to this theory: the taste of a man's ejaculate reflects his diet, including his use of alcohol and coffee. Female vaginal secretions are thought to reflect diet as well.

Many sexual problems stem from lack of energy. Orgasm, for instance, is a pleasurable release of energy. If the bodymind is struggling just to generate enough energy to survive, it will seek to avoid the energy discharge of genital orgasm.

Many sexual problems which are often thought to be psychological, and not just problems with orgasm, may be the result of low energy and little else. The so-called inhibited sexual desire syndrome that is common today may have a lot more to do with what is in the sex therapy candidate's kitchen than in his or her head.

In fact, the Society for Clinical Ecology (see *Appendix*) estimates that one out of every ten persons with a sexual dysfunction has their difficulty due to an allergy. Substances that can cause an allergic reaction range from the chlorine in drinking water to perfumes to oranges.

Supplements For Sex

You live in a toxic world. Supplement your diet with vitamins and minerals even if you are in good health now. You need to ingest a surplus of the vitamins A, the B group, C, E and P (bioflavonoids) for optimum sexual functioning.

Vitamin E, for example, helps the blood carry enough oxygen to the sex organs to achieve and sustain arousal. Phosphorus, calcium and magnesium cooperate to maintain sexual desire and health. Maintaining the proper proportion of these factors as a woman approaches menopause can prevent unpleasant symptoms.

Selenium helps maintain hormone response and is rarely adequate without supplementation. Manganese helps maintain normal blood flow essential to sexual performance and orgasm.

Zinc deficiency is a frequent cause of impotence in the male and a major contributing factor to prostatitis and prostate cancer. Premature ejaculation can be due to an undiagnosed case of prostatitis. Zinc deficiency in the female can result in inadequate vaginal lubrication.

Unless you take a zinc supplement the likelihood that you are deficient in zinc is high since the average diet supplies only a third of the amount after assimilation recommended by the National Research Council. Raw pumpkin seeds are a good natural zinc source.

Pollen, lecithin and garlic are also of great value. Pollen has helped men with prostate problems and women with menstrual problems. Lecithin assists in the production of sex hormones. Garlic, said to be ruled by masculine Mars, has a stimulating, circulating effect that boosts sexual well-being.

Many foods popularly believed to be aphrodisiacs do in fact contain vital sexual nutrients. Truffles and Chinese Bird's Nest Soup, for example, are extremely rich in phosphorous and oysters are by far the most concentrated natural source of zinc.

The nutritional factor in the achievement of orgasm by both men and women should not be overlooked. Pearson and Shaw report that taking niacin (one of the B vitamins) fifteen to thirty minutes before the sex act stimulates histamine release in the bodymind. This can intensify orgasm and may help men and women achieve orgasm who could not do so before. Try 50 or 100 mg to start.

Walker and Walker suggest taking 50 mg three times a day (150 mg of niacin total) plus 50 mg before sexual activity. They also report that high daily doses of vitamin C may increase sexual desire and intensify orgasms. Take plenty of the B complex, too, if you follow this plan.

Megadoses of magnesium orotate, potassium aspartate and bromelain have also brought success in the treatment of impotent men and preorgasmic women. However, the size of the doses involved requires that they be administered by a holistic physician.

Vitamin B-5 (calcium pantothenate) is said to improve sexual stamina. Some sources assign vitamin B-15 (DMG) aphrodisiac properties and general sexual curative powers. Max EPA may significantly increase sexual energy and activity. SOD may also be a major sexual aid as well as an overall body booster.

Aloe vera taken orally in capsules, as a liquid or gel is thought to be a sex stimulant and for some may supply quick aphrodisiac effects soon after ingestion. Pearson and Shaw report that reduced sex drive, enlarged prostate or prostatitis due to excessive prolactin in men may respond to 40 mg daily of GABA placed under the tongue. All of these substances are available at your local health food store.

If you would like to experiment with vitamin and mineral dosages, we recommend that you contact a nutritionist or holistic physician. This is a complex and sophisticated field. For instance, it is important not to megadose on fat soluble vitamins such as A and D and many minerals must be taken in limited quantities. It is recommended to take B vitamins together (most multivitamins contain the B-complex group) as an overdose in one may cause a deficiency in another. In addition, certain minerals require a specific vitamin to be present to operate correctly in your system and vice versa.

Nutritional factors do not operate in a vacuum. They work together in complex ways to help bring about that condition we call optimum well-being, sexual and otherwise. To give an example, in order for your body to make use of supplemental vitamin C at least five other nutritional factors, including vitamin B-6, vitamin B-12 and zinc, must be present in sufficient quantities in the body. In order for so-called aphrodisiac substances and supplements to live up to their reputations, numerous other nutritional factors must also be present in your body.

Ellen's Tiger Tonic   Blend a cup of apple juice, a frozen banana, two tablespoons of protein powder, a tablespoon of lecithin and a tablespoon of honeybee pollen for a delicious protein drink. Peel the bananas and place them in an airtight container before freezing them. You can also add nuts or one tablespoon of nut butter, such as almond. Pineapple juice or milk (dairy or soy) can substitute for apple juice. Add raw honey and wheat germ if desired.

Gypsy Potency Formula

For many thousands of years, men have sought to increase, prolong or regain potency. The Gypsy Potency Formula is a simple drink that has been credited with major rejuvenative powers. While there is no such thing as a quickie miracle potency formula, this gypsy secret is a wholesome runner-up that may surprise you with its potent effects.

Make a drink by combining cow's milk, honey and two or three egg yolks. Use the highest quality, most natural (raw if possible) milk, honey and eggs you can find. Drink this every morning. Some say the milk should be warm.

You may also want to add bee pollen, also said to be a potency energizer. Do this for two weeks to two months.

If your cholesterol is high, take Ellen's Tiger Tonic instead since it has no egg yolks. The regimen can be continued indefinitely by taking a spoonful of honey with a hot drink every day, making the full recipe only when your energy or sexual force is flagging.

Prostate Health

Prostate problems today include congestion, enlargement, infection and cancer of the prostate. Chronic prostatitis is a very common problem that can hinder sexual performance. Premature ejaculation is a typical symptom. Emotional factors, such as guilt or self-blame, may play a role.

You should certainly go to a qualified physician at the very first sign of any difficulty as well as going in for regular checkups. Here we would like to discuss holistic or natural approaches that can be used along with the healing plan prescribed by a conventional physician. Also, our research indicates that acupuncture with Chinese herbs can be effective in the treatment of urogenital and sex energy difficulties.

At the top of our list is wheatgrass. Make a juice from it and insert the liquid into the anus directly. The easiest way to do this is sitting on the toilet. A baby enema syringe is ideal. Then lie down on the floor with pillows to elevate the legs. Try two to four bulbs full one to three times a day.

Because the rectal canal is right next to the prostate, the wheatgrass is able to pass through the thin wall and gradually flush out infection or otherwise heal the prostate.

Pygeum tree bark from Africa, with its liposterolic compounds, is said to be remarkably helpful for problems of the prostate. Herb Pharm offers it in a concentrated liquid form.

Some sources implicate homogenized milk and dairy products as a major culprit in prostate problems. Only fresh, raw, guaranteed safe milk should be consumed then. Or, perhaps better still, cow's milk can be avoided completely and honey-sweetened soy milk substituted.

Aloe vera juice was used by the ancient Egyptians for healing. It has a powerful internal cleansing effect when you drink it. We find that mixing it with sparkling mineral water is the best combination for taste. The best brand of aloe vera juice in terms of potency and taste we have found is *Viva Vera* with micronized pulp.

If you are not drinking the wheat grass, the aloe vera will give you the internal cleansing that should go with the external cleansing through the anus. What you drink can definitely affect the prostate for good or bad. For example, drinking coffee or alcohol is known to irritate the prostate and may make symptoms worse.

Other healthful strategies include bee pollen, vitamins and herbs. While personal need varies, about 45 mg of zinc and about 150 mg of selenium are good to take daily since there is evidence that they help prevent prostate problems of all kinds. Unsaturated fatty acids have been found to help reduce an enlarged prostate gland in some men.

Raw pumpkin seeds are another valuable aid. A handful a day is recommended as a preventative or to help an imbalanced prostate condition. We also suggest raw vegetable juice drinks such as carrot and beet are suggested. Lemon juice or grapefruit juice may help. You may want to include yeast and wheat germ oil in your regular daily intake.

We strongly recommend a diet of organically grown food that is predominantly vegetarian. We say predominantly because some people do seem to require some light (non-red) meats such as fish or fowl. Also, when these foods are taken occasionally, even just once or twice a month, the task of obtaining all essential nutrients, which can be difficult on the strictly vegan diet, is greatly simplified. The addition of eggs and some dairy products (raw and fresh, of course), which is strictly speaking a lacto-ovovegetarian diet, also makes this much easier.

However, for those who refuse to eat meat or animal products as a moral decision, these options are not appropriate. While it does take a great deal of knowledge and work, such pure vegetarians, or vegans, are perhaps observing the healthiest diet of all.

Finally, we cannot stress enough the benefit doing sexercises regularly, especially Kegel exercises or the yoga variations, including the Stomach Lift. We theorize that the sluggishness that develops in the prostate and contributes to chronic problems can be largely eliminated by the internal massage that contractions of the PC muscle provide.

We suspect that this is particularly true when the PC muscle has been strengthened substantially after a month or two of regular exercise. For extra healing effect, combine the Kegels with affirmations like "I love myself" or "I love my prostate" or "My prostate is healthy and whole and functions perfectly."

Vaginal Health   The philosophy of positive attitude and proper diet can be applied to vaginal health issues as well. Many women have reported excellent results from the cleansing and healing power of wheatgrass juice or aloe vera juice introduced into the vagina or taken orally. The role of the emotions, in particular, must be remembered.

Of course, you should go to a qualified physician at the very first sign of any difficulty as well as for regular checkups. Our suggestions are designed to possibly supplement, not replace, the healing plan prescribed by your physician.

Leucorrhea, excessive mucus discharge, is usually due to improper diet factors. The increased mucus discharge is the bodymind's way of trying to eliminate toxic accumulations. Consumer foods, which lack healthy enzymes, are a major contributor.

Daniel Reid recommends whole lemon puree for this and other female reproductive system issues. Puree a whole lemon in a blender and add it to one cup of pure water with one tablespoon of molasses. Take this mixture once or twice daily. The molasses is optional.

Menstrual problems are often an indicator of imbalance in the blood as well as the endocrine system. For this, Reid also suggests the whole lemon puree, with the molasses definitely included. He also recommends one or two pints daily of fennel juice, mixed half and half with carrot juice. Fennel juice is said to strengthen the blood.

Vaginitis is another common problem. *Planetary Herbology* by Michael Tierra, which includes a wide variety of herbal strategies for women, offers a simple suggestion. For vaginitis or leucorrhea, he recommends one or two garlic cloves placed in the vagina. The clove(s) should be bruised and covered by muslin.

Taken as a douche, wheatgrass is said to relieve vaginitis. With its power to correct acid-alkaline balance and restore enzymes missing due to the effects of cooking or pollution, it is also an overall tonic for vaginal health. One great advantage is that it is inexpensive to buy or grow on your own.

Also, our research shows that acupuncture with Chinese herbs is quite helpful for vaginal and sex energy imbalances.

Menstruation is a sacred experience of power. Noted psychic Patricia Sun, for example, has commented that her psychic energy intensifies during menstruation. Not only in contemporary society but even in ancient tribal societies, this increased power threatened men, motivating them to exclude women having their period from gatherings.

For this reason, we agree with the ancient Tantric recommendation that couples try making love when the woman is having her period. Her energy will be stronger and she will be more sensitive. She should be on top so that the blood and energy are free to flow downwards.

Research by Viktoras Kulvinskas indicates that when a woman adapts to a wholesome, reduced protein, vegetarian diet her menstrual losses decrease significantly. Cessation of menses may even occur.

While there certainly are unhealthful conditions in which the menstruation ceases, what Kulvinskas is referring to is not an imbalanced state. Though the menstrual flow may diminish, the intensification of psychic energy tends to increase, amplifying its spiritual dimension.

Last but not least is what Betty Dodson calls "becoming cunt positive." Her approach includes self-examination with a mirror and fully exploring the art of *Selfloving*.

In our repressive society, women are especially inclined to incorporate negative valuations of their sexual organs. There is no doubt that this can have telling negative emotional and physical side-effects. It is important that women claim the power of having their own orgasms, of creating their own pleasure through self-love and *Selfloving* as well as with a man, be it in intercourse or not (see *Pleasuring The Yoni*).

As discussed in Prostate Health, we recommend an organic, vegetarian diet. For some women, diet will prove to be a much bigger issue. In general, women seem more sensitive to the effects of food than men in that they react more quickly and seem to purify more rapidly.

In contrast, though men may seem to handle toxicity well at first, often later on they develop serious symptoms that are difficult to eliminate. Therefore, a woman should celebrate her sensitivity and be glad that her form is less dense and more aligned with refined substances.

As with male urogenital disorders, we cannot emphasize enough the value of doing the Kegel clenches or Tantric yoga workouts. It is not just a matter of increasing pleasure. To a certain degree, they act as a preventative or a curative (see *Sexercises*).

It is said that wherever the mind is concentrated, energy and healing force will go. This is precisely how these sexercises work to heal at a subtle level. In the woman's case, especially, exercise is valuable as it tends to increase yang energy, enabling her to have more control over her sexual well-being and her ability to have orgasms.

DRUGS AND SEXUAL PERFORMANCE

A number of legal drugs that are prescribed for other needs are known to interfere with sexual pleasure and performance. These include tranquilizers, sedatives, barbiturates and certain sleeping tablets. Ironically, the Pill has been reported to lower sexual motivation in women. This may be a by-product of the depressive moods sometimes caused by oral contraceptive drugs.

Drugs that lower high blood pressure are the most frequent culprits, followed by drugs used to treat psychological difficulties. Even antihistamines can interfere with sexual capacity by blocking nerve impulses to the sex organs and glands. Marijuana, alcohol, cocaine and heroin can negatively affect sexual motivation and the achievement of erection and ejaculation, provided the dose is high enough and/or frequent enough.

Impotence is one of the frequently reported symptoms but it is not the only possible undesirable side effect. Other reported side effects include decreased sexual desire, difficulty in sustaining erection, inability to ejaculate, painful ejaculation, uncontrolled ejaculation, retrograde (into the bladder) ejaculation, decreased sexual desire in men and women and delayed orgasm or difficulty in achieving orgasm in women.

Alcohol is one of the most flagrant offenders. It depresses the action of the central nervous system. The all too obvious result can be an inability to achieve and/or maintain erection. Prolonged alcohol use is linked to male sex hormone imbalance. Caffeine and nicotine may also impair sexual function.

Women are far from exempt. Female desire and performance is also negatively affected by many drugs, including those present in alcohol, tobacco, coffee, prescription drugs and illicit drugs. Achievement of orgasm may then be, to an extent, diet dependent. However, because impairment of sexual performance in the female has been more difficult to demonstrate, studies have focused on health and reproductive risks.

For example, even moderate drinking during pregnancy can cause fetal alcohol syndrome resulting in facial abnormalities, low weight at birth and/or mental retardation. The caffeine present in coffee, tea, cola, chocolate and some over-the-counter headache remedies was implicated as a cause of benign breast lumps.

On the other side of the issue, the association of alcohol with sex as part of romantic ritual has a long history. Ancient Tantric texts suggest ingesting several glasses of wine in the course of celebrating sacred sex. Some people report that champagne, in particular, has an especially erotic effect.

Women taking birth control pills are likely to be deficient in vitamin B-6, vitamin C, zinc and folic acid. Smoking and aging in combination with birth control pills increase these deficiencies.

Some drugs are known to cause depression or mental confusion, which in turn hampers male sexual performance. Many of these same drugs are also thought to reduce sexual desire or delay or make orgasm more difficult for women.

Know which drugs your consort is taking. This includes oral contraceptive drugs. Drug interactions, with alcohol especially, are yet another problem. Be sure to review in detail the possible sexual side effects of every drug you are taking with your physician. The authoritative guide to drug side effects is the *Physician's Desk Reference (PDR)*.

If a prescribed drug is causing you trouble, ask to be placed on a different drug. Reactions are very individual. A drug that impairs sexual function in another person may not affect you and vice versa.

Of course, drugs are often only a contributing cause. Many of the conditions for which people take prescribed medications, such as diabetes, high blood pressure, hardening of the arteries and kidney disease, are also associated with sexual problems (see *Herbs For Lovers*).

ENERGY CENTERS The main energy centers of the body, called *chakras* in yoga, play an important role in Tantric lovemaking. We will occasionally refer to opening and working with energy via these centers. While the body contains many energy centers in addition to these seven located near the spine, these seven are considered the most important.

The seventh or crown chakra: cosmic energy, pure intuition, experience of oneness, goddess force gateway

The sixth or third eye chakra: the mind element, imagination, sixth sense (second sight), controls glands

The fifth or throat chakra: ether element, the ears, larynx and sense of hearing

The fourth or heart chakra: air element, the skin, hands and sense of touch

The third or solar plexus chakra: fire element, the eyes, feet and sense of sight

The second or sex chakra: water element, the tongue, sex organ and sense of taste

The first or root chakra: earth element, the anus, nose and sense of smell

Seven Steps To Heaven

There is a link between these centers and the glands they are physically near. Each center is also associated with certain psychological or life issues.

The root is related to survival and overall vitality. The sex center involves vulnerability, need, empathy, creativity and, of course, sex. The solar plexus keys us into self-assertion and power issues, especially top dog and underdog conflicts. The heart, along with being the home of the deep feeling core of self, focuses on love and acceptance, of self as well as other. The throat is tied to the challenge of telling the truth, including the expression of our creativity and ideas, though we risk rejection or criticism. It is also where we get involved in judging self and others.

The third eye and crown in the head do not have emotional tonalities, though they are felt or sensed to some extent by everyone. Via the third eye of awareness, we are able to see the nature of thought and go beyond divisions, but there is still a certain distance. We are still the observer.

Via the crown, though, the process of bodymind opening is completed. We rejoice in the cosmic flow. Open like the hollow bamboo flute, we celebrate the pulsation of the Great Breath as and through us. We are not merely in heaven. Heaven is in us.

Third Eye High   An ancient key to superconscious sex is to focus the eyes at the third eye trigger point between the eyebrows. Literally "park" the physical eyes at that point, allowing your awareness to flow into the third eye in the middle of your forehead. With practice, this region in the forehead (linked to the center of the brain at the pituitary gland) becomes open, sensitive to the inner touch and magnetic. Visions, altered states and the sexual-spiritual experience of blissful fusion, called Tantric orgasm, can be achieved very directly in this way (see *Third Eye Sex*).

A simple training exercise is to gaze at a candle flame. Then close your eyes and see the flame in the middle of your forehead or at the center of your brain. Concentrate on this light when you meditate or make love.

Esoterically, the source of life is cosmic light energy that descends through the crown into the bodymind. When it is reflected back up the spine (which happens instantaneously), it is known as Kundalini, the sacred life force that rises with extra intensity in response to sexual arousal, extreme emotions, crisis situations and meditation.

Climbing The Ladder   Sexual arousal automatically increases the energy going to and through these centers. In Tantric ritual, these chakras are stimulated in an ascending sequence. The liberated energy is then subtilized up into the third eye and crown (see *Tantric Ritual Sex*).

Whether or not the hoary Tantric formalities are followed, some couples climb the ladder of love step-by-step by combining the mantras, color imagery and musical accompaniment described below. Union in Yab Yum is optimal for this. The classic YabYum, which should be held for at least half an hour to insure results, can be modified. Probably the best solution is to back yourselves up with giant pillows, then recline in comfort and enjoy the ride up (see *Peaceful Positions*).

One of the traditional ways to bring the energy up to the third eye to attain visions and sexual-spiritual experiences employs these seed sounds from Tantric yoga: Lum for the root, Vum for the sex center, Rum for the solar plexus, Yum for the heart, Hum for the throat, Om for the third eye.

Some sources suggest extending the "mmm" as an "ng" sound. Lum, for example, is then pronounced "Lunggg."

You can also pronounce these with an "ah" sound if you wish. The sound for the solar plexus then, for example, would be Ram.

As you place your attention on a region, repeat the corresponding seed syllable and feel it sink deep into your bodymind, where it continues to resonate. Chanted with energy and enthusiasm, they have a powerful uplifting effect.

A less traditional approach is to visualize the colors of the rainbow like a pillar made of layers of colored light in and around the body. Red matches the root center, orange the sex center, yellow the solar plexus center, green the heart center, blue the throat center, indigo the third eye and violet the crown.

If you see different hues or shadings of color at some of these points than are given here, feel free to explore them. This meditation can be amplified by concentrating on the steps of the musical scale at the same time (see *Aural Sex*). Some practicioners even use colored lights to increase the impact (see *Appendix*).

Letting Go

Knowledge of esoteric details is not needed, however, to get wonderful results. Feedback from our students indicates that concern about such details can be an obstacle to spontaneity. It can also lead to a new kind of goal obsession: instead of being obsessed with having a conventional orgasm, you become obsessed with having a Tantric one.

Let go of what you know. Be surprised by the present.

It is better to stay several sessions with one technique that you like—the simpler the better, usually—and explore it thoroughly. If you want to go further with meditation on chakras and Kundalini, you will find resources in the *Bibliography* and *Appendix.*

Shiva, the patron saint of Hindu Tantrism, once observed "By practice, even without understanding, it will be made plain; your body will understand it long before your mind puts words to it. No amount of understanding without practice will work. It is not necessary that knowledge precede experience. Performance will produce knowledge."

Ultimately, the chakra system is rooted in the Heart, not the psychic heart in the middle of the chest but to the right of it. The published teachings of Sri Ramana Maharshi and Sri Da Kalki (Heart-Master Da Love-Ananda) are probably the best known sources on this.

Robert K. Moffett. *Tantric Sex.* New York: Berkley Medallion, 1974, page xvi.

EXERCISE FOR SEXUAL WELL-BEING

Exercise, like diet, is a basic ingredient in the total approach to lovemaking. Still, it is often ignored. Since we are each biochemically unique, there is no one set exercise plan for everybody. Each must work out his or her own optimum program for personal and sexual well-being. Be sure to consult with your physician regarding changes in your personal exercise habits, especially if you are just starting out on an exercise plan.

It is well established that regular moderate exercise improves health and sense of well-being. As a result, sexual health and well-being is also improved. However, it is not at all established that vigorous exercise programs, which do not appeal to everyone, are necessary for your total sexual fulfillment.

Since moderate exercise favorably alters the metabolism, exercise synergizes with food and nutritional supplements to maximize the benefits from both. Exercise has also been found to be a major factor in achieving weight loss. As an overweight condition can affect your sex life negatively, even down to the hormonal level, approximating your slim and trim ideal makes good sexual sense.

Research indicates that moderate regular cardiovascular exercise such as aerobics or running may increase the sex drive in both men and women. However, heavy exercise may have the opposite effect and actually decrease sexual drive. We found that this is true for us. Men who are early ejaculators due to overexcitability, however, may benefit from frequent intensive exercise for this very reason.

According to an article by Cook in *Playboy,* lovemaking in the hard style is not a good way to get your cardiovascular exercise. Though the heart may beat 120 times a minute or more, this is the result of hormonal changes. That's the bad news.

The good news is that European researchers have found that sexual arousal and activity elevate the testosterone level in the bodymind. Testosterone, of course, plays a major role in maintaining the sexual well-being of both sexes. Perhaps the best exercise for sex is sex!

There is another kind of exercise altogether. Neuroglandular exercise, which includes exercise styles such as hatha yoga and t'ai chi, is designed to balance and harmonize the human nervous system.

Neuroglandular exercise contributes to health and longevity by gently stimulating and balancing the nervous and glandular systems of the bodymind. Many positions of hatha yoga, for example, are designed to benefit specific nerve centers or glands. Special attention to breathing further energizes and balances the whole system as well as specific parts.

The ideal exercise program includes both hard, yang (cardiovascular) and soft, yin (neuroglandular) exercising. The proportion of hard and soft activity, though, should be based on individual needs and preferences. There is no universal standard for you to conform with.

Exercise is holistic when the mind is concentrated in the movements of the body. It is much easier at first to focus the mind in the body during the slow, serene movements of soft style exercises. With enough training this same focus can be maintained during the fast, dynamic movements of hard style exercises.

A little holistic bodymind exercise goes a long way. It is better to exercise only as long as you can hold your concentration, even if this means exercising less. Exercising without concentration scatters the mind, reducing benefits. Injuries are more common.

Making love is a form of exercise. To experience holistic lovemaking, unite mind and body during this exercise, too, whatever your preferred style(s).

Bringing mind and body together in physical movement is a giant step towards total wholeness. You will begin to enjoy total health, a oneness of body and mind that leads to oneness with the universe. It is this experience of oneness that is the ultimate goal of holistic exercise.

HARA Located about two inches below the navel and deep in the core of the body, hara is your vital center and the home of your life force. Hara awareness training is an excellent way to get more in touch with your body and with deeper levels of life force. It is the ideal place to ground and store energy.

To find hara (which means "belly" in Japanese), stand with your feet a little apart, your weight distributed equally over the soles of the feet. Close your eyes, relax and breathe slowly and deeply from your belly.

Allow yourself to respond to the pull of gravity and sink down while retaining your erect posture. Sway side to side, to and fro, around and around until you find this region in the lower belly.

Now focus there. Be centered there. Calm, deep breathing continues but now you feel that it originates in hara. Feel a warm glow there. Feel this warm energy spread to fill your whole body.

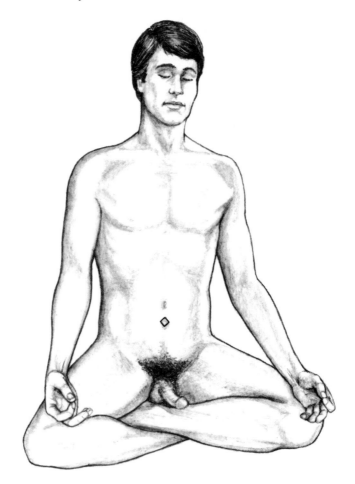

Now return to ordinary waking consciousness. Open your eyes. Remember this center. Remember hara in your daily activities.

Hara is the actual physical balance point or center of gravity for the body. In Zen and related styles of meditation where the rise and fall of the breath at the belly is observed, the mind is placed in hara.

This can be practiced as a walking meditation also. Non-thinking is maintained. After extensive practice, you develop the ability to maintain hara, to keep the mind in hara and not in the head.

Here is an experiment to do with a friend. Consciously breathe energy into your upper body and head. Puff yourself up, as if to instantly become a giant body builder. Ask your friend to stand in front of you and push your shoulder.

Now do the opposite. Let your upper body relax. Sink deep into your lower body and put your attention in hara.

HARA *above*
This is the vital center. Keep your mind in hara when you make love. You may experience a deep oneness with nature.

Give yourself a few moments. Ask your friend to push your shoulder.

Were you more balanced without hara or with hara? (If you answered without hara, try again.)

One easy way to cultivate hara is to sit in a kneeling position. Breathe deeply and slowly for a few minutes, concentrating on the exhalation. Make the exhalation as long and strong as you can. Do not be concerned about the inhalation. It will take care of itself.

Do this in the morning. In a few months, your hara will be strong.

Perhaps the most direct way to develop hara is to move about for five to ten minutes without make use of your arms in any way. When we hear that we should move from the hips, as is taught in the martial arts, we still tend to lead with the head. Instead, try walking, lying down, sitting, standing, kneeling and so on with your arms hanging loosely at your sides.

It is best to begin this technique on a forgiving surface, such as a soft rug or lawn, as you may tumble a few times. You will find that you are using your belly, back and legs in a new way.

Even a little practice leads to the experience of feeling that your legs are like strong roots, that your belly is your actual, natural center. You realize that it is possible to live from hara, from your own personal source of life.

It is but one step more to make love from hara, from your deep inner core rather than from your periphery. To keep your mind and breath in hara is a noble and rewarding way to make love (see *Taoist Circle Of Gold, Ground And Store Energy*).

HERBS FOR LOVERS

Herbs have been used to successfully balance sexual energy for thousands of years. Aphrodisiac herbs are warming and stimulating. Anaphrodisiac herbs are cooling and calming. Chinese herbs with acupuncture may be especially potent.

Certain well-known tonic herb blends, such as the commercially available shou wu chih, which includes tang kuei and ho shou wu, are said to be suitable for long-term use. These awaken spiritual energy as well as rejuvenating the body, sexual function included. Such classic tonic herbs are, perhaps, the ideal application of herbs for sexual fulfillment.

Traditional aphrodisiac herbs include caltrop, cannabis (illegal), dayflower, damiana, echinacea, false unicorn root, fo-ti-tieng, ginseng, goldenseal, gotu kola, Irish moss, kava kava, licorice root (female), lobelia, lupine, motherwort, oatstraw, peach leaves, peppermint, sarsaparilla, slippery elm, sundew, yohimbine (see our note of caution below). Anaphrodisiac herbs are said to include hops (it's in beer), sage, scullcap and star root.

Several popular Oriental products are reputed to have aphrodisiac properties. These include dragon brew, royal jelly, shou wu chih, tang kuei gin and tzepau san pian. Recommended teas include black warrior tea, heavenly root tea, two peony tea and small saikoto tea. Look for these products in natural food stores or Oriental groceries.

Some aphrodisiac or energizing herb combinations include animal substances, such as deer antler. We believe that the exploitation of animals for the sake of pleasure, though traditional in some countries, is not appropriate. Herbal alternatives are virtually always available. The ecological balance of our Earth requires the honoring of all life without exception.

Kava Kava

This delightfully mellow mood enhancer is the legendary love drink of the South Pacific. Unlike ginseng and damiana, kava kava is not effective taken as a tea. Said to be the gift of the god Tagaloa Ui, kava kava has been the major social intoxicant in the South Seas for centuries.

A member of the pepper family, the most available form of the shrub is the powdered root. Kava kava is currently being used to wean South Pacific natives away from alcohol. Several hundred years ago, the Islanders regrettably switched to booze when Christian missionaries proclaimed it "evil."

The scientific data on kava kava is limited. What research has been done indicates one very positive point—used in moderation, kava kava is completely safe. To experience toxic effects from kava kava use it is necessary to consume large amounts daily for months. There is evidence that occasional use of the kava kava drink is beneficial to health.

The legal chemical punch of kava kava comes from six resin-type unsaturated, closed-chain compounds (pyrones) found in the beverage. These pyrones slow down spinal activity without affecting the brain. The result can be an impressive variety of pleasant experiences—peacefulness, euphoric feelings, profound relaxation—all without any loss of consciousness. With larger doses it is reported that some

KAVA KAVA *above right* This sacred drink of natives known for their peaceful lifestyles and sexual freedom is not well-known in the West.

people also experience auditory and visual hallucinations and/or a delicious tingling in the sex organs.

One common observation is that kava kava warms the heart towards others, increasing mutual trust and respect. Although it is impossible to predict what you personally will experience, its reputation for reducing anxiety and acting as a muscle relaxant is probably well deserved. This unusual chemical makeup of kava kava can also make the tongue feel a little like it is anesthesized. This is a common experience and is considered to be totally harmless.

Making a tea from kava kava powder is not effective. The ingredients which give kava kava its kick are not water soluble. The natives get around this by chewing the plant for a considerable length of time before mixing it in coconut juice and then ingesting it. Western technology, however, provides an alternative to this time consuming task.

Just mix one ounce of kava kava powder with a few tablespoons of vegetable oil and a tablespoon of lecithin (liquid or granular) in a cup or so of water or coconut milk. A kitchen blender is quite handy for this. Blend this concoction until it resembles milk.

This is the little-known secret of successful kava kava drink preparation. You must either prechew it or blend it in this way to release the pyrones. This recipe for one ounce of kava kava powder serves two or more people.

Adam Gottlieb suggests making a resin of the kava kava and applying it to the surface of the penis or clitoris. The desensitization of the surface nerves that results is said to allow an extended sexual performance.

This method takes advantage of kava kava's anesthesizing property. Islanders put kava kava leaves on wounds to reduce pain and speed the healing process.

Gottlieb suggests extracting the resin type tar from the root (not the powder) in hot rubbing (isopropyl) alcohol and then evaporating the alcohol in a double boiler or heat bath. He advises placing a tiny piece of the resulting tar on your tongue and administering cunnilingus at the same time.

The woman's clitoris will react first with a sort of supersensitivity which, if tolerated, gives way, again according to Gottlieb, to some of the most incredible orgasms she will ever have.

The tar, by the way, does not taste bad at all. What results you will obtain no one can predict, but it certainly is worth trying. Be sure to make enough resin so that you can reverse roles, i.e., for fellatio. You can expect a numbing sensation on the tongue as well.

Alcohol will speed the absorption of the pyrones by the body. If you like the combination, add the milky blend you created to warm vodka, rum or brandy. If you have gone to the trouble of extracting the resinous tars, the ideal is to redissolve the resins back into, say, some warm brandy. As this kava kava–alcohol combo is said to be quite potent, do remember to be good to your body.

South Sea Islanders have long celebrated kava kava in the form of a sacred ritual. Undoubtedly, this reverent attitude enhances the experiences Islanders have with kava kava through what is known as the placebo effect or self-suggestion. In the ritual, a little kava kava is spilled on the floor as a gift to the god Tagaloa Ui before it is quaffed. The kava kava is served only in the finest goblets.

Traditionally, kava kava encourages social warmth and group harmony as well as an increased sense of personal well-being. The kava kava experience is said to be a subtle one for some people, requiring several occasions before the delights of kava kava are recognized. At any rate, the best advice is simply that you try it—in moderation, of course.

Damiana   Damiana is another of mother nature's sensual gifts. Some sources, including an occultist named Culling, claim great things for it. We have found it to be pleasantly relaxing and to induce a sensual mood. Herbal Kingdom Tea Company puts out an inexpensive, liquid damiana tea concentrate called *Aphrodite's Delight* that is convenient to use.

Damiana is also available as an herbal tea if you want to go a more conventional route. This one is for both of you and can be served chilled or warm.

Results are said to be best if the damiana is ingested about an hour beforehand. In general, women are reputed to be more responsive to damiana than men. Damiana with saw palmetto and juniper berries may be more potent. Some sources recommend it as a remedy for prostate problems as well.

Ginseng   Ginseng is reputedly able to help improve sexual ability by acting as a tonic to the glands and nervous system when used for an extended period of time. Highest grade ginseng can be quite expensive. An overall health facilitator, ginseng is considered a male tonic. Dong quai is the equivalent for the female.

We have found the *Four Ginsengs* put out by the East Earth Herb Company to be an excellent, all around ginseng stimulant in the easily affordable price range. They offer many quality products that may be of interest. Other good suppliers include Yellow Emperor and Eagle Eye.

It's good to take ginseng for a month or two, then discontinue it for a month or two. Some men take ginseng only a few months a year, claiming to gain full benefit and avoid systemic dependence as well. Just as with other stimulants, you can get hooked on ginseng. You may be able to feel the stimulation—like a mild coffee buzz, only deeper in your body and without the unnerving caffeine aftershocks.

Unfriendly "Aphrodisiacs"   Some naturally occurring substances that have reputations as aphrodisiacs can exact a bitter price. Spanish fly, which is prepared from the dried wings of *Cantharis vesicatoria* beetles, is poisonous and has been known to kill!

While its reputation as an aphrodisiac has received some scientific confirmation, yohimbine has been demonstrated in the laboratory to raise blood pressure dangerously. If you really want to experiment with it, just remember that the danger increases when yohimbine is combined with alcohol.

Yohimbine is available as an extract or in bark form. If you get the bark, make one cup of liquid by boiling one teaspoon for about ten minutes. Last we checked, yohimbine was rather difficult to locate—probably a good thing.

Jimson weed (*Datura stramonium*) can cause a coma lasting for days or death. Fortunately, there are alternatives to these well-known but hazardous substances. The ultimate aphrodisiac, of course, is your mind.

MEDITATION AND TANTRA   Why is sex so attractive to us? Is it, as some scientific views preach, merely animal instinct? According to Tantric views, sex is magnetic because we want the sweet taste of *samadhi* (higher consciousness), of light-love-bliss, of the transcendental, even if it is at first but a flash during sex. Meditation accepts that flash for what it is—a message about the nature of reality—and cultivates it into a transformed life.

The key that makes Tantric sex real Tantra and not, as one of our Buddhist meditation teachers put it, just "souped up nookie," is whether the person is really sincere about making an effort to go beyond the self or not. Getting a little loose, a little open feels good. And it's certainly healthy. But real Tantric sex blows your mind completely because it takes you beyond all of your conceptions of everyday reality—you taste the transcendental unity. Your life can never be the same.

Confusion About Fusion   The classic descriptions of the Tantric orgasm talk about a unitary or fusion experience. This is where it can get a little confusing. It is possible to have some sort of fusion experience via drugs, at a party, dancing, at a sporting event. The energies harmonize and merge and there is a moment where you feel like you are "one."

The "oneness" of any real Tantric experience, however, is radical oneness. It rips your mind off. It alters your view of reality. It forces you to reconsider the purpose of your life and who and what you are. It takes you closer to answering the question "Who am I?"

If your intent is to do Tantra, then the bottom line is that you need to have a regular meditation practice or similar self-discipline for self-transcendence that gives you the all-important reference point. Then your involvement in sex means you are bringing an enhanced awareness via meditation to your sexual experiences.

Levels Of Sex Energy   In yoga, it is recognized that there are three levels of energy: *tamas, rajas* and *sattva*. Sex that is crude, violent, selfish, unredeeming, where people are treated as if they are objects without feeling, is tamasic. As the sensitivity of the partners is undeveloped, they resort to gross stimuli in order to "get off." Tamasic sex is symbolized by the color black.

Rajasic sex, which most people would call good or great sex, is passionate, thrilling, romantic, exciting. As it has the qualities of fire, it is symbolized by red. While far superior to tamasic sex, it often leads to frustration unless sattvic consciousness is introduced as the relationship matures.

For example, a hot-cold involvement, as in the expression "the fire went out," may develop. A typical response is either to find a new partner or keep the relationship but have an affair. If the conflict further degenerates, then the classic love-hate relationship results. Tamasic behavior such as verbal or physical violence tends to dominate.

Sattvic sex, which is the Tantric or sacred sexuality path, incorporates the qualities of openness and space so that lovemaking is experienced as beautiful, meditative, healing, serene, flowing, peaceful, heart-felt, profound, blissful, harmonizing, mystical, spiritually beneficial. No longer a problem, sexual energy now contributes deeply to your personal growth path and overall sense of fulfillment.

Through sattvic, Tantric loving, the sex energy is harmonized with the spiritual life and its powerful energies made available for love, healing and self-transcendence. Sattvic sex is symbolized by the brilliance of the rising sun which, when it reaches its zenith, radiates a dazzling white brightness that burns away the ego.

In practice, most loving couples will find they tend to alternate between rajasic and sattvic lovemaking. They may even go through times when sex seems unimportant, only to emerge a few months later into a period of fiery passion where lovemaking is fresh and exciting again.

The intelligent desire to make love and experience a meaningful union should be allowed to arise from within as a spontaneous flowering. Rigid rules for spiritualizing sex, even if well intentioned, tend to backfire, obstructing the natural inner flow which knows the best way intuitively without thinking.

The Middle Way

Advanced Tantric sexual practices require a profound understanding and discipline of the mind and body that is usually based on many years of yogic practice. Such techniques are learned from a guru. Improperly performed, they are psychically as well as physically dangerous.

Such advanced practices, designed specifically for the quick attainment of enlightenment, are probably not suitable for most couples. However, if you would like more information, *Sky Dancer* by Keith Dowman and *Journey Into Consciousness* by Charles Breaux offer valuable insights from the Buddhist perspective.

Furthermore, complex, advanced esoteric sex practices such as these are not essential for attaining enlightenment. If that sort of Tantra is your path, you will know it. In fact, you will be unable to avoid it. If this traditional path intrigues you, the sections *Tantric Ritual Sex* and *Third Eye Sex,* based on teachings we received from Hindu Tantra masters, are sufficiently advanced for you to see if this way is for you.

On the other hand, meditation with the purpose of attaining a pure, one-pointed mind generally is required for achieving enlightenment. Sex is just a natural part of living as a human being. It is neither problem nor solution in itself. As one of our Hindu teachers, when asked by a seeker if he could be married, have sex and still get enlightened, replied, "Sex is only a problem if you have a problem with sex."

We feel that the middle way of love, ecstasy, awareness and harmony with nature, as described in *Sexual Energy Ecstasy,* is suitable for most couples. Once you are deeply in tune with this gently unfolding middle way of the Tantric loving couple, you will find that you receive instructions and experiences as your need for them arises. Love itself will become your guru.

Sacred Touch

Many techniques appeal to the mind and enable you to continue to mentalize sex. In contrast, mindfulness in the form of just pure touching, without accompanying conceptualization, does not foster further mentalization. Sex is not mental!

The value of touch has been widely acknowledged in the Tantric tradition, although this is not well understood today. In nondualistic Kashmir Shaivism, for example, it is taught that, of the five senses, touch is most directly related to the sex organs and higher consciousness.

Touch is said to emanate from a very subtle level of energy which is luminous, pure and neutral, what might be described as the inner breath, or even the touch of grace. Considered more intimate than the other senses, it is said to help move energy into the spine and awaken the sexual-spiritual force of Kundalini. At the same time, it has a centering, concentrating effect on the emotions which counters the usual tendency towards distraction and dispersion. Desire is fulfilled and higher states of consciousness are achieved.

The Joy Of No Body

The point of sex meditation or Tantric sex is that it will take you out of your head and down into your body and your heart. As Fritz Perls said, "Lose your mind and come to your senses." Tantra is all about learning to let go of the mind and discover your supreme Self hidden deep in your heart.

Paradoxically, by going deep into your familiar, physical body in a conscious, loving manner, as a yoga, you discover a deeper, truer body, a body that is pure presence and has no form. When you are lost in love, when you are swept away by the current of ecstasy during lovemaking, when you are melting into the clear light space above your head during the orgasm, when you are fused as one via the Tantric energy climax, you experience this.

Tantra is about the lighthearted joy of bodylessness, of formlessness. Admit it. During your really great orgasms, you completely lost track of who you are, of your body, of your partner—it all just simply melted away, overwhelmed by the power. Usually, we are very wary of this idea of having no body. But in Tantra we discover that it is fun!

Ultimately, lovers have as their nature joyous, open, luminous oneness. In Tantra, we go through the body to the source of the body, to the true body. By totally feeling the body, we actually taste a purity that is fully spiritual. Yes, the body is the temple, but we must go deeply into it and explore it completely if we are to find the inner shrine. Awake and aware, we celebrate the formless ocean of cosmic joy.

ORGASM AND ENERGY

Modern sexologists and psychologists have performed a great service by debunking the deep negative programming associated with sexual pleasuring and orgasm. However, they may have gone too far the other way.

Theories that tell us we are all the same arouse suspicion. Biochemical individuality is a fact. Why can't orgasmic individuality be a fact, also?

Female Sexual Orgasm

According to some sources, such as the ancient Chinese sex experts, a woman does not ordinarily lose significant energy via her orgasm. On the contrary, she gains energy and experiences the beneficial release of healing power. However, by repeatedly making love to men with whom she is in disharmony, or by forcing the orgasm rather than allowing it, she was believed to waste her vital force. Female *Selfloving* is consistently depicted in the erotica of the East, but male *Selfloving* rarely is.

According to Dr. Stephen Chang, the ancient Taoists had a saying: "Man shoots to death. Woman bleeds to death." The Taoists believed that the female orgasmic energy loss is insignificant in comparison to her menstrual energy loss. In their view, female orgasm is light and dispersed, akin to vapor or mist or fine perspiration. It is an event of great natural beauty like sunset or moonrise.

The potential loss of energy via the menstruation need not be an issue. Regular PC muscle workouts and other *Sexercises* are said to be very effective in retaining this energy, as are such practices as *Taoist Circle Of Gold* or *Elevate Energy*.

When sexual orgasm is exploited for the pleasure that usually accompanies it, the law of diminishing returns sets in. Orgasms and intercourse as a whole may become less satisfying, a source of confusion, even meaningless. One solution is to abstain from sexual activity and/or sexual orgasm until physical, emotional and mental balance are regained.

Another strategy for dealing with energy loss is the internal orgasm for women. Based on the *Elevate Energy* technique, the main difference is that you encourage energy up the spine when you relax the PC muscle lock and release the breath. It is also helpful to tuck the pelvis forward after retaining the breath. This straightens the spine.

The effective timing for the female internal orgasm is before the vaginal contractions but after you can feel the orgasm beginning to swell inside you. In other words, the energy has already begun to move. If your timing is good, and you have been practicing on your own, you will be able to step in and redirect the flow.

The muscular contractions of orgasm will then push the force up the spine instead of out the vagina, nourishing the master glands and centers in the brain. This will fill the whole body with pleasure.

According to ancient Chinese erotic lore, this technique can be developed to the point that it becomes a form of sexual vampirism. In this case, the woman is literally capable of sucking the life force out of her male partner when he orgasms.

Years ago, David encountered a lover, the daughter of a famous occultist, who used the technique in this way. It was not an intimate meeting. She seemed extremely hard to him, as if she was made out of a cold, grey, unfeeling metal.

The instant they were done making love, she glanced at the macho silver sports watch still strapped to her wrist and announced, "Sorry. Got another appointment." The appointment was next door with a friend of his. She was having sex with as many young men as possible—sometimes two or three a night—in order to prolong her life and beauty.

At first, he was angry at her for using him. Then he felt sorry for her. She was the loser, for she could not feel love. Eventually, her skin-deep beauty will vanish. Then she will have to face the ugliness inside—alone.

While this is not likely to be an issue in your case, it is perhaps valuable to know about this. We in the West tend to underestimate the power of these ancient techniques.

Naturally, it is possible for the male to practice a parallel exploitation using similar techniques. While this has been justified to some extent traditionally by the belief that the woman's energy is supposedly inexhaustible, this claim is belied by the fact that practicioners of this "yoga" are instructed to choose the youngest possible partners, preferably virgins, and to move on quickly, taking the "cream from the top," so to speak.

A long-term relationship with an older woman, that is, over 30, is discouraged, as her energy is said to be mediocre in quality and weak in strength. Even if this practice does lead to increased longevity, it is reprehensible and not in the spirit of true lovemaking.

The best circumstance, then, will be when both consorts participate in full knowledge in this type of internal orgasm technique. An additional benefit is that working together in this way leads to blissful, mystical experiences that bring lovers much closer together. By consciously cooperating in this way, the power of the technique is multiplied and the master circuit of psychic and sexual energy, the Circle Of Gold, is completed (see *Fusion Breath Sex*).

According to ancient Tantric belief, there are two types of women. The first type is inclined towards and prefers multiple orgasms, although she enjoys single orgasms, too. The second type finds the achievement of multiple orgasms more challenging, even quite difficult. However, the women of the second type, even when achieving multiple orgasm, usually find that they prefer having one very intense orgasm.

Some women do find that they prefer to conserve the orgasm as well, that having an orgasm depletes them. Some women find that *Selfloving* with orgasm seems to be accompanied by a noticeable energy loss. Possibly some women gain more when they withhold their own while taking in the energy of the male orgasm.

Consort chemistry can make a big difference. Orgasm with an incompatible consort may fatigue while orgasm with a harmonious consort truly inspires and energizes. Observations of the human aura during intercourse reveal that emotional rapport greatly increases the regenerative blending of energy fields.

Several mystical schools teach the student to regard the female consort as a generator or open channel of life-giving forces. Rather than viewing the female ability to sustain arousal and repeat orgasms as a threat, males were taught that helping her build up to and sustain a state of ecstatic delirium brought both of them healing and inspiration.

The outer limits of female orgasmic ability remain uncharted. While some women are still struggling to have their first orgasm, there are women who have learned to have a genital orgasm through fantasy alone, to have orgasm when gently and rhythmically rubbed or patted on unlikely locations like the head, arm or foot, or to have genital orgasm easily during intercourse even with a hair-trigger lover who ejaculates in a minute or two.

What is orgasmically appropriate for women? Women should feel encouraged to find what is natural for them and do it, whether or not it conforms to an established norm.

Male Sexual Orgasm

In the ancient Chinese Taoist tradition (see *Tao Of Sex*), it was believed that men experienced significant loss if they ejaculated more frequently than their age and overall state of health allowed. Books with detailed rules and instructions were popular. Harmony between the sexes was thought to be possible only when a man was capable of prolonged,

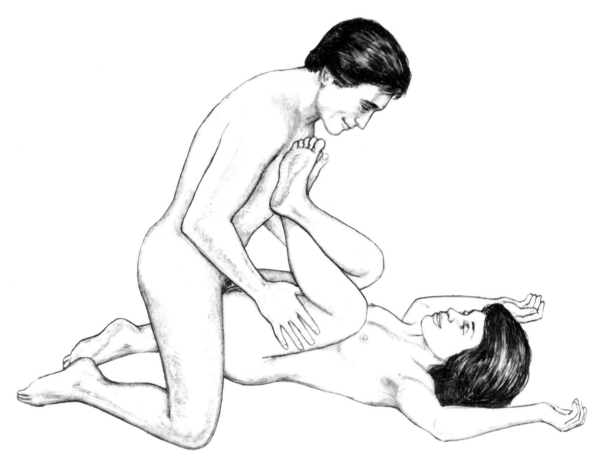

SHE CROSSES HER LEGS
above
This is easier than her legs
on his shoulders or her feet
pressed flat on his chest.
G spot stimulation and a
playful balance between
partners are the benefits.

leisurely intercourse, enabling the woman to climax to her
heart's desire.

For example, in *The Master of the Cave Profound* the
ideal method is for a man to make love very frequently but
to emit only two or three times for every 10 coitions. By
following this program, he is said to enjoy radiant health,
long life and inner peace.

In *The Secrets of the Jade Bedroom,* a less challenging
plan is suggested. Vigorously healthy males at 15 can ejaculate twice a day, at 30 once a day, at 40 once in three days,
at 50 once every five days, at 60 once each ten days and at
70 once in thirty days. Unhealthy males should wait twice as
long between emissions, e.g., at 30 once every two days.

The ancient Chinese prescriptions, in spite of their differences, do agree on four important points: the effects of
age, illness, seasons and frequent intercourse.

A man fifty or older should ejaculate no more than twice
per week. In times of sickness or extreme emotion a man

should avoid emission. The spring/winter rule should be followed, so that during the spring the man is free to enjoy a maximum frequency of ejaculation, but during winter he should avoid ejaculating altogether, especially if it is very cold. A man should make love as often as possible.

Contemporary research does offer some support for the Taoist ideas. For example, Winnifred Berg Cutler, co-author of *Menopause: A Guide for Women and the Men Who Love Them,* cites a number of strong studies that indicate a man's sexual hormones and virility start dropping in his 20s and go downhill from there. Ms. Cutler's concern is that there are a lot of frisky fiftyish ladies out there who can't find men with enough perk to play.

The male ejaculate is high in zinc and lecithin. These substances are found in high concentration in the brain. The ejaculate may contain other valuable nutrients as well. *Think And Grow Rich* devotes an entire chapter to seminal conservation, praising it as a great success secret.

Some contemporary men practice conservation instinctively via a sort of sexual energy "street smarts." This type of man may have no particular feeling for ejaculation conservation, yet intuitively prefers to avoid ejaculation when he is under a great deal of stress or simply working very hard. He reserves ejaculation for the weekend and for vacations.

Perhaps each man experiences an individualized cycle of true ejaculatory need. This need would vary a great deal from man to man. Many factors could determine a man's natural cycle of ejaculatory release, including heredity, age, vitality, stress level and lifestyle.

Irritability, low self-esteem, loss of self-confidence, sensations of loss or regret, depression, resentment towards or contempt for the woman or for himself and notable energy loss are some of the signs that may follow a very inappropriate ejaculation. Less dramatic and probably a great deal more common is a subtle but noticeable flatness in emotional tone or energy level following a forced ejaculation that may last for hours or even a day or two.

However, even these experiences have their silver lining. The discomfort that follows this deflation is not automatic. It is largely due to his unconscious struggle with this sudden yin condition.

When he relaxes and accepts, instead of distress he finds peace. There is an inertness about his inner state that enables him to go more deeply within, to stabilize in meditation. Contemplation of the void or emptiness is especially recommended.

Yoga teaches a practice of recycling semen emitted outside of the body through *Selfloving* or nocturnal emission. Make a ring with the fourth finger and thumb and rub the semen over your *Love Spot* and third eye point.

Any program of voluntary ejaculation conservation must be tailor-made. A man must listen closely to his bodymind. For example, a man on a severely toxic diet should improve his diet first.

Leisurely intercourse is better for conservation. A man should usually ejaculate after vigorous lovemaking to avoid overstressing his prostate gland, especially if he approached the point of no return.

A man who ejaculates according to his personal cycle of ejaculatory need experiences an invigorating renewal with ejaculation. To this fully celebratory ejaculation which is based on a man being very much in touch with his bodymind we give a different name, *ejac-elation*.

Orgasm—An Altered State

Our research indicates that working with the orgasm as an altered state of consciousness releases new energy levels and leads to breakthroughs in awareness. If the motivation for having a conventional climax at the time is merely to relieve tension, there does tend to be an energy loss. On the other hand, if the focused intention is to ride the wave of orgasmic bliss to a higher level of awareness, a positive, enhanced state of well-being results. Of course, a loving, understanding consort contributes greatly to this.

Also, as a result of sexercise training with the Thunderbolt Gesture, a sophisticated understanding of the movement of sexual energy develops so that even if physical emission of semen occurs, the essence that sexual yogis seek to conserve can still be retained and sent up the spine (see Conservation Chant in *Sound Sex*).

While physical semen does contain valuable nutrients, it is more importantly the carrier of psychic energy critical to the nervous and glandular systems of the body. When a man focuses on genital pleasure during orgasm, trying to make the expulsions as intense as possible, he is also encouraging maximum discharge of this subtle force, called *ojas*.

When the mind is used to divert the energy of orgasm up the spine to the centers of the brain, to expand it in a supercharged aura around the body or to shower it upon or radiate it to the consort, this essence tends to be recycled.

The belief system, attitude or state of consciousness that is associated with the orgasmic state has a very powerful effect. It is not so much what you do as how you do it.

PELVIC EXPRESSION

Singer Elvis Presley launched a musical career with his pelvis. Developing a loose yet dynamic pelvis can do the same for love lives. Pelvic awareness and freedom play a big role in making orgasm voluntary for both men and women.

Below you will find four good pelvic exercises. We have particularly enjoyed doing the first two to rock music. You can also take dance or movement classes, which may be the most effective approach. Bioenergetics training and various bodyworking methods are also helpful. *Total Orgasm* by Jack Rosenberg is a valuable guide.

Wear either loose clothing or no clothing at all. Make sure you will be alone or that whoever is with you is as interested as you are. Release your self-consciousness. Play your favorite music and let yourself go!

Pelvic Bounce

Pelvic bounces are done on the bed or on the floor. Like pelvic thrusts and circles, they can evoke powerful sexual feelings. Bouncing face down may be the closest thing to being a man on top in the missionary position that a woman can experience. Bouncing face up may be the closest thing to being a woman on the bottom that a man can experience.

To bounce face down, lie on your stomach with your palms flat on either side of your chest. Breathing through your mouth, lift only your pelvis and then let it down, so that it bounces gently against the floor or bed. Breathe through the mouth, exhaling sharply with each downward impact. A standard joke in our workshops is to say to the guys "Don't do this one when you have an erection!"

To bounce face up, lie on your back with your palms flat on either side of your buttocks, your knees bent. Breathing through your mouth, lift your pelvis a little and let it down, so that your lower back bounces gently against the floor or bed. Exhale sharply on each downward impact. You will naturally move your thighs up with your pelvis, so you will feel more whole body movement with this variation.

In our experience, bouncing face up lends itself to improvisation. You can bounce without impacting the floor with your back, doing a kind of limbo dance with your back lifted from the floor.

When you feel like taking a break, your first impulse will probably be to flop on the floor. Try holding a lifted up position like the one shown on the next page for a few seconds. Then slowly lower yourself down. Your experience of the openness and release that this exercise brings will now feel more complete.

Needless to say, don't do these exercises if you have a

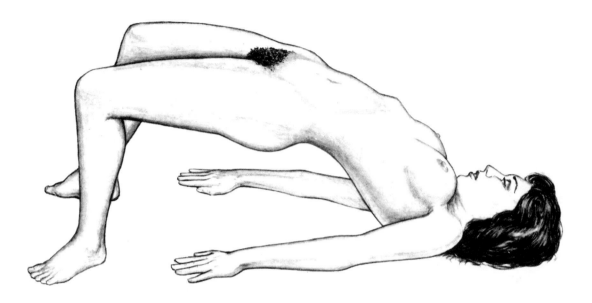

bad back or some problem with the pelvis. These movements are designed to be useful and fun, but are not intended to be therapeutic.

Pelvic Thrust *stand with your hands on your hips*

*pelvic thrusts
can be forward and back*

*or circle to the right
then circle to the left*

*exhale as you thrust forward
or circle forward
and inhale
as you pull backward
or circle backward*

*keep your weight low
really get into it . . .*

*do this for a bit
it's really fun to do to music*

PELVIC BOUNCE *above*
This is lots of fun. You
don't have to go as high as
the woman shown here.

*now for something even better
really cock your pelvis back
then snap it forward*

combine this with an inhalation
as you cock your pelvis

then exhale a sharp "Whooh!"
from the mouth
as you release it forward

dispense with the hands on the hips
if you like

this coordination of
pelvis in with breath in
and pelvis out with breath out
is really valuable
especially for men

it may feel unnatural at first
but it isn't

this is the way the pelvis and the breath
work best together

you may find that you tend
to hold your breath
this is a common experience
when you discover this is happening

just let it go
and keep on going

The Cat

The Cat *(Marjariasana)* is one of our personal favorites. While there are many other fine yoga poses and stretches, including Upward and Downward Dog, the Camel and the Sun Salutation sequence, the Cat has a certain sensual flavor and beauty that we find unique.

Beginning on all fours, inhale, letting your back sway. Bring your shoulder blades up and in. Lift up from your sterum. Your head follows.

Now exhale. Arch your upper back, tucking the pelvis in and under. Bring your chin towards your chest.

This sequence can be performed up to 10 times for one cycle, then repeated after a brief rest. For a variation, when the back is lifted on the exhalation, draw your diaphragm up and in and pull your anal muscles up and in. Keep this pose as long as it is comfortable.

The Cat brings flexibility to the spine and is excellent for

CAT *opposite*
A wonderfully sensual solo exercise, the Cat is one of our favorites. After mastering the basic movement, concentrate on complete breathing.

the back, the pelvis and genitals. It also assists in digestion, which in turn will improve the performance of the nervous system.

The Cat is also recommended for pregnant woman, who should do the Cat with their legs wide apart. They should avoid the variation mentioned above.

Regular practice of this simple exercise leads to a deeper understanding of the principle of expansion and contraction, inhalation and exhalation, yang and yin.

The Butterfly   The Butterfly (*Baddha konasana*) is a sitting stretch with the legs in front and soles of the feet together. It is an experience of unfolding rather than mere muscular stretching. Working with a partner may help, increasing the feeling of intimacy.

Newcomers to this pose can sit with a pillow or folded blanket under the buttocks, the back to a wall. When you are finished doing the posture, always use your hands on the outside of your knees to bring them slowly back together.

Open the knees to the side and join the soles of the feet together. Intertwine the hands or clasp the hands together under the toes. If you can't reach the toes, then hold onto your ankles.

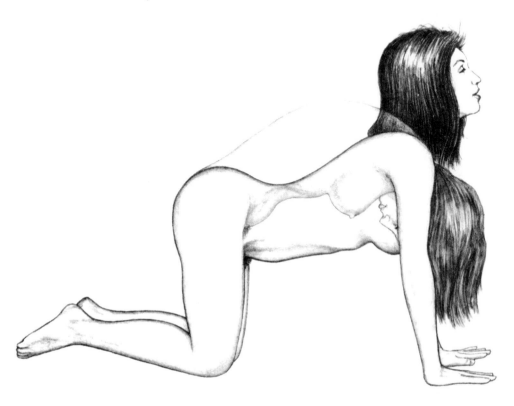

As you press one sole against the other, expand your chest lifting from the sternum. Keep your shoulders down and your head in line with your spine.

As you inhale, your head should rise. If you find it difficult to hold your hands under your feet you can grasp a sock or strap. This will allow you to add an extension to your arms so that you can feel your chest expand and open wide. Then you will naturally feel your belly expand and begin to breathe deeply from there.

Many make the mistake of trying to force the knees down, as if this is aerobics. You will find that your knees come down without any effort. If you are in pain, place a pillow under each knee, just high enough to ease the pain. All that is needed is to open your chest and breathe deeply. You will feel yourself opening like a sunflower to the sky.

A partner can help with this experience by resting their hands gently on your thighs from the front. Or they can do the pose with you with your backs touching.

You may also want to try the Butterfly lying down. A simple, quite restful version is to place the buttocks flush against the wall. The outer edges of the feet are supported by the wall higher up, of course.

Whatever way you choose to enjoy it, the Butterfly is a delicious private opening to be savored from within. It is not necessary to think of surrendering to a partner. Surrender to yourself. The openness will follow easily.

Enjoyed in this way, the Butterfly reveals that yoga is very much about the breath. As the body opens, unfurls, uncurls, so does the sexual energy. This is the natural way.

The Butterfly is said to offer many health benefits, including help with genital and urinary imbalances, sciatica, and menstrual irregularity. Pregnant women who do this pose every day for just a few minutes are said to have little pain at childbirth and to avoid varicose veins.

PLEASURE, HEALTH AND THE ANUS

The anus is a taboo and secret place. An area where many nerve endings are concentrated, it can be a source of great pain or pleasure. Many people need to be sexually aroused before the anus feels like a pleasure center. Though greatly neglected, the anus is a significant erotic zone.

At the same time, it said to be associated with stored fear and anger due to our very early conditioning. The next time you get angry, shift your awareness to your anus. You may find it is clenched like a tiny but rigidly powerful fist.

There is also a connection between the anal region and the cardiovascular system. Hence the ancient Egyptians used retention enemas not only to cleanse the anus and the colon but to heal the heart as well.

Releasing Tension   Tension in the anal region is largely unconscious. However, when the anus releases, sexual performance and pleasure often increases for both men and women. Sensitivity of the clitoris or penis may be heightened.

Since there are valid hygienic concerns, the best approach is probably to use latex gloves (available direct from sex product supply houses). Immediately after you are done, discard the glove(s). As an added precaution, you can rinse your hands with alcohol.

Feces usually cannot be found in the rectum except just before excretion. As soft feces may be present, however, anal douching is appropriate if your partner is concerned.

You can help each other heal the anal region through gentle, caring massage. Start with the buttocks. Use a small amount of vegetable oil. If you don't own a massage table, have your partner lie on the floor, not the bed.

Sit to the side of your partner. Use firm pressure to move your hands in circles from the outside of the buttocks inward. Follow with the thumbs in alternating strokes going up the buttocks. Complete with the beginning stroke.

After this warm-up massage, apply plenty of lubrication and, with a suitably covered finger, slowly enter. Once your finger is inside, you can gently rotate it or wiggle it.

Some may prefer the use of a vibrator or dildo instead of a flesh finger. Any sex toys used with this area need to be seamless and have a flared base. Any object used that is more than four inches long needs to be very flexible as it must easily accomodate the curve of the rectum.

The recipient should always feel that he or she is in total control. Go as slowly as they wish. They set the pace. Be sure they know this.

The initial response of the anal muscles may be to spasm, as if defending themselves. This is a natural response. Simply remain gently in place. Allow this response until it subsides. It is very common.

Encourage the receiving partner to be as relaxed as possibly, breathing deeply and making sounds of release as needed. They can think of relaxing, melting, letting go, nurturing their inner child. Buoyed by your warmth and support, their experience will be most pleasurable, and may lead to a deep breakthrough.

Opening Up

For men, especially, opening up to a gentle finger in the anus can lead to a wonderful new realm of sexual responsiveness. A quivering stimulation by the exploring finger all over the prostate area can be the key that allows the first experience of the deeper, more internal orgasmic release, as the prostate is much closer to the core of the body.

Indeed, the man may discover that for the first time he feels like a full participant, not just an outsider or observer.

Enjoying anal stimulation may make him a better lover, as anal relaxation is a key to ejaculation control, sensitivity to pleasure and emotional opening. Also, the root of the penis, at the front of the anus, is easily stimulated in this way, leading to yet more erotic sensitivity.

Feelings of vulnerability are very common after this experience. Women especially may find that opening in the anal region leads directly to getting in touch with repressed rage. It is not that these emotions are stored only there, but relaxing and opening this region tends to trigger awareness of such feelings.

As with anything else experimental, take this process very slowly. Verbalize as you go: "How does this feel?" "My God, I never realized how strong the PC muscle is. I can really feel it!" Encourage a dialog at first.

Relaxed caressing of their whole body beforehand helps considerably. If pain develops, the experience should be stopped immediately.

An excellent time to begin discovering your anal region on your own is in water, during a bath or shower. Just a simple caress of your anal region is beneficial. If you are comfortable with the idea, gently move your finger into your anus.

Allow the anal sphincter muscles, both inner and outer, to contract and expand around it. Breathe deeply to connect with your anus.

Anal arousal for pleasure usually focuses on the rim of the opening. This is where the most nerve connections are situated. Stimulating the anus has been known to lead to orgasm for both men and women. Due to the prevalence of AIDS, we cannot recommend anal intercourse or rimming (oral love of the anus).

If you like using a vibrator, select an attachment and use it *only* for anal loving. Specialized attachments are available that match the natural curvature of the anal canal. Consult Jack Morin's unique guide *Anal Pleasure & Health* if you would like to go further (see *Appendix*).

POMPOIR POWER The voluntary control of the circumvaginal muscles during sexual intercourse is known as pompoir ("pahm-*pour*") in the Tamil language of Southern India. According to authors Herbert and Roberta Otto, a popular mythology developed around this ability in the United States between 1930 and 1950. Popular sexual literature made much of this ability under the name "snapping pussy," which in the South was called "snapping turtle."

The Arabic world had a word for a woman who had developed and mastered her circumvaginal muscles for the purpose of enhanced lovemaking. She was called *kabbazah,* "holder."

If you've ever had the experience, from either end, then you know just how appropriate the label is. Women of Ethiopia and Southern India, in particular, enjoyed renown as kabbazahs. All in all, the skill was at one time more common the world over than it is now.

The Benefits The erotic intensity of a pompoir-powered union in any style, hard or soft, should not be underestimated. Pompoir is a profound contribution to the entire spectrum of lovemaking that yields a new erotic universe. Dependence on male thrusting alone to reach the heights of erotic glory is like trying to win a foot race on one leg.

For women, this training can be a very rewarding experience. In pompoir the penis can be fondled, caressed, gripped, massaged, milked, licked, inundated and rippled as a whole or in sections. But don't think that the fun is all only his. The experience is uniquely arousing and satisfying for you, too.

You will be able to achieve genital orgasm more easily by clenching, especially when you combine it with breathing in or out. In fact, some women report they can achieve orgasm via clenching in a kind of "no hands" *Selfloving*. This skill is enhanced by an intense yet relaxed concentration on the physical sensations and, for some women, letting go into sizzling erotic fantasies.

The gripping action of pompoir can be combined with thrusting, giving you the best of both worlds. Far from being an exotic trick, pompoir is the female counterpart to the male's thrusting ability. Men are born with penises but a certain amount of practice is usually needed to move a penis with real finesse. Likewise, women can train their vaginal muscles and develop the art of pompoir.

According to prominent sex therapist Bryce Britton, conditions that may be avoided or even eliminated by doing

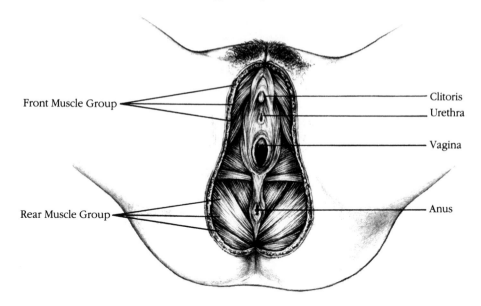

Front Muscle Group

Rear Muscle Group

Clitoris
Urethra
Vagina
Anus

pompoir development exercises include vaginitis, cystitis, incontinence, constipation, failure to orgasm and infertility. On a personal health basis alone, do the exercises.

Using pompoir you may also experience many delights and psychological benefits as well as the health benefits mentioned above. You may become more orgasmic, experience more pleasure through your vagina, improve your sexual health, become more self-confident sexually and in daily life.

As your vaginal sensitivity increases, you may find that soft style lovemaking is more enjoyable. For example, lying motionless together after he has entered is more satisfying, especially with an impromptu squeeze now and then. When you do start moving, squeeze as he enters or leaves. As erotic intensity builds, movements of exquisite slowness bring intense pleasure. Be sure to try this when you are on top.

Mentally focus on the pleasurable feelings. Concentrate on the rich sensory details. Visualize the vaginal muscles in action. You can even relive the sensations in your imagination when you are alone. According to Britton, you are actually developing new nerve connections.

The Training   There is nothing mysterious about how to develop the pompoir skill. The Kegel exercises or other sexercises practiced daily for a few months will develop virtuoso ability in most women. Once the muscles have been trained, it doesn't take that much to keep them in shape.

Britton suggests visualizing a sequence of rings inside the vaginal tunnel. This can be three, six or nine rings, as long as they are divided into groups of three.

Feel and see these rings get smaller as you tighten the muscles. Then expand them to normal size as you relax the muscles. Practice with an object inside, such as a dildo, for valuable feedback. Eventually, it is good to practice with your partner's penis resting inside of you.

Distinguish between sensations in the front, middle and back thirds of the vagina. Also go around the clock, placing your attention inside your vagina at the top, along the right wall, at the bottom and along the left wall of your vagina.

Discover where your sensitivity is the greatest. If your partner is practicing with you, ask him to flex his PC muscle again and again. Explore the resulting sensations.

By learning to distinguish your PC, or circumvaginal muscle, contractions front to back and back to front, you will develop the renowned pompoir skill. Then, according to Hindu erotology, you will be a queen of love. Our experience indicates that this is not merely poetic license.

The Key   The key to pompoir skill is that there are two circumvaginal muscle groups involved. The Root Lock and the Thunderbolt Gesture of yoga develop these muscles groups separately first and then coordinate them (see *Sexercises*).

The first group is the outer front muscles near the clitoris, which includes the bulbocavernosus, ischiocavernosus and urethral sphincter muscles. The second group is the inner rear muscles near the anus, which includes the pubococcygeus, iliococcygeus and levator ani muscles. These two muscle groups create the female pelvic floor.

They are not so neatly separated as this analysis suggests. The pubococcygeus (pew-boh-cox-uh-jee-us), or PC, muscle stretches from the pubic bone to the coccyx. The point is that these muscle groups can be independently and voluntarily controlled.

The full pompoir action is a sequential or simultaneous contraction of the two muscle groups. The movement can be from front to back or from back to front or both at once. This action has most often been described as a milking, sucking or massaging motion.

The *Ananga Ranga* of Kalyana Malla describes a two-stage process that is based on the woman's ability to focus. The first stage is simple contraction and release so that a penis or other cylindrical object in the vagina will be firmly grasped. The second stage is the famed milking motion.

CIRCUMVAGINAL MUSCLES
opposite
Anatomy is rarely appealing but this diagram gets the point across—she has very powerful love muscles that can be trained, with heavenly results for both of you.

SAFER SEX   Today, of course, AIDS is a major concern. The threat of AIDS has lead to deeper commitment in some relationships. To other couples it has brought pain and sorrow as young lives and deep loves are lost. The impact of AIDS varies greatly from one person to the next, but all agree that we need to be well informed and stay up to date as new information becomes available.

There are many ways of being together described in this book that a couple can do without genital union or the exchange of bodily fluids. Indeed, it is possible to have a deeply satisfying climax without genital stimulation. Neither kissing nor removal of clothing are necessary for this kind of energy orgasm, sometimes called Tantric orgasm, to take place.

Some couples have found great fulfillment in the sexual celibacy style. Because performance and disease are not issues, a deep intimacy is easily reached as you hold and surrender to each other. Some couples discover that this leads to a wonderful ecstatic experience that is equal, if not superior, to conventional sexual satisfaction.

Safer sex today means using condoms, and using them correctly. The water-based lubricant Astroglide® is highly recommended. Also, the spermicide nonoxynol-9 will offer extra protection.

You can eroticize your use of condoms. Make the condom a part of your ritual as you prepare to make love. Give it a funny name and laugh at the silliness of it. Or make the use of a condom a special experience.

We know a couple who calls the condom "Mr. Dickie's raincoat." Another couple does a chant to the goddess of love as they pass a crystal over the condom to "raise its vibration and allow the free exchange of subtle energies."

As of this writing, there is no cure for AIDS. Do take the time to become as fully informed as possible—and to inform your partner(s) as well. It could save your life.

Of course, AIDS is not the only sexually transmitted disease. Please take the time to be informed about other health risks of sexual contact. Remember, even though intercourse with a condom is safer, it is still not totally safe sex.

Safe Encounters by Whipple and Ogden, *Terrific Sex in Fearful Times* by Peters, *The Condom Book* by Everett and Glanze and *The Complete Guide to Safe Sex* by the Institute for Advanced Study of Human Sexuality are good sources of information. There is even an audio tape available called *How to Talk With a Partner About Smart Sex* by Zilbergeld and Barbach. Please see the *Appendix* for more resources.

SELFLOVING   Masturbation is an ugly sounding word with negative connotations. In spite of today's supposed sexual sophistication, you can still find "self-abuse" listed as a synonym for selfloving in the dictionary. We prefer "selfloving," the innovative term developed by Betty Dodson.

Onanism, from the story of Onan in Genesis, is another insensitive synonym. Onan was punished for spilling his seed—during *coitus interruptus,* in fact—rather than fertilizing an available female. Though this attitude may have made sense when survival of the race was at stake, in today's overpopulated world it does not.

However, just to call masturbation selfloving does not eliminate the negative programming. You may be surprised at how helpful it is to actually give yourself permission to have pleasure and enjoy selfloving. This can be done in the form of affirmations or even a little ceremony that you create for yourself.

Guilt and shame about selfloving is less about masturbation and more about your attitude towards sex. As a private, uninhibited opportunity to explore the sexual and sensual potential of your own body, the positive power of selfloving actually opens you up to being a better, more enjoyable partner when in bed with another.

While the importation of Eastern attitudes towards sex has certainly brought a degree of enlightenment, there is also a hidden hazard. These Tantric and Taoist systems bring with them a rigid philosophy of conservation of the sexual energy, which is sometimes expressed in vividly paranoid terms. Consider this Taoist advice to men, designed to encourage semen retention: "Making love is as hazardous as taking a walk on the brim of a vast abyss filled with razor-edged swords." Surely such advice is going to inhibit surrender!

Whether sex is with self or with another, we are in fact consorting with the life force, which is our actual lover. But the usual notion is different.

When we are supposedly with the other, we are not in fact with them. Then, when we are physically alone selfloving, we tend to feel ashamed and abandoned. We miss the enjoyment, for we tend to think we should be with a partner.

The Benefits   Selfloving, Dodson elaborates in *Sex For One,* is good for many reasons. It offers a way to relieve tension and fall asleep. It offers a way to feel good that is self-sufficient and under our control. It provides an outlet for people who do not have partners. It is the best training for learning how to have an orgasm and also how to control the arousal that leads to orgasm. It can enable a partner to have orgasm when the stimulation via intercourse is insufficient. It can keep a couple together when one partner is no longer interested in sex. It can relieve menstrual cramps.

Selfloving gives teenagers a way to have their orgasms with no risk of pregnancy. It is a beautiful way for a couple to share. It can be a powerful form of dynamic meditation, complete with brain waves going not only into alpha but delta as well. It is perhaps the most direct way to develop a deep and lasting appreciation of our sex organs and physical being, healing our body image. Last but not least, so important in a world with AIDS, it is the primordial way to have safe sex.

In The Mood Here are a few factors to incorporate in your selfloving. Set up the environment as you would for lovemaking. This includes putting the phone machine on. Have your favorite oil or lotion on hand, a towel, a mirror so you can watch yourself easily, a big comfortable pillow to lean on and your favorite music.

Retune your thinking to view the act as literally a gesture of self-love and empowerment. Most important of all, take your time.

To help get in the mood, start with a warm bubble bath (for men, too). Then do some stretching, perhaps the pelvic workouts or yoga. Try dancing. Reflect on the importance of loving yourself. Place one hand on your genitals, the other on your chest at the heart and affirm "I love my genitals, I love myself."

Maintain deep complete breathing while selfloving. Kundalini Kegel or *Elevate Energy,* even just a few PC muscle clenches, are good here. When the time comes for sexual arousal, feel free to use any means (do not use a vibrator in the tub or shower, of course!).

Play with the affirmation "You love me" while selfloving. You may find that the "you" is actually you, that what you really need is not love from someone else but love from self. The love you get is the love you choose to let in.

You can even open directly to Love without thinking of a specific person. "I am open to love. Love is all around me. Love surrounds me and fills me. I am filled with the bliss of love. I am totally fulfilled [full filled]."

For those with a devotional bent, here is another approach to creating a sacred atmosphere. On a small but attractive table or box, place a red and white candle, rose, sandalwood or jasmine incense (if you like incense) and the picture of a god or goddess (in a protective plastic pouch) that you relate to.

If you are into mythology or Eastern religion, you may have connected with such a being or symbol already. Here is a new way to invite them into your self (see *God And Goddess*). Make love to them as you make love with yourself.

Whether the stimulus is a pornographic magazine, book or video or the memory of a passionate partner encounter, it is good to let go of the external source or at least become somewhat independent of it. Use your erotic stimulus, a magazine picture, for example, as a trigger. Once you get going, switch over to a detailed, self-created fantasy that incorporates the imagery, sights, sounds, smells and setting suggested by your stimulus.

Inner Lover   As you tenderly stroke your lips, imagine that it is the lips of your fantasy lover. As you play with your breasts or chest, imagine that it is the hand of your fantasy lover that caresses you. As you play with your clitoris or penis, imagine that it is the hand or genitals of your fantasy lover that arouses you. You will quickly become stimulated to orgasm.

The art of internalizing the lover becomes easier with practice. One way to develop your ability to fantasize is to review your favorite personal erotic memories in detail. In this way you will develop skill at evoking sense impressions using your mind's eye, its ear, nose, tongue and skin, too. Just as a writer must emphasize the sensual detail in a story, you will find that the more specific your memory or fantasy, the more powerful it becomes (see *Dream Lover*).

The ultimate level of practice with the imaginary lover(s) is, perhaps, to reactivate the feeling of orgasm from memory or imagination alone, without physical stimulation. Then the pleasure of orgasm can be accessed to some degree at virtually anytime.

This can also be achieved via training with a mystical symbol (such as a circle with a dot in the middle) and an opening sound (like *"Aaahh"*). This task is made easier when the eyes remain closed and the process is approached as a meditation. Remember, the orgasm is a conditioned response.

Strangely enough, there can be performance stress even when selfloving. For men, it is the tendency to "jerk off" and rush the act, to "get off" quickly and grab a little tension relief. For women, the demand can be to have an orgasm right off, to have a better orgasm or a multiple orgasm, or perhaps simply to have an orgasm.

FEEL THEIR TOUCH
overleaf
It is easy to see how the expression "fertile imagination" came to be.

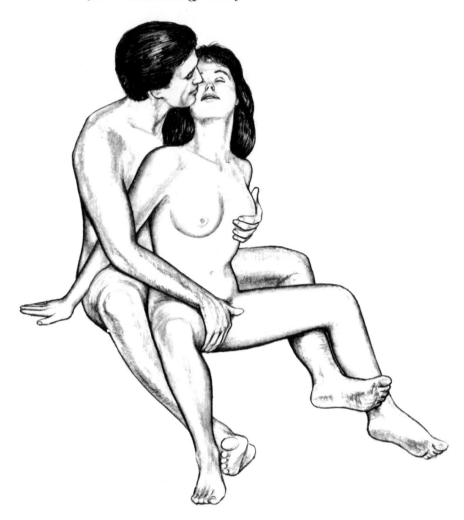

The G Spot—
Hers And His

As the clitoris is a woman's main sex organ, the Gräfenberg or G spot has become another potential source of confusion and performance stress. While every woman has the G spot or urethral sponge region, women experience this area differently. Unstimulated, its surface area is small and often hard to locate. After a woman is sexually aroused, it swells to between a dime and a half-dollar in size. Then it can be felt as a firm area some two inches in along the front wall of the vagina. Women vary enormously in their response.

Some claim that G spot stimulation leads to a deeper climax that is more satisfying than what they are able to achieve through clitoral stimulation alone. Yet many women, including some leaders of female sexual liberation, claim they haven't been able to find it or, when they did, it was no big deal. *The G Spot* by Ladas, Whipple and Perry gives excellent instructions on how to find and stimulate it. A vibrator with a G spot attachment may help (see *Appendix*).

The male parallel is the prostate gland which can be indirectly stimulated through the perineum between the testicles and anus or directly through the anus (use a surgical glove or finger for safer, or just plain clean, sex). An important pleasure center, it accounts for the thrilling throbbing at the base of the penis that men feel during ejaculation (see *Pleasuring The Lingam, Voluntary Orgasm For Men*).

An added advantage to stimulating this Prostate Point area is that it delays ejaculation and prolongs pleasure. Pressure on the prostate relieves some of the buildup of fluid which leads to the sense of ejaculatory urgency. The prostate is called the *Kunda* in Kundalini yoga and the ancient texts extol its virtues. A man can certainly stimulate himself here during selfloving (try the G-Spotter from Good Vibrations).

Take it easy at first. Indeed, it is not necessary to have orgasm when you are selfloving. The most important thing is that you are spending quality time with yourself (see *Pleasuring The Yoni, Voluntary Orgasm For Women*).

Mutual Selfloving Yet another alternative is mutual selfloving. While we discuss stimulating another elsewhere, we want to emphasize the delight of watching your consort stimulate themselves. Not only can it be powerfully erotic, you may find that you learn a great deal about what they enjoy and how they like to be stimulated.

David was a bit hesitant the first time. Not any more. It is a beautiful event to share and witness.

Selfloving And Tantra Selfloving has many levels and styles. For example, in *Masturbation, Tantra and Self-Love,* Margo Woods describes a technique using selfloving that she learned from her Tantric teacher.

For three months, selflove every day. Bring yourself to the brink of orgasm at least three times. Each time you reach that point, on an inbreath pull the energy up to the chest to the feeling center of the heart.

Generally, it is recommended that you conclude with orgasm. The only exception would be if you have become very adept at transmuting the sex force, which only you can know.

This technique is designed to quickly bring altered states of consciousness, opening to love and transformation of negative emotional states. At a practical level, Woods experienced healing in the types of relationships she attracted.

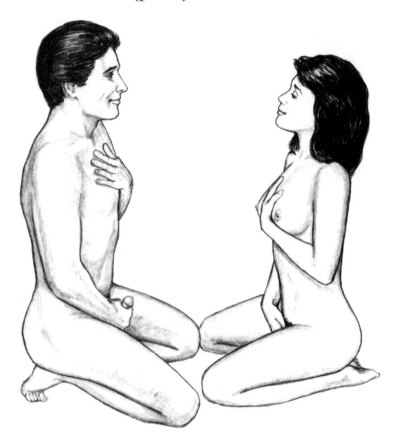

MUTUAL SELFLOVING
above
We learned new ways to
give pleasure to each other.
Validation that it is OK to
selflove when you have a
consort was a nice bonus.

As her body image changed, she also lost weight. More and more, she loved herself for herself and was no longer seeking pleasure from food. She had found the source of pleasure was in herself.

The solar plexus and third eye are also suitable points for focusing your near peak orgasm energy. Drawing the force up your spine to the solar plexus will help you increase your store of energy. Taking it up to the third eye leads to visionary or flying or other expanded space type experiences.

Of course, to open to more love, draw the energy up to the heart. To help you concentrate on the heart center or third eye point, place saliva or a dab of clove or peppermint oil on the breastbone or at the space between the eyebrows.

Remember, just because you take the energy up doesn't mean you can't go ahead and enjoy the pleasure of conventional orgasm. In effect, you can have your cake—conserve the sexual energy—and eat it, too.

If you are into the extremes of sex energy conservation, know that before you decide to give up conventional or-

gasms you need to *fully* explore and be very comfortable
with your erotic self first.

Do the Root Lock, Kundalini Kegel or *Elevate Energy* to
move the energy up, then eventually go ahead and have
your climax. Our experience has been that when the sex
energy is spread throughout the body and not concentrated
in the genitals (successfully transmuted in a given session),
you will know it! There is no question of frustration or
holding back or denying yourself. You feel complete.

What you do want is to have fun. What you don't want is
to be stuck with undischarged, hot energy that doesn't know
where to go (which may result result in health problems if
natural release is denied over a long period of time).

It is valuable to recognize that one of the benefits of the
Sexercises in this book and similar workouts is that they lead
to a direct experience of sexual pleasure that is based on
opening to self as source.

Conventional, direct stimulation of the genitals is only
one form of selfloving. Just as with partner sex, what you do
to prepare and get in the right mood will turn self-conscious
masturbation into an uninhibited celebration of selfloving.

SEXERCISES

Sexercises, of course, is a combination of the words "sexual"
and "exercises." Sexercises are designed to maximize sex
muscle strength and control.

Weak flabby muscles cannot do their job well. Your arm
muscles can do their job fairly well because you use them
every day. Your sex muscles, though, are rarely used in your
daily life. You use them to hold in urine or feces until you
can get to the bathroom. That's about it.

The monarch of the sex muscles is the pubococcygeus
(pew-boh-cox-uh-jee-us), or PC, muscle. This muscle contracts at the rate of one every .8 seconds in both sexes during
orgasm. The anal muscles also contract.

The contemporary rediscovery of the great value of these
muscles for sexual health and pleasure is credited to a Los
Angeles physician, Arnold Kegel. He developed the famed
Kegel (*kay*-gill) exercises in the 1950s. It may not be news
that you can exercise your sex muscles. The popularity of
Kegel exercises has seen to that. But do you know that the
Kegel exercises are a rediscovery? Effective sexercises have
been practiced in China and India for thousands of years.

The ancient experts viewed the human bodymind as a
bucket full of energy with holes in the bottom where life

energy leaked out. These holes are the urethral opening, the anal opening and, in the woman, the vaginal opening also. It was believed that when these sex muscles were sufficently strengthened through exercise they sealed the bottom of the bucket.

The Eastern sexercises were developed in cultures that placed less emphasis on the genital orgasm. Currently, sex experts tout the development of the PC muscle and other sex muscles as a way to achieve, intensify, prolong and control genital orgasm in both sexes. Neither approach is better in itself. When less emphasis is placed on getting the orgasmic payoff, though, other personal gains, such as emotional growth or health benefits, may become more noticeable.

Whether or not you focus on having orgasms is not the real issue. That is a matter of personal style. It is also worth noting that some men and women have observed that these sexercises have a significant rejuvenating effect.

In our seminars, we ask how many regularly do Kegel or yogic PC muscle exercises. Usually, only a few hands go up. Given the endless emphasis on exercise in this culture, this seems surprising. Perhaps it is guilt about sex, perhaps it is the fact that it is not obvious (until you make love!) that you do these sexercises, as they do not give you big breasts or bulging biceps.

Addicted to appearances, we fail to become artists of love. As the paint brush is to the painter, these sexercises are to the love artist. They are not crude mechancial gestures but symphonies of the bodymind that lead to self-generated waves of bliss. For those so inclined, these methods lead to the awakening of Kundalini, the mystic life force, and the arousal of and union with the cosmic lover within who leads us beyond inner conflict to happiness.

Kegel Exercise   Before you start Kegel muscle squeezing, it is most important that you locate the exact muscle involved. The anatomical name of the so-called Kegel muscle is the pubococcygeus muscle. It's called the PC muscle by many people who work with it.

Where is your PC muscle? It stretches between your legs, from your genitals and your anus. It is part of the pelvic floor in both sexes.

The standard way to find your PC muscle is to stop and start as you urinate. Do this several times. There—you've found it! Women may need to keep the legs open wide so that the muscles in the buttocks don't add confusing signals (see *Pompoir*).

Another way is to pretend you've got to hold back a bowel movement and tighten your anal muscles. Or you can try the direct approach. Insert a well-lubricated (use saliva, vegetable oil, KY jelly or Astroglide®) finger into the anus and squeeze. You will feel the anal muscles as well as the PC.

Men should stand in front of a mirror and make their penis move up and down as they squeeze their PC muscle. Women can delicately place their index and/or middle finger in the vagina and squeeze. The vagina will grasp them, perhaps quite firmly. It may even push them out. The PC muscle itself can be felt in the vagina as a ribbed muscle about one and a half inches in.

Do not use the stomach muscles to do this. Once you get the hang of it, you can do "Kegels" writing, reading, walking, sitting, working, watching TV, listening to music and so on.

You may find that a tightening of the muscles in the stomach and thighs happens no matter what you do at first. This is common. But after the first few days or weeks, when you've completely isolated the muscle, these extra contractions should be hardly noticeable.

Once you have definitely found the PC muscle, start with quick or short Kegel squeezes. Contract the muscle 20 times at about one a second or faster as one session. Do two sessions your first day. Gradually build up to 75 twice a day. When you can comfortably do 75 quickie Kegel contractions twice a day, add sustained or long Kegel movements.

Long Kegel squeezes are equally simple. Instead of holding the muscle contraction for a count of one, hold it for a count of three. Start with 20 of these per session, two sessions a day. Build up to 75 each session twice a day. Take your time. Avoid straining. The PC muscle is just like any other muscle. If you overdo it, it will become sore.

You will have built up to 300 reps a day. However, once the PC muscle has been strengthened, a maintenance regime of 150 per day in one three-minute session should be plenty. Make these focused, committed clenches. Concentrate deeply on the physical sensations. You may find this easier if you close your eyes.

Learn to relax between contractions. Without this relaxation the muscles will not grow as quickly. Relaxation is as important to your control as contraction. If a man learns how to relax these muscles during sexual intercourse, he can last much longer.

It may help to breathe in time with your clenches or to count breaths. You may be holding your breath and not even realize it.

Some people include the bearing down maneuver in their daily work outs. After first tightening, then releasing the PC muscle, push down and out gently as if trying to have a bowel movement.

This is the same sequence that you would use for sexual arousal and control. You will feel the action of your stomach muscles and anus as you bear down. We call this a "push out" (see *Voluntary Orgasm For Men*).

A useful variation is to do sets of reps that pair long Kegel clenches with strong push outs. Try doing these after you've developed good PC muscle strength.

While doing Kegels to music can be fun, not all music is suitable. The most important thing is the rhythm. We find that "Union of the Snake" by Duran Duran is a good example of a popular song with the right kind of rhythm as well as a relevant message (snakes are a symbol for sexual energy and Kundalini).

Men can easily add weight training to their Kegel practices. After achieving erection, place a small wet towel on your erect penis. Move this towel up and down. You can increase the size of the towel. Some men even use sandbag weights. A participant in one of our workshops told us that young men in his high school held locker room contests to see how many towels they could lift.

Women can work with cylindrical objects that provide solid resistance.

Use the power of visualization. The great bodybuilder Arnold Schwarzeneger worked out using precise mental images to guide the growth of his muscles.

Women can see their vagina as a tunnel made up of several muscular bands that can contract or expand at will. These circular bands of muscle are seen growing in size and strength with each contraction.

Men can imagine that the PC muscle is a steel cable running between their legs which they can tighten or loosen at will. The steel cable should be seen as growing thicker and stronger with each repetition.

You can affirm as you clench. With a quick Kegel clench say a short positive affirmation such as "Yes" or "Love." With a long Kegel clench you can say a longer affirmation. In the *Ananga Ranga,* women are training in the arts of love are advised to repeat "Kamadeva," the sacred name of the Hindu Cupid, with each clench. Another mantra, said to have great esoteric power, is "Kling."

Don't be surprised if the exercises arouse erotic feelings while you're doing them. This is part of the fun. Whatever your approach, develop your ability to focus your attention on your sensations and feelings for maximum results and enjoyment.

Indeed, you may feel waves of bliss that have nothing to do with your environment at the time. They are not caused by an outside stimulus. They are internally generated. You are awakening your natural inborn pleasure potential.

Sexercises are, in fact, an autosexual act that can lead to a profoundly transforming union of male and female within yourself. Naturally, the more interested you are in your mystical potential, the more likely such experiences will be.

The benefits of the Kegel exercises are numerous. These include getting more in touch with your genitals and sexual feelings, improving the blood flow to these areas (which can be quite healing in itself) and making orgasm more voluntary.

Women can use it to firm up the muscles of the vagina after having a child. Kegel exercises have enabled many pre-orgasmic women to become orgasmic. Muscle strength, sensitivity and control gained through Kegel contraction exercises are known to make genital orgasm during intercourse or *Selfloving* more voluntary and more intense. Coordinate the Kegel clenches with breathing, visualization and concentration for maximize results and control.

Men can use it to delay ejaculation. Intensely contract the PC muscle, then fully relax it. Contraction when on the verge of ejaculation or nearly so, however, is likely to bring it on.

After two months of dedicated practice, you will probably have achieved mastery over your PC muscle. If you have—you will know by the results in bed—you can maintain good PC muscle tone with occasional workouts. Virtuoso status, though, is achieved and maintained only by working out weekly, if not daily.

The Chinese Deer Exercise

In ancient Chinese health theory, the sex glands are the stove that heats the bodymind house. Feed the stove plenty of wood (keep the sex glands energized via lovemaking and sexercises) and the house will stay warm and full of life.

The Deer exercise is an ancient Chinese health practice. The muscles around the anus are contracted. This gives the sexual muscles a good workout. The anal contraction is coordinated with other techniques. These techniques help move the heat from the sexual stove to other parts of the body.

Actually, this distribution of energy takes place automatically. The overflow from the awakened sex glands goes up to the thymus gland. The thymus gland shunts the energy up to the thyroid, pituitary and pineal glands.

Depleted persons need to strengthen the sex glands first. After they have stoked the sexual stove by doing the Deer exercise consistently for several weeks or months, the heat will begin to spread, energizing and revitalizing. A cold stove heats nothing, not even itself (see *Tao Of Sex*).

Female Deer Exercise

First the Deer exercise is performed in two steps. Later these steps are combined. If possible, practice it right after waking up and just before going to sleep. If not, then do it once a day. However, if you are pregnant, do *not* practice this exercise, not even for one day. Taoist sexology forbids it.

Sit naked on a flat surface, such as your bedroom floor, with your legs stretched out before you. Bend either leg and place the heel in your vagina so that it presses firmly against your clitoris. If this is not comfortable, place a hard ball there instead. The pressure should be consistently firm.

Now bring your other leg close to your body. Raise the foot of this leg and rest it on the calf of the leg already in position. Insert the toes between the calf and thigh. If this is too difficult, place the other leg in front of you. Sit as erect as you can without straining.

The most important thing is to be comfortable. A small pillow under the buttocks and a folded towel between the ankles may help. If you practice yoga, you may know this position under the name *Siddha Yoni Asana*.

Arousal may take place, which can be encouraged. This can be performed as an elaborate *Selfloving* exercise, the self-stimulation caused by the heel being the first stage. But this is not at all necessary.

Rub your hands together quickly in order to create as much heat as possible. Put your hands on your breasts and feel the heat from the friction. From a central position, the *Love Spot,* move your hands upward and outward and continue circling around gently massaging your breasts.

Maintain the pressure of the heel against your clitoris as you do a minimum of 36 circles and a maximum of 360 circles. A pleasant warm feeling may be experienced at the breasts or genitals. This is a good sign. You are accumulating energy.

This movement is said to have a healing effect on the breasts. According to Dr. Stephen Chang of San Francisco, lumps or cancer may be avoided or even eliminated. It may reduce the size of the breasts. The opposite direction may enlarge the breasts but have the opposite health effects.

To perform the second part of the exercise, drop the hands to a comfortable position and maintain the gentle but firm clitoral pressure. The second part requires you to contract the vaginal and anal muscles. Hold this as long as you can without straining, then relax. Contract and relax these muscles as many times as you are can with ease. The correct feeling is that you are trying to suck air up into your vaginal and anal openings.

Take it easy. Don't overdo it. You may experience a delightful feeling that flows from the genitals to the top of the head. This indicates that your pituitary and pineal glands are being fed by the sexual glands.

After about a month, the muscle contractions will be easy to maintain. Begin combining them with the breast rubbing. The contractions can also be performed separately. Contractions may be easier to learn if the muscles involved are seen as fists which you are clenching.

Concentrate your mind on what your body is doing. You may be in the habit of letting your mind wander as you exercise. Total concentration during these exercises leads to levels of sexual power and pleasure that most never know.

Many benefits are claimed for this technique. Among these are the prevention or elimination of hemorrhoids, menstrual irregularities, vaginitis and infertility. It will improve sexual performance and may add healthy years to your life. You will develop *Pompoir* power. It may increase your physical beauty and sexual and personal magnetism. However, you may first experience a cleansing phase as toxins in your system are released.

The Deer exercise is designed to naturally and safely stimulate secretion of the hormones essential for personal and sexual well-being. As a result, you may find that you menstruate less heavily or even that your menstrual cycle ceases. According to Dr. Chang, this is a benefit as vital nutrients and energy that would otherwise be lost in the menstrual blood are reinvested.

If your menstruation stops or decreases and you want it to continue as before, simply discontinue the exercise. In fact, missing even one day can be enough to return you to a menstruating condition.

Male Deer Exercise   Benefical hormonal stimulation is also the goal of the male Deer exercise. Like the female Deer exercise, the male Deer exercise is first performed in two steps. Later these steps are combined. If possible, practice it right after waking up and just before going to sleep. If not, then do it once a day.

Perform this exercise naked sitting, lying down or standing. Choose the most relaxing position for you. If you practice hatha yoga, the sitting pose *Siddhasana* is ideal.

Rub the hands together so that friction and warmth are created. Then grasp the scrotum by itself or together with the penis with the right hand. Rest the scrotum in the center of the palm.

Circle the left palm just below the navel 81 times in either direction. A warm feeling will develop.

Then reverse the hands and the direction. If the left hand moved in a clockwise direction before, now the right hand moves in a counter-clockwise direction. Do 81 repetitions in this direction also. You can imagine a fire building in the genitals if you like. This is step one.

To practice step two, you can remove your hands or keep them in place. Now contract your anal muscles. The correct feeling is that you are trying to suck air up into your anus. To tighten is not quite enough. Suck in with those muscles. This effectively contracts the PC muscle also.

Remember to relax completely between contractions. Hold each contraction as long as possible. Do as many of these long contractions as you comfortably can. This is step two.

After a month of practicing the anal contractions daily, if not sooner, you will have mastered the anal muscle contraction. Now combine the two exercises into one. You may feel a pleasant sensation rising up the spine or other pleasant sensations. This is the result of the anal muscles tenderly squeezing the prostate gland as they contract.

Concentrate your mind on what your body is doing. You may be in the habit of letting your mind wander as you exercise. The importance of concentrating on these exercises cannot be emphasized enough.

This exercise is said to prevent or eliminate prostate problems, hemorrhoids and infertility. It sensitizes the penis. It may even increase the size of the head of the penis. Regular performance of this exercise is said to improve or eliminate impotence or early ejaculation.

A man may bring himself to the verge of orgasm and then apply the exercise. Presumably, since more hormones have been rallied, this is more beneficial. However, the discipline required may be prohibitive.

Ejaculation is not part of the exercise. This version, however, is thought to be extremely effective in cases of impotence if performed faithfully every day for a few weeks or months.

According to Taoist sexology, you are literally making deposits in your life force savings account.

On the other hand, repeated non-ejaculation after being on the verge has been known to lead to congestion of the prostate. The tendency for some men is to go from the extreme of frequent ejaculation to that of no ejaculation. Better is the middle way of moderation, based on health and energy level.

Yoga Sexercises

These exercises provide the same health benefits to the genital and excretory organs. Like the Chinese exercises, they are part of a comprehensive system of bodymind exercise. Nonetheless, you can benefit considerably from the Tantra yoga techniques given here without participating in the whole system. You will find sources for more information in the *Appendix* and *Bibliography*.

The yoga sexercises described below are the Horse Gesture *(Aswini Mudra)*, the Root Lock *(Mula Bandha)* and the Thunderbolt Gesture *(Vajroli Mudra)*. They combine controlled muscular tension with voluntary inhalation and exhalation of the breath, producing rapid results. Maximum efficiency and peak energization is achieved when the anal muscles become so strong that they can be locked in place as other more specialized exercises are performed. Unlike the Kegel and the Deer, these techniques work the anal and urethral (urinary) sphincters separately.

Never do any yoga breathing exercise—these exercises included—to the point of discomfort or dizziness or light-headedness. Never do any yoga exercise while on drugs. Wear loose clothing or none. Practice early morning or late evening, especially if the air is bad where you live.

Ideally, practice on an empty stomach. To further enhance biomagnetism, it is said that you should exercise on top of a natural-fiber blanket or a pad consisting of a layer of wool covered by a layer of cotton.

A good sitting position for many people is the "easy Burmese" (or "easy Lotus") illustrated on page 110. Sit on a folded pillow or rolled up towel so that you can feel the contractions of the PC and anal muscles clearly. Later you can dispense with the pillow or towel if you wish.

The Secret Of Anal Locking

The secret of anal locking is knowing that the anal sphincter actually consists of not one but two sphincters or rings of muscle, an inner ring and an outer ring. Correct performance of the Horse Gesture and the Root Lock means that both rings are fully contracted at the same time.

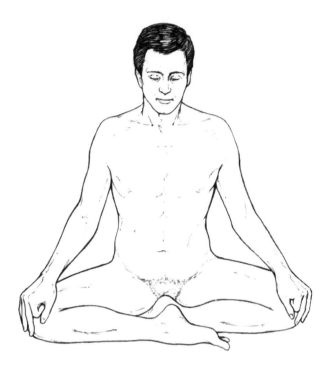

The inner sphincter is located less than an inch up the rectal canal. To verify the two sphincters for yourself, begin by very slowly contracting the anus from the outside going in. You will feel some tension but probably not enough to grab your attention. Continue tightening. At a place just a little higher, you will suddenly experience a distinct, much more powerful contraction of the pelvic-anal floor. Now you have contracted the second inner ring. Contraction of the second inner ring is particularly important due to its multitude of nerve connections with other organs.

Horse Gesture

The first ancient yoga sexercise we will explore is the Horse Gesture (*Aswini Mudra*), so named because of the horse's control over the anal sphincter muscles. The Horse Gesture is step one in the yoga sexercise training program. It is practiced as a preparation for the Root Lock. During the Horse Gesture, we specifically contract and relax the anal sphincter muscles. Note the emphasis on concentration and conscious control.

EASY BURMESE *above*
This is much easier for Western people than the famed Lotus pose. The pelvis opens gently and you stay in touch with the ground.

Sit comfortably in a chair with your spine straight. The feeling of your buttocks against the seat of the chair provides feedback that will help you more rapidly identify and control the correct muscles. A thin pillow on the seat may also help. Place your feet flat on the floor, your hands at your thighs, palms skyward. Or, lie on your back with your knees bent, your feet about a foot apart, the small of your back flat on the floor. Close your eyes and relax.

o   Variation One: Inhale deeply but comfortably and hold briefly. As you slowly exhale, contract the anal sphincter muscles, pulling the anus up and in.
o   Variation Two: Inhale deeply but comfortably and hold. Contract the anal sphincter muscles as rapidly as you can. Exhale.

Full concentration on the anal sphincters is what distinguishes the Horse Gesture from the other two exercises. Remember to focus on feeling these muscles relax after tensing them. Conscious relaxation of the muscles actually increases muscle strength as well as enhancing sensitivity to pleasure.

The Horse Gesture is said to prevent or eliminate hemorrhoids, enlarged prostate, fallen uterus and menstrual difficulties. It is also reputed to develop penis thrusting power and vaginal holding power. Skill at isolated contraction of the anal sphincter rings increases control over ejaculation and enhances orgasm.

Begin with five repetitions and increase as desired. Once you have clearly identified the two anal sphincter muscles for yourself, you may practice in any position as long as the spine is kept straight.

The Horse Gesture is a preparation for the Root Lock and the Thunderbolt Gesture. You may discontinue it once you have mastered the art of locking the anal sphincters. However, the tendency is to rush ahead to the Root Lock long before the Horse Gesture has been fully mastered.

If you have mastered the Horse Gesture, you are able to feel a distinct locking sensation due to the increased strength of these muscles. You will have no difficulty sustaining a powerful contraction of both anal sphincters.

Root Lock   The Root Lock (*Mula Bandha*) also concentrates on the anal sphincters but goes on to spread the contraction through the pelvic floor. To get the feeling right, remember a time when you had to hold back feces or hold in an enema. The benefits of the Root Lock are reported to be similar to those of the Horse Gesture.

Sit as before. Become aware of your anal area, first by feeling how the floor or chair below you is pushing up on your rear, then by focusing your awareness precisely at the anus. You may wish to close your eyes in order to feel the sensations more clearly.

Take in about one-half of your lung capacity. Swallow this air if it is comfortable for you to do so. As an alternative to swallowing or in combination with it, gently bend the chin down and in slightly.

Concentrate on retaining the air deep within. Now, very gradually, tighten your anal sphincter muscles as much as you can. Always include the internal anal sphincter muscle.

If these breath locking techniques are uncomfortable for you, just breathe naturally and focus on the muscles.

Now expand the contraction from the anus through the pelvic floor to the genitals. Women will feel a definite jerking or quiver in the labia. Men will feel a definite tug on the testicles.

Still holding the breath, relax the anus, pelvic floor and genitals totally. The order is not important, but encourage a feeling of letting go, as if the muscles were melting like butter in the sun. Now sniff a small amount of fresh air and then exhale evenly and completely. You have completed one Root Lock. Follow the Root Lock with the Thunderbolt Gesture in the training program described below.

Thunderbolt Gesture

Whereas the Horse Gesture works the anal sphincters alone, and the Root Lock works the anal sphincters and the pelvic floor, the Thunderbolt Gesture *(Vajroli Mudra)* specifically exercises the urethral sphincter. To identify your urethral sphincter with accuracy, drink a quart of water. As you void the resulting flood of urine, stop and start the flow fifteen to twenty times. You have identified the urethral sphincter. In fact, some lovers routinely perform starting and stopping the flow as a way to exercise the urethral sphincters.

Sit as before. Now place your attention at your urethral sphincter. Take in one-half of your lung capacity. Swallow this air or otherwise contain it. Now squeeze your urethral sphincter just as if you were stopping your urine flow while simultaneously drawing your lower belly up and in. Pretend you are trying to literally pull your sex organ up into your pelvis. Now relax the entire contraction completely.

Do as many urethral-lower abdominal contractions and relaxations as you can on a single breath. As you do so, encourage the sensations of sexual thrill to flow from the pelvis to the nerves in the spine to the brain, especially the pituitary gland region.

When you can contract no more on the one breath, relax the urethral sphincter, pelvis and lower belly completely, sniff a small amount of fresh air in and then exhale evenly and completely. You have now completed one Thunderbolt Gesture.

The Thunderbolt Gesture is said to benefit the urinary and genital organs as a whole. In particular, the ability to hold urine is improved. Women may find clitoral responsiveness heightened. Men may find the strength and rapidity of their erection increased.

Here is the Thunderbolt Gesture self-check:

○ For women: delicately put your index finger and/or your middle finger in your vagina. Do the Thunderbolt Gesture. The vagina will grasp your finger(s) lightly if not firmly.

○ For men: stand nude before a mirror. Do the Thunderbolt Gesture. The end of your penis will jerk or lift.

Tantra Yoga Training

Follow this training program after mastering the Horse Gesture. Always do the Root Lock and the Thunderbolt Gesture in every session. Do the Thunderbolt Gesture after the Root Lock. Start with 10 of each.

Add five or more a week. After approximately three months time you will be doing the recommended maximum of 60 repetitions per day.

You may wish to experiment with the amount of air you take in. You may find the exercises easier to perform as well as more effective if you take in three-quarters of your lung capacity or even your maximum intake.

For people who are not comfortable with breath retention exercises, an alternative practice is to build up to 75 rapid Kegels emphasizing the anal muscles (Root Lock) and 75 rapid Kegels emphasizing the urethral sphincter muscles (Thunderbolt Gesture) per day plus only three breath retention repetitions.

These last three are held as long as possible, emphasizing a firm hold on all three areas of muscle contraction (anal, pubococcygeus and urethral sphincter muscles). They can be approached deeply and slowly, as a meditation.

The entire series only takes a few minutes. It's a great way to start your day!

Relaxation is as important in these exercises as contraction. Be sure to completely relax the muscles involved as you release after each contraction. Think the word "relax" at the areas involved. You will find that this not only increases your benefit but insures a stronger, firmer contraction following the relaxation phase.

As you become more skilled with the sexercises of yoga, seek to distinguish between the muscles of the anus, pelvic floor and urethra. Sensitivity and control are just as important as strength.

The concentration point for the Kundalini, the mystic sexual-spiritual force, is said to be at the middle of the perineum just inside the body for men and at the cervix for women. As you perform the Horse Gesture and the Root Lock you will become attuned to this region. Then even thinking of this area brings an invigorating release of energy.

Kundalini Kegel Sit in the "easy Burmese" or other comfortable position with a folded towel under your buttocks and perineum or on a chair.

As you do your Kegel contractions or Root Lock repetitions, imagine that a warm, loving light is blazing at the Kundalini concentration point in the cervix or perineum. Encourage this pleasurable feeling of warmth and light to expand.

Feel this soft, warm energy rising up and filling your bodymind. Then extend it outwards, dissolving the boundaries of your bodymind in a sea of radiant, blissful energy.

To visualize this energy does not necessarily mean that you see it clearly, as if watching a movie. It may only mean that you feel or sense it there. If this is easier for you, then work on going with the feeling rather than on getting a vivid visualization. Melt into this feeling of graceful, expanding energy and become one with the ocean of life around you.

You can combine this meditation with an affirmation such as "I am light," "I am love," "I am bliss," or simply "I am." Also, you can do it with the Tongue Press (press your tongue against the soft palate towards the back of your mouth) and *Shambhavi Mudra* (roll your eyes up and back to focus on the third eye trigger point between your eyebrows). Both of these techniques encourage the energy to move upwards.

Recall an especially memorable orgasm or some other time when you felt greatly inspired and uplifted. This is the feeling that you are seeking to generate consciously here. At such times, the Kundalini is more alive, kindling your consciousness with positive, luminous waves of energy. In essence, you are learning to make love to yourself. That is the spirit to use with this technique.

You may experience a deep feeling of self-love or blissful contentment when you do this meditation regularly. You are discovering yourself as source.

The key to this meditation is to concentrate on and in the

KUNDALINI KEGEL
opposite

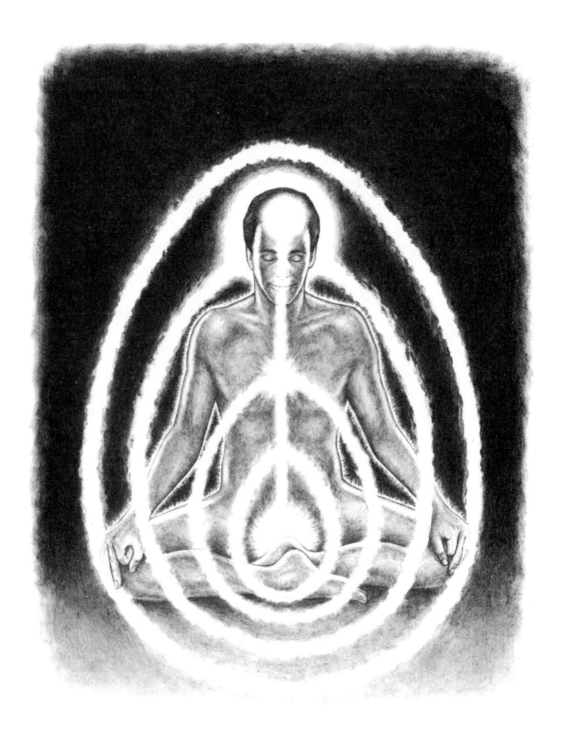

soft center of whatever sensation has developed from doing the Root Lock. This deep concentration is the key. The spreading of the energy will naturally occur as you relax the body more and more and sink down into the sensations (see *Elevate Energy*).

Stomach Lift   Another yoga exercise with notable sexual applications is the Stomach Lift *(Uddiyana Bandha)*. The Stomach Lift may alleviate constipation, menstrual problems and digestive difficulties. It is also said to prevent or correct hemorrhoids, prostate problems, lack of libido, infertility, impotence and early ejaculation. The sexual benefits, though substantial, tend to be underplayed in conventional yoga guides.

Neuroscientist and yoga expert Keven Kingsland has observed that this technique stimulates the central nervous system resulting in strong alpha rhythms. It is reported to increase insulin secretion. The abdominal brain is also toned up, enhancing the reticular activating system.

The Stomach Lift is thought to help reverse the direction of the energy so that it ascends up the spine to the psychic centers in the brain. This leads to a refinement of pleasure and the ability to access higher levels of bliss and awareness.

Perform the Stomach Lift first thing in the morning before eating. This is a powerful exercise, so don't push yourself. If you experience dizziness, stop immediately, as this is a sign you are trying to do too many repetitions for your skill level. Although some yogis do 1500 a day, taking a few minutes each morning to do 25 repetitions is a sensible goal for most of us.

While the Stomach Lift can be performed sitting down, the standing position with the legs apart and slightly bent at the knee is best for learning and mastering this technique. Place the palms on the thighs. Lean forward and round the back slightly.

Completely empty the lungs. Do this as quickly as possible to give yourself more time before you have to breathe in. Breathe out through your nose, then with pursed lips to maximize exhalation.

Keeping the lungs free of air, relax the stomach wall. Then slightly lift and expand the rib cage. The diaphragm and stomach will then rise up into the vacuum you have created.

Hold this position for a few moments. Then release the wall of the stomach gently. If you let it go too suddenly, the inhalation will rush in noisily. This can also happen if you try to hold the outbreath too long.

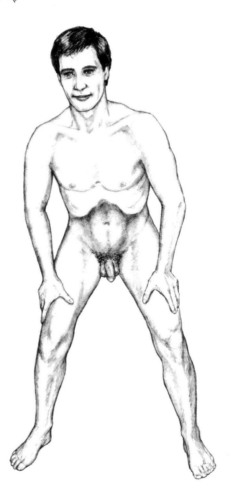

There are two approaches. You can hold the retraction in
for about five seconds, release it, breathe normally, then
repeat. Five of these equals one set. The second approach is
to do five of these quickly on a single exhalation. One of
these equals one set.

Start with three sets per day for the first month. Then go
to four sets the second month and five sets the third month.
Five sets a month is a good maintenance practice. You will
quickly feel the heat, energy and well-being generated by
this powerful practice.

The Stomach Lift should not be be performed by people
with heart problems, ulcers or by pregnant women.

Churning of the abdominal muscles *(Nauli)* is the advanced form which may be performed during or after sexual
intercourse to recycle sexual energy as well as part of a
regular health routine. Naturally, the Stomach Lift can be

STOMACH LIFT *above*
Its sexual benefits are
not well publicized.

performed for sexual energy recycling as well. *Nauli* involves isolating the vertical, straight abdominal muscles, the recti abdominis. Mastery of the Stomach Lift is a definite prerequisite for this exercise. Instructions for *Nauli* can be found in some hatha yoga books, usually with reference to the benefits for the digestion, metabolism and bowel action.

Root Lock, Thunderbolt Gesture and the Stomach Lift are part of a complete, systematic Tantra yoga program that is designed to awaken the internal energy—Kundalini—for spiritual development (see *Appendix* and *Bibliography*).

Study with an expert teacher is recommended. However, many hatha yoga teachers have only a passing familiarity with these practices, as they are considered specialized and advanced. It is wise to consult with your physician before taking on such practices, regardless of your present state of health.

Other Sexercises

There are many other exercises which benefit the genital and pelvic areas. These include kicks to the front, side and back and pelvic lifts, standard for aerobics classes. Swimming while kicking vigorously is also good.

Upward and Downward Dog stretches, which are taught in most yoga classes, are excellent. Camel, Locust, Cobra, Plough, Spinal Twist, Forward Bend and Shoulder Stand, all superior for sexual well-being, are also popular hatha yoga positions (see *Pelvic Expression*).

Yoga, stretch and dance classes offer great workouts for the pelvic-genital region as well as overall health and mental benefits. To really benefit from these exercises, take a local class on a regular basis from an inspiring teacher.

SEXUAL ENERGY RECYCLING

When something is recycled, it is returned to its source. The wheel, or cycle, is turned back to the beginning of its circular path. There is some evidence that in human beings the sex energy cycle has two stages. The first stage begins in the brain, at the pituitary and pineal glands, and ends in the sex glands. The second stage of the cycle, the actual recycling step, returns energy to these master glands in the brain. This second step is often neglected.

Though health, diet, exercise, positive mental attitude and other holistic health factors play a major role, the most important single factor is your attitude towards sex energy in general and genital orgasm in particular. Positive results are achieved by developing a respectful, even reverent attitude towards this exciting form of creative energy. Whether you are celibate or making love or *Selfloving* with genital orgasm daily, your attitude will be the factor that decides if the reality of sex energy in your life will be a blessing and a blossoming. Allowing for the individual variations that do exist, your state of mind probably determines your benefit or loss via sexual thoughts, feelings and activities, especially orgasm.

Our belief is that each man and woman is a completely unique individual with his or her own sexual energy path to follow and his or her own unique orgasm needs. These change, too, as the man or woman changes. There is no right or wrong way to manage sexual energy. There is only the individual response which, ultimately, is valid precisely to the extent that it contributes to personal well-being.

It may be that how you have your sexual orgasm makes a greater difference to your personal energy than whether or not you have it. Do self-centered consorts who exploit their orgasms for surface pleasure drain themselves of energy? Do ecstatically intimate, vulnerable consorts gain energy via their unselfish orgasms?

Energy is spent via other kinds of sexual activity as well. It takes energy to think about sex, look for sex, worry about sex and so forth. Sexual energy can be channeled into art, business, religion, service. However you choose to manage your sex energy, attitude is all-important.

The Benefits The ancient sexercises were designed to return energy and essential biochemical ingredients, including hormonal substances, from the sexual glands to the hypothalamic-pituitary region and pineal gland, both located in the brain. The hypothalamic-pituitary region is responsible for the stable functioning of the sex glands, adrenals and thyroid, all of which play essential roles in maintaining sexual well-being, and of the other glands as well.

Although the role of the pineal gland is less clear, it is also known to play a vital role in the maintenance of sexual and emotional well-being. To return the vital factors to the hypothalamic-pituitary region and the nearby pineal gland, is, in biological terms, sexual recycling.

The ancient experts believed that these sexercises could add many healthy years to our lives. Is there any scientific evidence to support the belief that these practices may in fact promote healthful longevity?

Though the causes of aging and senility remain unclear, substantial evidence has accumulated indicating that it is precisely these parts of the body, the sex glands and the

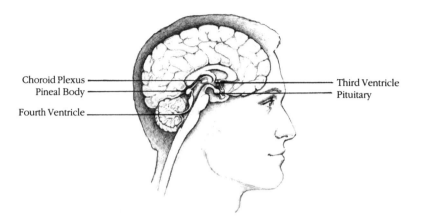

Choroid Plexus
Pineal Body
Fourth Ventricle
Third Ventricle
Pituitary

hypothalamic-pituitary region, which contain the so-called aging clocks. Life extension researchers Pearson and Shaw, for example, report that male pattern balding is partially due to certain male hormonal activity that stays dormant until an internal clock gives the signal. The Leydig cells of the testes, which produce testosterone, are the prime suspect for the location of this particular aging clock. That male hormones must somehow be involved is shown by the fact that castration stops male pattern balding.

A prominent research scientist, Dr. W. Donner Denckla, believes that the pituitary gland secretes an unidentified death hormone. It has been proven in the laboratory many times that removing the pituitary and/or hypothalamus from the brains of animals will extend their lives. Eels, mice, salmon and female octopuses have demonstrated an impressive longevity after having the pituitary gland or equivalent removed.

The ancient sexercises were traditionally practiced as part of a comprehensive bodymind rejuvenation program, such as the Chinese internal exercises or the Indian hatha yoga. These programs systematically stimulate the glandular and nervous systems from within.

Sexual stimulation releases hormonal factors that have a very positive effect. For example, rheumatologist Dr. George Ehrlich reports in an article in *Forum* magazine that many patients experience up to eight hours of relief from arthritic pain after sexual intercourse. To recycle sexual energy is to tune in to and purposefully take advantage of the wonderful benefits of sexual stimulation.

To experience the benefits of recycled sexual activity, be physically active. Cardiovascular exercise, such as aerobics,

PINEAL AND PITUITARY
above
These are the master glands.

is recommended in lieu of these older methods if they are not practiced. Many sexual problems, especially in women, are the result of insufficient available energy. Regular exercise of any kind increases energy.

Positive Attitude

Successful sexual energy recycling is the result of self-awareness, sensitivity and positive mental attitudes. Your attitude towards orgasm is particularly important. Do you view orgasm as a convenient thrill with no purpose or value other than push-button pleasure? Or do you view the genital orgasm with a touch of awe, wonder, celebration, magic, even sacredness? Our experience has taught us that *how* we have our orgasms largely determines the potential aftereffects, such as fatigue or energization, irritability or inner peace, dullness or inspiration.

One of the benefits of conserving the genital orgasm together can be that your desire for each other remains at a high pitch. You may enjoy a feeling of erotic intensity and intimacy unlike anything you've ever experienced before.

You may feel the energy charge build up, intensifying your pleasure and sense of unity. When you do share genital orgasm, it is a special event. You can easily prove this to yourselves by making love without genital release, then making love hours later or the next day. Hungry for each other, you share the erotic thrill at peak intensity.

Full Circle

A dazzling array of techniques have been developed to assist in the recycling of sexual energy. You will find many of them in this book, including the sections *Elevate Energy, Sexercises, Tao Of Sex, Taoist Circle Of Gold* and *Third Eye Sex.*

It is useful to keep the technique and the ideology of the system in which it was developed separate. We suggest that you keep in mind that motivation is destiny, that love really is the answer.

The energy path of ascending and descending energies, which we call the Circle Of Gold, is fundamental to the Taoist and complete Tantra yoga practices. However, what you are doing via such practices is returning to self energy that is vital to your quest for wholeness instead of wasting it on lesser pursuits outside of yourself. Naturally, through dual cultivation, caring consorts intensify these effects.

Your recycling technique during intercourse can be as simple as breathing deeply and completely, feeling the energy fill your whole bodymind. Perform your PC–anal contractions, drawing the energy in and up with your inhalation. Will this energy to ascend to your crown. Complete the cycle·

as you release this living energy to your consort with your exhalation.

There are many other excellent techniques covered in *Sexual Energy Ecstasy*. Our experience, though, has been that the extreme detail of the bodymind technologies of the East, their multitude of centers and methods, can be a distraction. Through meditation and self-enquiry, discover the already whole Self within.

After all, according to Tantra, you are already there. You are where you want to be here and now—this here, this now, this very moment. The problem with maps is that they make you think you are separate from your destination.

Every technique is a springboard, a jumping-off place. Don't stay stuck on the shore. Take the plunge!

The golden circle of love-light-bliss illustrated symbolically as fire and water in *Fusion Breath Sex* is, ultimately, a symbol of your primordial wholeness, of perfect union of male and female principles, of *Shiva* and *Shakti,* of your intrinsic enlightenment.

Your true Self lies in your heart. Above all, remember that you are the answer. Therefore, find out who you are!

TAOIST CIRCLE OF GOLD

This is an easy variation of an ancient Chinese Taoist method for recycling sexual and life energy. It combines the Tibetan "Backward Flowing" method with the Taoist Microcosmic and Macrocosmic Orbits. Offering the proven benefits of tranquillity and healing meditation, it helps strengthen and balance the sexual energy enabling prolonged, invigorating, awakened lovemaking.

This technique is taught by Justin G. Stone, a teacher of meditation and T'ai Chi. You can record these instructions yourself and play them back as a guided meditation.

With your eyes closed, sit with your back straight. Rest your tongue against the roof of your mouth just behind your top front teeth. It can touch your teeth slightly. Breathe through your nose.

In your mind, see yourself on a fluffy white cloud. This cloud billows up around your hips. Now this cloud lifts you. You are light as a bubble as the cloud lifts you into an endless blue sky. Higher and higher you climb, effortlessly, lifted as if by a giant hand.

Right above you, you now see a giant waterfall of warm, shimmering light. The light is a radiant gold, like the sun. As you move closer to the waterfall of liquid light, you feel the mist from the waterfall. Now as you move even closer you move right into the waterfall of golden light.

You can feel the cascade of golden light flooding over your head. You float higher and higher into the waterfall and the golden liquid is an avalanche of light flowing down and over the top of your skull.

Now this light actually enters your skull in a place behind your eyes. Now you hear the sound of water, like a flowing stream.

Now this moist radiant light is flowing down to your nose, now your mouth, now your chin. The warm golden light flows down your neck to your shoulder and chest. Every cell of your bodymind is warmed and excited by the touch of this golden light.

Now it trickles down from the chest to your belly and finally to the special point, the storehouse of this golden life energy, that is located one or two inches (or about two fingers widths) below your navel. From this internal point, called T'an T'ien (Tanden or *Hara* in Japanese), it separates to spill down the outside of both legs at the same time.

The friendly, warm golden light has now reached the soles of your feet. You can feel how moist the light is and how it thrills every cell of your bodymind as it touches them.

Gradually the warm, moist golden current flows up the inside of both your legs at the same time. Slowly it reaches your knees. Eventually, it enters the genital area and moves to the coccyx (tailbone) where once again it is a single flow.

Now this warm golden current is at the small of your back. Then, from the small of your back, it flows up the center of your spine to the middle of your back. Then it moves to between your shoulder blades, down the outside of your arms over the middle fingers to the centers of the palms, and then back up the inside of your arms.

Now it moves back to your spine between your shoulder blades and up to your shoulders, your neck and to the base of your skull. Now, at last, it flows to the top of your skull and cascades down over the top of your head. Your skull and brain are washed by this warm golden force.

Repeat this cycle again.

Now repeat this cycle for a third time. Only this time, when you get down to the special point about two inches below the navel, the T'an T'ien, which is your storehouse of this warm golden life energy current, let it rest there for several minutes.

Strive to feel the force there with great intensity. Just sit in full awareness of the light in your T'an T'ien.

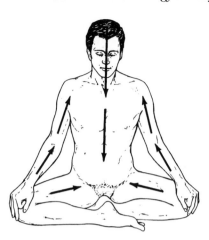 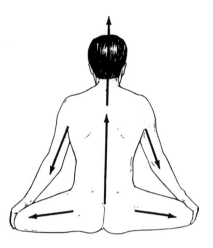

Just feel. No thinking. Just feel this golden warmth and force resting in your special place of power.

Now, after this period of quiet meditation in T'an T'ien, take the light back up your legs and up your back and arms. Only this time, as you go up the back, slowly inhale and take the breath with the light up to the top of your skull.

This can be even easier if you coordinate moving your eyes up with the breath and the light. Your eyelids remain closed, though.

When the light has reached the top of your head, hold that breath, with your eyes raised up, for a few seconds and allow all of your skull to be radiated with this light.

The light now goes slowly forward, pouring over the top of your head. You begin exhaling slowly, gradually lowering your gaze. When the breath is completely exhaled and your eyes are completely lowered, that's when the warm golden light should reach your T'an T'ien.

Once again, this time holding the exhalation, you sit silently feeling the warm golden light there. Not thinking. Just feeling.

This concludes the basic Circle Of Gold meditation technique (see *Elevate Energy, Hara*).

Practice Pointers   Here are some useful tips. Simple and straightforward, the Taoist Circle Of Gold is a "feel good" meditation that should give you positive results right away. It does not require a knowledge of the esoteric anatomy, yet it is powerful and safe. The key is to practice it regularly.

The Circle Of Gold can be started from the soles of the feet or from the base of your spine (the coccyx or tailbone).

If you start it from the coccyx, first draw it from the T'an T'ien through the gap between the legs to the base of the spine, for T'an T'ien is where the warm golden life force makes its home.

The beginning part when you approach and enter the waterfall of warm golden light can be repeated each time you begin the Circle Of Gold at the top of the head. So you would approach and enter the cascade of golden light in your imagination each time the light has gone up through the back, neck and head and is ready to pour down over the top of your head again.

Take care that the light moves very slowly. Try to feel that each cell of your bodymind is basking in the warmth and radiance of this precious golden light as the light passes through on its journey through your bodymind. This warm golden light is none other than the concentrated life energy known by various names such as Chi, Ki, Mana, Prana, Vitality, Life Force, Shakti, Orgone Energy, Bioplasma.

Remember, keep your eyes closed (or half-closed, half-open) and your back straight.

Emphasize the pouring of the warm golden light over the top of the head and the sitting with the feeling of the light in the T'an T'ien. Note that you always conclude the meditation by resting in the T'an T'ien. This insures that the energy does not get blocked or scattered. Remember, T'an T'ien is the energy storage battery of the bodymind.

Try the Circle Of Gold for 10 to 20 minutes morning and evening for starters. According to the Chinese tradition, you should do three or nine cycles or a multiple of nine.

Once you get the hang of it, you can start coordinating the eye, breath and warm current with the first cycle. But you don't have to. The key to success is "easy does it" and have fun!

Another appeal of this process is that it encourages your creativity and artistic input. You are free to embroider or change the visualization to match your personal imagery.

After a few weeks of solo practice, you will be sufficiently adept that you can do the Circle Of Gold while making love. Then you can dispense with floating in the clouds. Concentrate on the circular flow of warm golden light and its stabilization in the T'an T'ien *(Hara)*. Naturally, the fun— and the benefits—are increased when you circulate this loving energy together.

Even if you begin dual cultivation, continue with your private practice. Some of the benefits from lovemaking take 72 hours to be absorbed, which your solo efforts will assist.

TAOIST CIRCLE OF GOLD
opposite
Here is how to visualize the flow of energy down the front and up the back. This Taoist yoga moves the life force through the whole body.

This technique is believed to increase and balance the sexual drive and to bring healing energy to any part of the bodymind that needs it. Another benefit of this meditation is more tranquillity.

However, according to Buddhist meditation tradition, doing only this kind of meditation can lead to the subtle trap of being attached to tranquil states. Once your mind starts to calm down, include an insight type of meditation such as vipassana mindfulness or the enquiry "Who am I?" to gain liberating wisdom.

TECHNOLOGY FOR LOVERS

Biocircuitry is a simple but universal principle: by externally linking certain of the body's energy centers, you skillfully enhance the flow and balance of the body's natural energy.

The Copper BioCircuit™ consists of two separate copper screens attached by a length of wire to a copper handle. After placing the copper screens on a comfortable surface, you lie down on your back on the screens. You then close your eyes and relax for at least 20 to 30 minutes. Typical experiences includes deep refreshment, waves of energy, tingling sensations and so on (see *Complete Circuits, Appendix*).

Experienced users of the BioCircuit™ have found that the tool offers several sexual benefits. Men have reported that it is an excellent way to recover energy after orgasm.

One man who suffered from a sense of continuing energy leakage after orgasm reported that lying down on a Copper BioCircuit™ immediately after lovemaking resulted in a powerful recharging effect as well as a deepened rest or sleep. The usual sense of energy loss, which could continue into the next day or so, was not experienced.

Another exciting application is physicalizing fantasies. When lying in a BioCircuit™, mental imagery becomes much more vivid, lifelike and sensual. One well-known holistic health specialist conducts hypnotherapeutic sessions to connect the client to her "inner mate," a subconscious resource in the form of a sexually attractive other who is an always available source of erotic inspiration, affection and affirmation. When the client lies in the BioCircuit™ during the session, the vividness, sensuality and actual levels of sexual arousal are dramatically increased over the sessions which rely only on imagination and hypnotic suggestion.

Because it is a solitary activity, like floating in a samadhi tank, lying on the BioCircuit™ isn't directly arousing unless accompanied by active sexual or otherwise arousing imagery. However, since the BioCircuit™ has the ability to render you more centered and energetically balanced, it should bring new levels of subtle delight. Energetic control during sex is increased, which means that orgasm can be more voluntary as well as more pleasurable.

Yet another Tantric application is that of being genitally pleasured by your consort while you lie on the BioCircuit™. Our *Spreading* technique is ideal here. Energy is increased, relaxation deepened, sensitivity enhanced, all the basic ingredients of a profoundly satisfying erotic peak experience. We encourage you to experiment with this arrangement.

ULTRA–INTIMACY

The advice of the Greek philosophers—know thyself—applies just as much to lovemaking as it does to work, money, food, relationships and the pursuit of personal truth and happiness.

Along with the increase in personal power and creativity that Sexual Energy Ecstasy lovemaking produces goes the responsibility, or response-ability, of emotional maturity. What you say and do will have a noticeably greater impact on others, especially your consort(s).

You will find that you are more deeply affected by your consort(s), due to the intense bonding that takes place via Sexual Energy Ecstasy practices. Ups and downs and game playing that may have been acceptable to you before will not be acceptable to you now. You will need to identify your key motivation(s) for participating in the sexual act.

Can you be honest with yourself? Identify your motives, your emotional motives especially. Sex is very much an acting out of your most typical emotional states.

Know what it is that you are after. Simply be very, very honest with yourself. Do what you like to do without harming others in the process.

Well before making love, say relaxing on the couch, air out your anxieties, frustrations, doubts, fears. Talk about your emotional garbage. Don't take it to bed with you.

If you become sexually attracted to someone, consider discussing it immediately with your consort. What we have found is that we always feel closer to each other and the attraction for the other person quickly fades. While you should certainly follow your own intuition and stay within the guidelines of your relationship, our experience suggests that having an affair begins with failing to be honest, allowing separatist fantasies to thrive.

Emotional states are contagious and can be transmitted during sexual communication. Not only that, what you hold in when you are with your consort in the living room will hold you back from ultra-intimacy in the bedroom, and perhaps hold your consort back as well.

What are your secret fantasies? Share them and play them out. Trust and joy will develop. Let nothing be hidden. Let everything be sacred.

According to the ancient code of Tantra, the healthiest action to take is always whatever it is that you *deeply* want to do. Just do not knowingly harm another or interfere with their spiritual growth. Everything is allowed, then, provided you follow this unique variation of the well-known Golden Rule: "Do *exactly* what you want to do and defend the right of others to do the same."

Aware of the repressive effects of society, Tantra took the opposite position as an antidote. It is important for people to know that spiritual life, that being a lover, is not all just rules and regulations.

Remember the joy that is your root. Nothing is denied. You are free to experiment. Enjoy yourself!

Paradoxically, this is not a license for indulgence. All actions are to be pursued with awareness. Indeed, the principal sin is ignorance.

Tantra does not want you to sleepwalk through your life. Staying awake means taking risks, being different, being yourself.

Ecstasy is actually a revolutionary act. People who know how to fully enjoy themselves are true voluntary consumers. They need only be themselves to be happy. The pursuit of happiness which, by definition, never ends, does not fascinate them.

Lovers make love. They do not chase fantasies, for the pursuit is based on a sense of lack here and now. Only one who is already full will overflow with desire to the degree of devotion.

Your attitudes and beliefs about lovemaking, the opposite sex, the same sex and about orgasm also play a major role in what you will experience while making love. Ultra-intimacy and sexual relationship satisfaction in the fullest sense are direct by-products of knowing yourself.

Tantric sex, Sexual Energy Ecstasy, ultra-intimacy is a mirror.

Can you see your face?

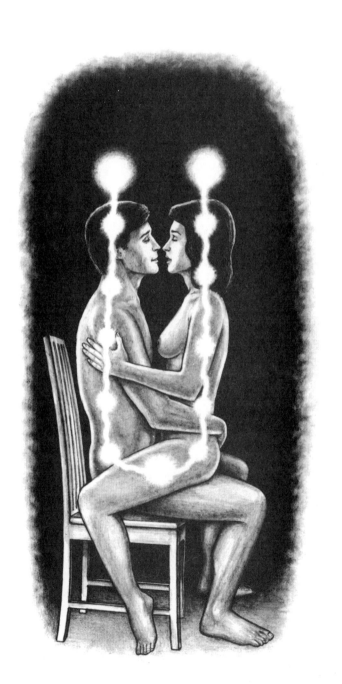

For
Play

**HARMONY
SIGNS**

*we will be specific
compatibility is describable*

here are some of the signs

first, and most important, peace

*when you are together
do you at times
rest in a pool
of stillness
of quiet clarity?*

*do you at times
feel a great peace
a sigh of whole-body relief?*

*do you at times
feel that you are
at last
home?*

*you will know
with effortless certainty*

*drink deeply that kiss
red dragons dancing
release the healing juice
quaff it well
lick your lips
roll the tongue, dragon bold
within the oral cavern*

*like a wine taster vastly experienced
you will know if the wine of that lover
is the answer to the questions
asked by your body day and night
in their saliva
the essence of their chemistry
an answer beyond the brain's devices
of fantasy and fear*

*the taste of his or her skin
is like reading a life diary
written with invisible ink
electromagnetic effigy*

personality is spread
like oil on a canvas
there for the discerning
a man's armpits
the nape of a woman's neck
everywhere are lighted shrines
open to worshippers whose key
they will unlock
(truly, the nose knows)

smell is the mystery
master of the brain
so direct is its message
so subtle its caress
you will be lost at once

emotional chemistry
beyond the body
revealed by the natural odor
of man and woman
a good whiff is enough
to tell bad from good
discover your destiny together
or apart
with your nose
(not your head)

never force the union
of earth and sky
dawn and dusk

the magic of the twilight
where all is possible
including happiness
and perfect balance of the sun and moon
is only found
eyes wide open

soixante-neuf, 69
completes the great circle
energy is freed
by your eagerness
take the time to taste
the lap of your lover
the code of your communion
is written in the flowing juices

MAITHUNA *right*
Khajuraho, India,
11th century A.D.

electricity is king
in the land of lovers
some couples who pursue peace
sacrifice chemistry
they avoid conflict and no longer attract each other

some couples have chemistry
but no peace

better to have both

peace is the father-mother of love
chemistry is the glue of ecstasy

if you two would last
listen to the song of your secretions
your biological messengers
answer the royal request

force not the form

friend or lover
both or neither
it makes no ultimate difference

you are your true lover
you are your best friend

close your eyes and listen
with your whole bodymind

your heart is a radio
is he or she playing your tune?

IT'S THE THOUGHT THAT COUNTERS

The supreme discipline is to live in the present, even under such appealing circumstances as making love. Even then, we are distracted from the present by our thoughts as they regurgitate the past and fictionalize the future.

Beyond the curtain of everyday thinking mind lies a fabulously rich realm.

"Yum. That ice cream was good!"

Did you really experience the ice cream? The ice cream was there, were you there?

What was the texture of the ice cream? How soft or hard was it? Could you sense the coldness and crispness of the ice *cream? What was the color of the ice cream? How did this color vary? How did you hold the spoon? Did you see the spoon dig into the ice cream? What kind of sound did the spoon make as it penetrated the ice cream? What did the very first bite of ice cream taste like? The second bite? The last bite? As the last bite of ice cream taste faded away, what taste replaced it?*

Everyday thinking mind creates mirages. We think that we are eating the ice cream. In fact, we are eating our thoughts about it. Go back to the last time you ate ice cream. Chances are you missed the ice cream's uniqueness. What you experienced then was mostly replays of your ice cream memories and displays of your ice cream expectations.

We usually experience our experiences through the subtle screen of our thoughts. Unless we pay very close attention, the artificiality of experiencing through a screen of thoughts goes unnoticed.

We think thousands of thoughts in the time it takes to consume a bowl of ice cream. Most of them have nothing at all to do with ice cream. Our minds wander in the nowhere lands of annihilated past and fantasized future. The purity of ice cream experience, of sense experience in general, is polluted by irrelevant, irreverent thoughts.

Exactly the same problem is encountered in lovemaking. For most people, though, lovemaking is more important than eating ice cream.

How to make love in the sensory present?

How to make love in the realm beyond the curtain of thought?

Don't try to eliminate thought. Thoughts appear naturally, like leaves on a tree.

Instead, shift the mind into neutral gear. Just like a few fluffy white clouds drifting in the brilliant blue of the summer sky, occasional thoughts float in and out. This tranquillity is most easily developed through deep relaxation before or during lovemaking.

Thoughts are a natural phenomenon, like clouds. The clouds in the sky of mind are no more a problem for us than the clouds in the sky of earth are a problem for the sun.

Sometimes, the clouds of thought mass together, creating a thought storm. What did you do that last time you were caught in a thunderstorm? You probably sat down and waited it out.

A thought about impotence or about not having an orgasm is not a problem. Only when impotence thoughts or no orgasm thoughts mass together and make a thought storm do they seem to become a problem. Then the sky of the mind looks troubled and dark. The thunder of anger, the cold wind of fear, the snow of loneliness, the hail of doubt make their appearance.

Sometimes, in spite of our best efforts, thought storms appear. This is fine. A thunderstorm viewed from a good vantage point is a beautiful, awe-inspiring show. Thought storms are no different. All it takes is a good seat a safe distance away. Then we will enjoy the free show.

When a thought wants to come in, don't argue with it. Let it in. If a thought wants to stay awhile, let it stay. If it wants to leave, let it leave. Thoughts appear, persist and disappear. Thought storms appear, persist and disappear. That is their nature.

MAKING LOVE IS A TOUCHING EXPERIENCE

To stay in the sensory present as you make love, remain aware of change. Totally be at the points of contact between skin and skin. Be one, literally, with the sensations themselves. Stay at the intersections of sensory greeting.

Sensory moments begin, grow, peak, fade and end, only to be replaced by new sensory moments. Make love in the shadow zone of endless physical transition. Make love in the raw reality of mindless bodyfullness. Leave the sensation of self behind.

Drink the unfiltered sense experience. Add nothing to the raw sense data. Be sensitive to the kaleidoscope of changing details at the interception of flesh by flesh. Allow the smouldering sea of subtle sense activity to sweep interpreting thought and self-consciousness away.

When touching or being touched, make that touch fill all awareness in that moment. That touch, or, more precisely, the field of sensitivity where toucher and touched intercept to create touching, is the total universe. There is found an infinity of sensory nuance. When the curtain of thought is drawn aside, this is the natural way of experiencing the senses.

At the cutting edge of sensation lies a realm of indescribable beauty that has no equivalent in the mind. Words cannot describe it. The everyday thinking mind cannot comprehend it. It is a mystery beyond belief. It is the miracle of direct experience. Reach out. Be all that you can be by being only what is. Be the sensory present reality itself. Go beyond touching and being touched. Go beyond confining labels. Be the touching itself.

Just touch.

FOR PLAY   The act of making love has a beginning, a middle and an end. *For Play* is about the beginning, *Swept Away* the middle and *Climax* the end. These correspond roughly to the phases in the Masters and Johnson model of sexual intercourse, excitation, plateau and orgasm/resolution.

You have seen "for play" spelled foreplay. In that spelling, it refers to erotic stimulation with a very definite goal: genital union with orgasm. Playing with each other with that goal in mind is fine, but it is not the only way to play.

Instead of playing for orgasmic payoff, play for play.

Duplicate the mood and energy of happy children at play in your lovemaking.

If genital union didn't exist at all, how would you behave? Just being together would be the goal. Touch itself would be the climax.

Instead of you deciding when it is time for foreplay to end and genital intercourse to begin, why not let your genitals decide?

Act as if the penis and vagina have minds and wills of their own. Rest penis on vagina. Let them make their own introductions.

If they decide to go ahead, then you will. But if they don't, you won't. This "as if" game can inject a startling zest and freshness into your lovemaking, but you must stick to the rules.

There are simple skills that smooth out the rough spots in your relating, ways to set up your lovemaking environment, strategies to draw out the best in a person without taking advantage of them. This is relaxed, intelligent, skillful effort. This, too, is for play.

When you were a teenager, did just a touch or a look from the object of your desire drive you crazy? To return to this whole-body total eroticism that starts with a glance and builds and builds and builds is for play, too.

You are not giving up anything, you see. You are taking in everything, and giving yourself the time and place and space in which to enjoy it.

You are just having fun—right now—playing for the play of it.

ACULOVING   Acupressure or shiatsu massage before lovemaking is one of the most precious secrets of the Oriental lovecraft. Oriental courtesans have offered this service with great success for many centuries. These women were trained in the art of giving a whole body acupressure massage. Before his massage, the man was completely bathed and scrubbed by the courtesan. Some of the most prized courtesans were also trained in *Pompoir.*

According to acupressure principles, healing energy is stimulated throughout the bodymind, and deep relaxation is created. The internal organs are also massaged, so that the person feels relaxed and renewed inside and out. For a more Western approach, see *Erotic Massage.*

Hand And Foot Massage   Acupressure expert Michael Blate, director of the G-Jo Institute in Florida, suggests massage of both hands or both feet. This takes about 20 minutes. Now allow your consort just to be in that relaxation, even if they seem lost to the world. Within 30 minutes they return, refreshed, revitalized and, perhaps, wonderfully ready to make love.

This kind of massage works best with the attitude you are giving a deeply relaxing, healing experience. Odds are that if they do want to make love to you, this approach will bring that sooner or later, and with the best possible results.

We like to use oil for manual massage of the hands, feet and big toes. Our favorite oils are almond or canola with a few drops of lavender. We avoid petroleum-based oils.

Some may prefer the high-quality water dispersible massage oils which prevent linen stains and are easily rinsed off. Jojoba, while too viscous for body massage, is a delight for genital lubrication. We prefer vitamin E cream or aloe vera cream for facial massage.

If you are massaging the hands, massage both hands entirely, including the wrist. Do one entirely, then do the other. Do the palm, the back of the hand, the fingers, between the fingers, everything. If you are massaging the feet, massage both feet entirely, including the heel, the area just below the ankle and the Achilles tendon. Genital and urinary organ stimulation points are located at these spots.

For optimum results, press as deeply and firmly as you can without causing pain. Knead each tiny bit of surface area, penetrating deep below the skin. The first few times you do this it may be helpful to imagine a grid of tiny squares over the hand or foot, creating a multitude of minute massage areas. Take 10 minutes or more on each hand or foot. Knead each zone thoroughly.

Though hand and foot massage are remarkably relaxing, they are also very simple to perform. A foot massage with a little lotion (we especially like *Sunshine Herbal Foot Lotion* with wintergreen oil) is almost always welcome. In fact, we

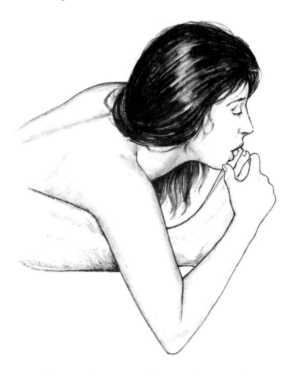

cannot emphasize how much joy this simple gesture can bring to your consort.

Big Toe Massage   A quick way to evoke a calm energy in your consort is the big toe massage. This can be performed by sucking with the mouth as if the big toe were a man's penis. While we like to call this Big Toe Fellatio, we want to stress that the recipient can be a woman or a man. Acting out the fantasy that the big toe is a sex organ will be fun for some, though.

The sensations may be felt all through the body, right to the top of the head. The stimulation may feel incredibly good, so good, in fact, that the sensations could be compared to a continuous low-grade orgasm.

Special stimulation points for the pituitary and pineal glands are located in the big toe. The pituitary stimulation point will be found in the middle of the big toe pad. The pineal stimulation point is slightly up and to the right of the pituitary point. The location of these points varies from one individual to another. Massage these points gently using a circular movement with your thumbs.

BIG TOE FELLATIO
above
Said to be a replica of the whole body, the big toe is called a *marma* or power point in Tantra. A massage style from India just does big toes (feels great!).

Positive identification is found by pressing firmly in the general location. You may use the eraser end of a pencil. The precise locations will feel tender to the recipient.

Pituitary stimulation harmonizes the physical dimension

of sexual response; pineal stimulation harmonizes the emotional dimension.

A thorough big toe massage evokes a subtle aliveness in the whole body. Five minutes on each big toe is a complete massage in itself. Be sure to do both big toes.

Of course, you can suck on and massage all ten toes. Tired of oral genital sex, i.e., 69? Suck on each other's toes at the same time and enjoy "20."

Foot Washing   An ancient tradition that we would like to see revived is washing feet. Most of us would like a full body massage before lovemaking but that takes a lot of time. Or it may feel like too much work. Washing feet requires very little effort and can be performed fully clothed (minus shoes and socks, of course) as a preliminary to lovemaking or as a caring gesture that is complete by itself.

Bathe the feet first in warm water. After drying them off thoroughly, anoint the feet with oil or cream. Gently rub the oil or lotion in. Allow the warm feelings that you have for this person to flow out through your hands. Exchange roles if convenient.

The psychological implications of washing the feet of another person may include respect, humility and service. Washing the feet can be a part of a ceremonial preparation for making love (see *Doing It Rite*).

But these implications don't have to be explored. The tender sensuousness of the experience makes it one not to be missed. Next time, instead of or along with giving them a bath or massage, wash their feet. Washing feet is relaxing and energizing for both the giver and the receiver, which makes it an ideal preparation for making love.

Face Massage   The face, ears and sexual organs are also rich with nerve reflex points. Massage of these areas benefits the entire body. Ear massage is a technical skill beyond the scope of this book. However, many people find a gentle massage of the upper inside halves of the ears invigorating. Avoid the ear canal, of course. Genital acupressure massage is discussed in the *Tao of Sex* section.

Facial massage releases the mask of facial tension that tends to develop in social interactions. Dropping this facial mask may noticeably increase social and sexual responsiveness. Men who tend to ejaculate early and women who have not been orgasmic during intercourse may especially benefit from letting go of the facial tension mask.

Before beginning the facial massage, ask your partner to

clench their teeth and scrunch their face towards the tip of their nose in a tight ball. Have them concentrate with eyes closed on the tip of their nose, hold for a count of five, then release.

Rub their cheeks, nose and forehead gently up and out to the sides with your fingers or palm. Upward motion counters the downward pull of gravity, aging and negative emotions.

The temples respond well to a gentle circular motion. Knead the scalp and the base of the skull for additional energy and release.

Conclude by firmly but very gently pressing the depression at the top and towards the rear of the skull (the fontanelle) for a count of three. This powerful acupressure point releases the face, head and neck at the same time. Caution is advised when stimulating this last point.

Also very relaxing is a warm towel over the face, as any man who has had a shave the old way knows. A warm wet towel over the lower back (the kidney area) may stir the libido as well as relax. Sometimes a cold pack is effective there instead. You can follow up the foot washing with a foot massage.

Acupressure Massage   Everybody has personalized tension stash areas. They may not be located near a standard erotic zone. For example, people stash tension in the jaw, neck, shoulder, upper and lower back, thigh and calf. Find the secret tension hideaways and you may not only guarantee a great time together, you may have made a friend for life. It's better to be a little too gentle than too firm when dealing with potentially painful areas of the body like these tension stash spots. You can find these areas out by asking your consort where they store tension as well as by gentle probing as you massage.

Below we describe more massage movements that make use of quite a few sexual acupressure points. Acupressure to some of these points can be self-administered. Some aculoving areas are effective for just men or women, but most are effective for both. Therapeutic applications, such as dealing with persistent impotence or frigidity, are beyond the scope of this book.

The ideal style, perhaps, is gentle and playful. Just the same, you may achieve some startling results. Your consort can inhale deeply just before you begin a technique, then exhale as the pressure is applied.

Repeat each point several times before moving on to another one. Unless you are incorporating these aculoving areas into a leisurely whole-body massage, it is better to stimulate just a few areas but very thoroughly.

The arms and hands are extensions of the heart. You can send love through your hands at will (see *Love Spot*). If the idea of sending "love" seems too abstract, focus on giving a warm, good feeling through your touch.

The back or feet are good places to start. Being touched there feels safe to most people. Finish with the medulla oblongata point. Since the effects of aculoving massage may take a few hours to reach their peak, experiment with timing the massage for maximum benefit.

Acupressure is a powerful tool to be used with discretion. Do *not* press on an area that is healing or scarred. If your partner has any of the following conditions you should *not* give them acupressure stimulation: (1) If they are pregnant. (2) If they have a chronic heart problem, particularly if they have a pacemaker. (3) If they are heavily intoxicated with alcohol or other drug(s), including powerful prescription drugs.

This mini-guide outlines an acupressure massage for the whole body. Specifically designed to enhance sexual well-being, it starts at the medulla oblongata point behind the head and ends with the soles of the feet. The location, a massage technique, the sexual benefit and whether the technique is designed for men, women or both are described for each aculoving area.

○ *Medulla oblongata:* press the hollow in the base of the skull with thumbs or rotate middle fingers to energize entire male or female body

○ *Thyroid gland:* apply firm pressure with ball of thumb in front of neck above clavicle on either side to increase female sexual response

○ *Wrists:* massage the entire wrist gently, especially the area down from the thumb, to enhance male or female sexual response

○ *Thymus gland:* gently massage the valley between the breasts on either side above and below *Love Spot* to emotionally and sexually warm the female

○ *Breastbone:* gently massage the bony region between breasts to improve male sexual ability

○ *Nipple tips:* a delicate feathery touch here brings increase of male or female sexual desire

○ *Liver:* press fingertips of both hands under edge of right rib cage to relieve liver-anger-sex connection and improve male sexual function

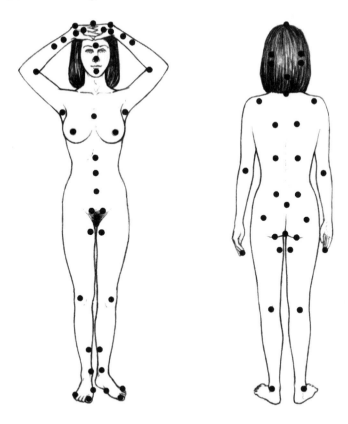

○ *Solar plexus:* press with fingertips of both hands in the pit of the stomach right below breastbone to delay male ejaculation or boost and balance female sex drive

○ *Navel:* press with fingertip to relieve loss of sex drive due to congestion for male or female

○ *Adrenal glands:* press gently but firmly with your fists on both sides just above kidneys (between thoracic vertabrae 11 and 12) right above where the adrenal glands are located (under the lowest ribs) to increase female sexual stamina or uplift male emotion

○ *Sea of energy:* press with fingers about two inches below navel on midline to directly stimulate sex glands and increase energy for male or female

○ *Pubic:* gently massage along top edge of pubic hair line to stimulate male or female sex drive

○ *Symphysis pubic:* rotate finger or thumb or gently rub a little below pubic hair line where pubic bones meet to relieve male constipation, stimulate the bladder and sex drive, and increase testicle sensitivity

○ *Penis control:* press with third finger beneath pubic bone just above penis to delay ejaculation

ACULOVING POINTS
above
So many points, so little time. Try working on just one area at a time. After you find a spot, close your eyes and feel it with your hands.

○ *Inguinal region:* press palms with heels of palms in towards genitals on high inner thighs to gently arouse female or some males

○ *Lower back area:* create friction by moving palms in circles, then go up both sides of spine to warm kidney region and increase sexual desire and relaxation for male or female

○ *Lumbar:* press thumbs in space on each side of spinal column between each of the five lumbar vertabrae just above the sacrum to stimulate male or female internal organs and sexual drive

○ *Sacrum:* apply fingertip or thumb pressure to inverted triangle of bone at base of spine to delay male ejaculation or boost and balance female sex drive

○ *Gluteal fold:* massage gently where the buttocks and legs meet to increase male or female sexual vitality

○ *Cleavage of buttocks:* massage gently between cheeks near the end of the tailbone to increase male or female sexual vitality

○ *Buttocks:* a gentle and penetrating massage motion here is relaxing and arousing for male or female

○ *Valleys of buttocks:* a penetrating kneading motion in the valleys of cheeks close to hips helps produce rapid erection following ejaculation

○ *Governing vessel one:* gently massage area around tip of tailbone to stimulate sexual heat and performance for male or female

○ *Anus:* massage gently around rim and just inside rectum to relax inhibitions of male or female consort

○ *Perineum:* a gentle circular rubbing motion or stationary pressure at this nickel-sized area midway between rectum and genitals stimulates male or female sexual heat and performance

○ *Triple yin:* firm pressure next to shin bone three inches above inside ankle bone favors full female arousal

○ *Kidney one:* firm pressure with thumb or finger in middle of foot soles just below ball of each foot energizes overall, sexual vigor included, for male or female

AURAL SEX "If music be the food of love, play on," wrote the Bard of Avon in his play *Twelfth Night.* Like Shakespeare, many people enjoy making love to music. As a background, music generates mood, stimulates fantasy and suggests rhythms and kinds of movement.

Light headphones can be worn while you make love. Even if you are not such audiophiles, wearing headphones is delightful when you are on the receiving end, such as during fellatio, cunnilingus or a massage.

Rock and roll is one obvious choice because of the explicit sexual themes and hard driving rhythms. Rhythm and speed vary enormously from song to song. The connoisseur will create a customized cassette. Here is a sample sequence of classic rock selections with the same basic beat: "Don't Stop Till You Get Enough" (Michael Jackson), "Heart of Glass" (Blondie), "Urgent" (Foreigner), "Gimme All Your Loving" (ZZ Top) and "Hit Me With Your Best Shot" (Pat Benatar). You can design your tape to begin serenely with a sweethearts soft pop sound and build up to a hard rock crescendo. Funky dance music and Jamaican reggae offer some delicious sounds. Instead of making your own tape you may want to buy workout music, e.g., aerobics records. These collections provide a strong consistent beat. Make sure you get the music without an instructor's voice.

Some of our romantic favorites from the classics include the Strauss waltzs, *Bolero* (Ravel), *Afternoon of A Faun* and *La Mer* (Debussy), *Scheherazade* (Rimsky-Korsakoff), *Rite of Spring* (Stravinsky), *Romeo and Juliet* (Prokofieff), *The Four Seasons* (Vivaldi) and *Fantasia On A Theme By Thomas Tallis* (Ralph Vaughan Williams). If you are looking for intensity, try Wagner. We also like Ravi Shankar's sitar music, African drum music and calypso music.

Put on a recording of the ocean and get swept away. Many record stores carry environmental recordings. Perfumes can be coordinated with the natural setting depicted by the sounds. For instance, the perfume called *Rain Forest* adds when listening to *Ultimate Thunderstorm.*

We highly recommend *Oceanic Tantra, Tantric Wave* and *Tantric Wave Ritual* (Kutira Decosterd). The latter, a narrated musical journey, is an ideal introduction to Tantra.

Listen to relaxing, inspiring music before or while you make love. We find that *Starborn Suite, Spectrum Suite* and *Crystal Suite* (Steve Halpern), *Wave #1: Inter-Dimensional Music* (Iasos), *Lemurian Sunrise* (Steve Kindler and Paul Warner), *Ambient 1: Music For Airports* (Brian Eno), *Silk Road* (Kitaro), *Mountain Light* (Rob Whiteside-Woo), *Dance of the Hi-Tech Shaman* (E. J. Gold), *Rainforest* (Robert Rich), *Colors of Light* (Karunesh), *Midnight Blvd.* (Dancing Fantasy) and *Music For Zen Meditation and Other Joys* (Tony Scott, Shinichi Yuize, Hozan Yamamoto) are ideal for this purpose. Steve Halpern's *Spectrum Suite* and *Crystal Suite* deserve special attention for providing well-designed musical meditation journeys up the seven *Energy Centers*.

The sensual "Moments In Love" from *The Best Of The Art Of Noise* is perhaps the closest thing to New Age erotic music we have heard. More energetic but quite enthralling are the electronic classics *Oxygene* (Jean Michel Jarre) and *Rainbow On Curved Air* (Terry Riley). The modern classical compositions *The Photographer* and *Mishima* (Philip Glass) conclude with what may be the best descriptions of orgasm in contemporary music.

In the area of Hindu music, G. S. Sachdev's flute in *Classical North Indian Ragas* beautifully expresses longing and subtle romantic feelings. *Jai Ma Kirtan* from the Mount Madonna Center offers charming devotional chants to the Goddess. *The Sound of Tamboura* creates a uniquely soothing background with its warm, hypnotic drone. We recommend as an effortless preparation for Tantric lovemaking *Experience Yoga Nidra,* a guided deep relaxation experience combining an ancient Tantra yoga method taught by Swami Janakananda with music by Roop Verma.

Certain music is ideal for *Extrasensory Sex*. Though the selections just mentioned would be fine, our special choices of music for *Extrasensory Sex* include *Angelic Music* (Iasos), *Himalayan Bells II* (Karma Moffett) and *Tibetan Bells II* (Henry Wolff and Nancy Hennings). These pieces are uniquely cosmic in effect.

Some people have found *Extrasensory Sex* to be "boring" due to the low stimulation level. Listening to evocative exotic mood music counteracts this tendency.

Record your favorite music on one side of a 90-minute cassette tape, so that you can enjoy 45 minutes of continuous sound. You won't have to get up to flip the tape over. Or use an auto-reverse tape deck or CD player.

In order to provide accurate and up to date information regarding the use of music for enhancing sensuality and sexual experiences, including attaining states of altered consciousness, we interviewed Steven Halpern, Ph.D., a widely respected composer and expert in the New Age music field.

Ellen: Steven, are there scientific principles involved?

Steven: There are two main physiological laws involved. The first is that your body is literally a human instrument. Your entire body responds to sound, not just your ears. Moreover, it vibrates in different frequencies in different areas, much like the strings of a piano. Most importantly, it plays better when it's in tune. Just as with a violin, where you tune the strings so they vibrate "in phase," as sensitive lovers we align and attune our chakras.

Related to this is the law of entrainment: the natural rhythm of our breath and heartbeat may be easily overridden by the beat of an external rhythmic stimulus.

David: What is the effect of popular music?

Steven: Pop top-40, disco, heavy metal and rap all accentuate the grosser aspects of resonance and entrainment with a lot of low-pitched frequencies that resonate in the first and second chakra area and a thumpus non-interruptus rhythm (all too often now the product of a robotic drum machine rather than a flesh and blood drummer). While this certainly has its place, it would be a shame to miss out on the higher harmonics of sonic eroticism. But for extended lovemaking or listening sessions, not just any music will do!

Most music is too "busy" and demands our attention, even if in the background. We've been culturally conditioned to respond to certain patterns of chords, melody, etc. If it gets familiar and too easily recognizable, it gets boring. And who wants to get out of lotus posture to change the mood music?

Ellen: How can we tell if a certain piece of music is good for us as a background to making love?

Steven: Look for music that caresses you rather than kicks you. *Watch your breath.* Notice if you and your partner are breathing more evenly and slowly. Are you breathing in synchronized patterns?

Notice how the music feels all over your body. Your entire body responds to sounds, especially at the acupuncture points.

Certain compositions, like those in my Anti-Frantic™ series, allow your body to make its own decision and choose the rhythm that is most relaxing and natural. Most people's bodies choose a similar pulsation that relates to a fundamental overtone of eight cycles per second—which just so happens to also be the dominant frequency of the planet Earth herself.

David: How does the right kind of music enhance couple dynamics?

Steven: Two bodies that are in sync with each other are more sensitive to each other. This increases sensuality and pleasure potential for a romantic close encounter of the intimate kind.

To go to higher levels, such as in Tantric practice, in musical terms to raise both of your energy states up another octave, explore the subtleties of a chakra-alignment duet.

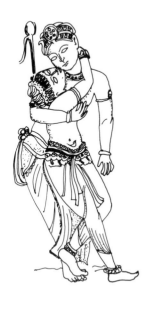

DANCE OF LOVE
above
After a sculptured doorway,
Rajivalochana Temple,
India, 8th century A.D.

Synchronize your breathing, and focus on each chakra, one at a time, starting at the root chakra.

You might begin with a few seconds per center and graduate to longer periods of concentration. Soundtracks such as *Spectrum Suite* and *Crystal Suite* were composed explicitly to support and enhance this meditation. They actually include the color visualization that goes with each frequency change.

Ellen: Any other sound advice?

Steven: As you tune in to what feels good for you, you'll take more responsibility for the response-ability of your physical and supra-physical bodies. Treat yourself well— bring more high quality sound into your life. Choose your music consciously, and remember to clean and demagnetize your tape deck. Stay tuned . . . and enjoy!

Since music is so important, at least for some couples, the placement of the speakers is very important. We suggest that you place your stereo speakers on stands in the far corners of your bedroom. If the head of your bed is against one wall, your speakers go in the corners of the opposite wall.

An inexpensive setup designed by composer Brian Eno may add to your bedroom pleasure. A third small speaker is placed behind the bed to create a quadrophonic-type musical environment in which the sounds seem to surround you. This speaker should be connected to the red (positive) junctures on your amplifier. If this speaker is too loud, add a potentiometer of 6-12 ohms and 10 or more watts. For more information, see the back cover of Eno's album *Ambient #4: On Land*.

BOUDOIR BASICS   Here we offer inexpensive suggestions designed to enhance your bedroom's ambiance. These holistic boudoir bonuses recreate the psychological and electromagnetic conditions that prevail under more idyllic settings, such as making love in the forest or on a tropical beach. Subtle environmental cues and stimuli play an enormous role in sexual response. Without much expense or effort, you can fine tune your bedroom and enjoy the benefits of a personalized boudoir that radiates vitality and relaxation.

Nature's Way   An abundance of negative ions is thought to be relaxing and may improve many aspects of sexual functioning, including potency, reproduction, breast milk production, menstruation and sexual performance and enjoyment. Excessive positive ions may be associated with increased stress and may have a negative effect on sexual functioning in some people. Negative ion generators produce billions of negative ions, restoring the ion balance to that found in healthful natural settings.

If you have sexual health or performance problems, place a negative ion generator close to the genitals so that the negative ions stream directly on them. Try this in daily 20 minute sessions for two weeks. Research in Italy and Russia suggests this procedure may help, but by law no claims can be made for it, of course.

Keep your television somewhere other than at the foot of your bed. According to pyramid power expert Dee Jay Nelson, the pyramidal shape of your television picture tube produces a mildly debilitating radiation. Nelson used a copper sheet to cover the screen in his laboratory. A thick piece of wood may do the job.

Orient your bed so that the head faces magnetic north. Place a wool blanket under cotton sheets on your bed. Both steps should enhance your available bioelectromagnetism.

Use natural fabrics on your bed. You will help the pores of your skin breathe. You can avoid possible skin irritation and/or allergic reactions.

Far better than a bed pillow for support under your consort's buttocks while you are making love is a crescent-shaped pillow. Beautifully embroidered crescent pillows can be found in stores that carry Indian imports. Don't ask for these pillows as accessories for making love. They probably won't know what you're talking about. Inflatable plastic pillows that serve the same purpose are also available.

Some scents are traditionally thought to be reliable in the bedroom. These include musk, patchouli, sandalwood, jasmine, rose, ylang-ylang and juniper as an essential perfume oil or an incense. If you want to explore the more subtle effects of oils, be willing to pay a little more for "first quality" essential oils (see *Appendix*).

Fresh flowers in the boudoir do a lot more than decorate. The red rose not only offers its special fragrance; under its outer lips the vagina resembles nothing so much as a partly opened rose. The color of the hibiscus flower as well as the flower itself has long symbolized ultimate sexual fulfillment in the Orient.

A robe the color of hibiscus (scarlet) is considered ideal for the female consort to wear before lovemaking. This is one inexpensive way to incorporate the power of color in your love life. What about the bedroom itself? You will not have to repaint your bedroom walls and redecorate. Thanks to the miracle of lighting, virtually any bedroom can be quickly transformed into a seductive, eductive cove of comfort and sensuous communion.

Turn On Your Love Light   When Edison and Swan developed the incandescent lamp in 1880, they changed the way people would make love in the twentieth century. The household electric light bulb sends out a pallid yellow light with just a dash of orange in it. This type of lighting tinges human flesh with grey, white and yellow tones that are, to say the least, unflattering. Since, scientists tell us, the brain gets 75 percent of its sense data via the eyes, a change in the way you light your boudoir may light up your love life as well. Light is known to affect the pineal gland, which plays a major though as yet unclear role in our sexual lives.

One option is to go primitive, that is, pre-Edison. Candles are reliable. Small and large colored glass containers, available from religious and occult supply shops, offer some of the advantages of colored lighting. Their intensity is less but candlelight flatters the human body by making it look more fluid and smooth. Some people prefer the illumination of a beeswax candle or kerosene lantern. Coals in a brazier are another option. A brazier has the advantage of also being an incense burner. Frankincense and myrrh can be bought as little chunks and tossed on the coals. The fireplace is another popular sensuous light source. Your natural light sources may give off a slightly eerie blue light which adds surprisingly to the erotic mood.

Pre-electric light sources are not the only way to brighten up your bedroom activities. Back in the days of swinging, a San Francisco hostess consulted with a color expert on how to perk up her sex parties. He suggested magenta, a blend of red and purple. The expert advised magenta lighting in every socket and beneath the furnishings as well. He also made her promise that for the first couple of hours of the party only non-alcoholic refreshments would be served. In the orgy that followed nobody bothered to break out the booze.

The magenta tone can be approximated by blending the light from a red bulb and a purple bulb. You may be able to find a magenta plastic light filter or achieve a magenta tone by combining red and purple filters. However, other color tones are also very effective. Inexpensive professional gel filter material is available from theatrical supply houses.

If you purchase only one colored bulb, your best choice is almost certainly amber. Keep the watts low. Orange adds a vibrant glow to the skin, but amber does this and adds a luxurious softness to the appearance of the skin.

Cool tones, such as green and blue, are erotically effective. This goes contrary to conventional thinking which assigns red the sexy color status, but you will see for yourself if you experiment with the cool tones.

Actually, red is too much of a good thing. Under a red light skin tones have an artificial appearance and glands and emotions are said to become overstimulated, resulting in unstable arousal and unprovoked angry conflicts.

Purple and ultraviolet lighting offer a uniquely enthralling effect. Hindu sexual yoga texts claim that certain shades of purple or violet are the color of the female sex energy. In some rituals, a rich violet light is shone upon the female consort's genitals before intercourse begins. The shade of red unique to hibiscus flowers is also used.

You may want to experiment with several lights. You can combine cool lights, warm lights or a cool light and a warm light. You are also able to vary their brightness by choosing light bulbs of different wattage. Author Howard E. Smith, Jr. suggests blending a bright green light with a dim red light.

The psychological illusions created by colored lighting are impressive. Under blue and green lighting, men reported that their consort's breasts not only appeared larger but actually felt larger when touched. Under the same lighting women saw men's penises larger than life. Tests conducted on college students revealed that red illumination hastened erection while green illumination slowed it down.

Oils and powders are yet another way to play with the effects of lighting. Oils increase contrasts. Powders soften and smooth out the visual drama.

One excellent source of colored light bulbs is *GE Party Bulbs*. These inexpensive all-purpose bulbs are available in a wide variety of hues and wattages. Floodlights are available in a variety of colors. Ultra-violet lamps are easily purchased. However, don't look directly into the U-V light. This shouldn't be a problem, as you will be looking at each other instead. Full-spectrum lighting is now available also as well as holistic colored lighting products (see *Appendix*).

Your basic boudoir is complete with a short table for food and drink. Fruits, bread, a flask of light red wine, vials of damiana and saw palmetto berry liquid essences and some fresh spring water will nourish and invigorate without weighing down.

CHARGE UP   One very effective way to charge up with energy before making love is this method developed by practical mystic Betty Bethards of the Inner Light Foundation. It combines alternate co-breathing with positive energy imagery. Don't be concerned about how clear or vivid your mental image is. You may not see anything. You may just have an impression or feeling of it. That's enough.

Achieve genital union. Sit in YabYum on the bed, floor or in a chair (see *Peaceful Positions*). Put your attention at the point of genital connection.

Visualize a sphere of golden light the size of a beach ball there. Take a moment to build and enjoy this beautiful image.

Either consort may begin the breathing. Let's say the man begins. As he exhales, he imagines that he is thrusting this light from the genitals up her spine to the top of her head. As he is exhaling she is inhaling. As she inhales, she imagines that she is drawing that same light from the genitals up her spine to the top of her head at the same time.

Now, when she exhales, he inhales. She sees the light going down her spine, through the genital juncture, and up his spine to the top of his head. She thrusts the light with her exhalation as he draws the light with his inhalation. When he finally thrusts the light back through her, he will send it from the top of his head, down his spine, through their genitals and up her spine to the top of her head.

You may want to make a gentle noise as you inhale and exhale so your partner can be sure of where you are in the exchange. Or you can hold hands and squeeze as you exhale. Remember to breathe as fully and as completely as is comfortable for you. Take five minutes or less to Charge Up.

The Charge Up is ideal preparation for *Extrasensory Sex*. When Charge Up is complete, lean back and relax into the Seesaw (see *Peaceful Positions*). We suggest YabYum first because you can hear each other breathe.

The Charge Up can be elaborated to include visualization of the psychic centers that are along the spine. This can be as simple as thinking of the solar plexus, heart, throat, forehead and top of head as you bring the energy up or down. Try to really feel your inner channel through your breath (see *Energy Centers, Fusion Breath Sex*).

Another variation is to hold your breath when you inhale to and through your crown. As you pause for a moment, see and feel the energy explode into space through the top of your head. Then, as you exhale, pull the energy back down through your body and give it to your partner.

CHARGE UP *opposite*
This playful yet powerful exchange of energy is not as difficult as it sounds.

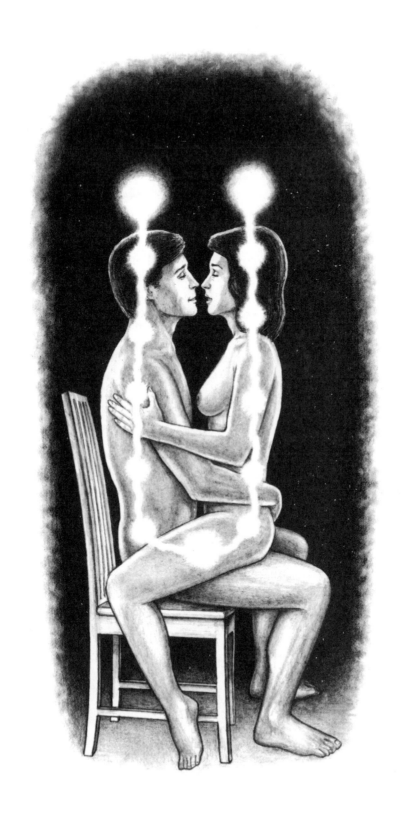

DO IT RITE   The words rite and right are semantic cousins. The basic purpose of a ritual is to help you feel and be right with the world and right with yourself. Back when ritual was big, it was believed that if you did not do each required rite (ritual), or if you did not do each rite right, then life might do you wrong. In the old, old days, doing it right meant doing it rite as well.

Ritual—
A Sly Method   The chief value of ritual for us moderns is that it can still penetrate our carefully cultivated cool. In the face of ecological destruction and social turmoil, we turn off. We can watch only so many depressing TV news programs and read only so many violent newspaper headlines before we submit with relief to a mild self-administered emotional lobotomy.

It takes courage to recognize this desensitization. To not just have sex, but to make love, to meet heart core to heart core, is the very opposite of self-insulation. Making love requires that most precious and rare yet uniquely human response, deep and sincere feeling. But to feel or not to feel is not the question. Men and women who can no longer feel are somehow no longer human.

What is needed is a way to cut through these emotional straitjackets and get to you and me where we really live. But how?

Direct confrontation, as you might find in an encounter group, is one way. But sexual intercourse already tends to be a little tense and confrontative. A sly method is needed, one that gets to the gut through the back door.

Is there a strategy that is pretty, friendly, fun, entertaining, enchanting, clever and sly all at once? Is there a way to sneak in through the basement of the human psyche and take control of its gas, water and power? There is. The name of this time-honored strategy is ritual.

Of course, sexual ritual isn't for everybody. But before you dismiss the idea, think about our contemporary sexual rituals like candlelight dinners and romantic tropical vacations. Sexual ritual in the privacy of your own home as a prelude to sexual union is just as much fun.

The key is to feel a blend of wonder, reverence for life and carefree playfulness. Some consorts worship each other as god and goddess to get in this mood.

A Western Ritual   Here is a simple but powerful ritual based in part on the traditional Tantric ceremony, adapted for Western consorts. Doing an easy sexual ritual together is a great way to get to know each other. It can put new life in an old relationship.

Prepare your environment sensually, with texture and color. Keep romance foremost in your mind as you decorate. Include some flowers, especially rose or hibiscus. If possible, place a powerful negative ion generator in the room and turn it on before beginning. Natural settings generally have the right negative ion balance, especially if near water.

Bathe or shower separately. Cold water can be surprisingly invigorating. Anoint the body with natural essential oils. An expensive French fragrance is also acceptable.

Prepare a table with flowers and fruits, bread and wine or a favorite light beverage. The table should be a height that is suitable for eating while sitting on cushions.

Candlelight or kerosene lantern light is preferred. No standard light bulbs allowed.

Have no music unless at the very beginning. However, a long-playing tape designed so that the musical selections are closely choreographed with your ritual steps may be used. Another alternative is a very neutral, long-playing background tape that will mask distracting outside sounds. This applies mainly to urban dwellers. The natural, mysterious quiet of the late evening is one of the reasons for the traditional late timing of sexual rituals.

Assure no interruptions: no telephone calls, no appointments, no kids, no other things to do for the next three to four hours.

You might want to read love poetry or make a verbal declaration (or confession) of affection and good will before beginning. Make your declaration sitting facing each other as you hold hands and look in each other's eyes.

One ritual step which can be very effective is to do the Root Lock exercise together as part of the ceremony any time before the ritual meal.

Massage with a sensually fragrant oil like ylang-ylang is a fine preparation. Washing each other's feet would be especially appropriate as well as relaxing (see *Aculoving*).

You may also wish to limber up with some hatha yoga stretches or other relaxing, energizing movements. You may want to go through a stress reduction or whole-body relaxation routine or listen to an inspiring cassette tape.

Perhaps you want to follow the example of the Orient. The female consort dances for the man. She may dance so beautifully that he is lifted above his tensions and anxieties. She takes on the appearance of a goddess to him. Far from being a coarse seduction, both lovers reach an elevated plane long before the transcendental delicacies of intercourse are tasted. Of course, the man can dance, too.

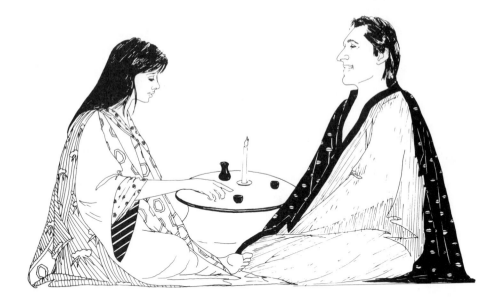

The man enters the boudoir first. Dressed only in an elegant robe, he sits at the table contemplating the delights of the goddess he will soon be enjoying.

Eventually, she also enters. She is also dressed in a stunning robe, one which he has never seen before.

Silently, they may share a light meal together along with a glass of wine. Sharing a peach with sincere sensuality works great as a non-alcoholic alternative.

She slips her robe off first, very slowly. He admires her several minutes. Do not rush this stage. He should savor every detail of her flesh as it is revealed inch by inch as if he had never seen her before. Then he takes his robe off, also very slowly. In turn, she admires him.

Now, finally, they touch. Still no words are spoken. They may massage each other. They may worship each other's sexual organs, manually or orally. This stage prepares the sexual organs for intercourse. Do not overstimulate here.

Sexual union takes place, preferably with the woman on the man's lap. The man can sit on a pillow or have his back supported or both. He can half-recline. But she is on top. These are all variations of the classic YabYum position (see *Peaceful Positions*).

A Taste Of Tantra   In the classic Tantric form, the couple remains motionless in sex meditation, the attention focused on their own or their partner's third eye (see *Tantric Ritual Sex*). This may be with arousal through PC muscle stimulation, as in *Kabbazah Sex,* or without, as in *Extrasensory Sex*. The physical stillness and non-action, in this tempestuous context, are part of the yoga.

Mind and feeling elevated in this way, the sexual union becomes a sublime experience that reveals the heights of human potential. While this practice initially proves more difficult than expected for many couples, due in part to boredom, for those who persist the results are often extraordinary. In fact, it may be those couples who have already shared a wide variety of sexual experiences together and have achieved a degree of satiety that will be most available to this transcendental alternative.

Be creative, be yourself and, above all, be light and easy. It is good to take preparing for the ritual seriously, but once you have started be playful, have fun. You may find that the best ritual is one you design yourself. Completely personalized, it caters to you with your preferred stimuli.

The ideal ritual mood is that you are already there. You are already in a fabulous heaven world where the two of you reign supreme as god and goddess. Free of cares, fears and doubts, all of which are the fare of mere mortals, you have chosen to meet together in this elegant way as an expression of the richness which you already possess in great abundance.

The basic premise of ritual is to increase available energy, increase available emotion. However, the quality of the feeling tone is far more important than the quantity of emotional energy. Intense passion in itself is no guarantee of happiness; indeed, according to Eastern spiritual teachings, that which has become hot will eventually turn cold (spicy lovers who become bitter enemies).

In the advanced Tantric Buddhist rituals the meditative skills of generating compassion, perceiving the emptiness of experience, even of bliss, and detailed visualizing of self and consort as deities are required so that the ensnaring hooks of intense passion do not blind the practicioners. That such skills need to be developed to an extraordinary degree is emphasized again and again. The more conservative approach to Tantric sex is to reduce the passion-stimulation component while increasing the awareness component, a strategy that is optimized in *Extrasensory Sex* and other externally passive but inwardly dynamic meditative styles.

It is not without reason that the ancient sources describe mystical sexual practices as literally playing with fire. Fire can heat your house—or burn it down.

On the other hand, we in the West live in a unique environment. Saturated by sexual stimuli through books,

WESTERN LOVE RITUAL
opposite
The main point is that making love is an art. The art of love, like many forms of art, has a ceremonial element.

magazines, movies and television, we need to approach the issue of sexuality consciously, boldly and directly. We are all Tantric yogis and yoginis—whether we like it or not—in the sense that we must deal every day with sexual energy, with what it is and what we want to do with it.

This fact of life, combined with the widespread exposure to modern depth psychology, has introduced us to new ways of working and playing with the sex energy. We are discovering for ourselves that alertly and purposefully investigating sex energy can lead to self-knowledge, enhanced relationships and enriched living. Sex is here to stay, so we may as well make peace with it. We can start by becoming its friend.

Ritual offers an opportunity to focus and refine the feeling tone or mood you usually bring to sexual expression. Utilizing artistic elements such as music, dance, color, symbolism, sensual massage and poetry, the raw material of sex attraction is converted in alchemical fashion into the glorious love-bliss enjoyed by the gods and goddesses, utterly free of problem and conflict, capable of illuminating the mind, the milk of paradise. Instead of sex just being something that happens to us, we take control at a new level and learn to ride the tiger of sex energy to new heights as we develop sensitivity to its deeper pulse.

When creating and doing a ritual such as this, then, it is best to concentrate on creating the right mood. Keep it light and loving, a gift of the moment. Look for deeper levels of meaning if you wish, but the real key is to brighten and uplift the mood as much as possible, to achieve the mood of open-eyed wonder and innocence typical of a happy child.

The heaviness and seriousness that accompany much of our sexual behavior are largely toxic by-products of negative mood habits that became linked with sex energy through early guilt and fear conditioning. There are few elixirs more enthralling than feelings of joy and love, the ecstasy of sexual energy sandwiched between, shared by consorts who yearn to open their hearts and be one.

DREAM LOVER   Would you like to meet your dream lover? Now you can. Instead of relying on Hollywood, take matters into your own hands. Create an exquisite imaginary lover, ideal and perfect in every detail. Give your imaginary lover the perfect body and generous nature of a god or goddess. With your imagination, you can make him or her exactly as you would like them—literally a dream come true.

Everything Is Allowed

Allow them to do and be anything you like. They will always be by your side and always love you. You can do anything to them, even humiliate them any way you like. Though they are the most beautiful being you have ever seen, you can make them your slave and submit them to the most outrageous or exotic fantasies. Likewise, they will do anything to you that you want, limited only by the vividness and richness of your imagination.

Far from being an unhealthy self-indulgence, your imaginary perfect lover acts as an escape valve. Our problems begin when we try to stop life's natural urges. Expressed safely in this way without hurting anyone, we can have our cake and eat it, too. We have safely channeled anti-social actions away from where they could really hurt a living, feeling person by acting them out on the mental realm.

Your dream lover may also provide you with feelings of love and acceptance, with courage, with advice and insight. They can be your radiant guide, your cosmic lover, your ideal companion and anything else you can dream up all rolled into one. One advantage of using an Eastern figure is that his or her body has many arms with which to stimulate you. Of course, your two-armed dream lover will have the capacity to sprout extra arms any time you like.

You can easily take your dream lover with you into your dreams. As you go to sleep, look at your third eye or imagine a brilliant red dot at your throat. See your dream lover in your mind's eye. Ask them to take you to an out-of-this-world paradise, a temple of spiritual wisdom and healing or on some other fantastic journey (see *God And Goddess*).

Do not be surprised if your dream lover takes unexpected forms. In fact, this is a gift. Affirm that you are deeply loved and appreciated. Allow your dream lover to take the ideal shape for you that best expresses unconditional love.

At the same time, you must ask for what you want. For example, working with a dream lover is an excellent way to learn more about the higher dimensions of sex.

In one recent dream lover session, for example, David asked specifically for a Tantric sexual guide. A pretty, young English woman with flaxen hair appeared. Her heavy, dark blue cloak with a high collar up to her ears reminded him of the uniforms worn by nurses a century ago.

"I asked for a Tantric guide," David said, thinking her dressed inappropriately for the part.

"The name is Brigitt," she briskly replied in a strong Cockney accent. "I can teach you about the Tantric climax all right, but none of that tiddling in the grass."

With that, she flung her cloak off. Underneath she was dressed in shimmering light of many colors. In a flash, she joined with him face to face in the YabYum posture. Without the physical barrier, they merged easily, so that her body completely overlayed his. They were one body, yet two. Thus ensconced, she taught him her technique for raising the sex energy (see *Fusion Breath Sex*).

During such a union the movement of energy is easily accomplished. You are already in your energy bodies. You need only focus your attention to feel the power.

The story does not end there. David looked up "tiddle" in an unabridged dictionary. It is an obsolete word meaning "to fondle."

Guided Session

To embark on a session with your dream lover, find a relaxed position and roll your eyes comfortably up towards the third eye focal point between your eyebrows. This is your inner movie screen. Once you are absorbed in your private movie, you may notice that you are actually seeing it just behind or in front of the middle of your forehead.

It may help to establish what you are wearing (a comfortable toga with purple borders, for example), your surroundings (a dazzling turquoise stone temple that looks down on the ocean), your position (reclining on a soft, luxurious, green couch), the weather (warm and balmy with just a hint of cool sea breeze), the sky (light blue with a few fluffy clouds) and so on. Details such as a drink in your hand, the temperature, color and flavor of your liquid refreshment, the color, shape and texture of the goblet as you grasp it, the silky smoothness and exotic embroidery of the couch you are lying on and so forth help considerably.

It may also help to talk to yourself mentally, to literally talk yourself into and through the experience. "Ah, this is the finest wine I have ever tasted. So delicate yet robust. These Mediterranean grapes are great!" At some point, as you become fully absorbed in the experience, the self-talk drops off by itself.

We can continue this journey, if you like. As you gaze in front of you, you notice that there is a tall open gate there. Suddenly, with a flash of light, he or she appears. At first, it is difficult to make out the details of their appearance. Gracefully, they walk towards you. You are able to see more and more detail.

Even if their appearance remains fuzzy and vague, the thrilling impact of their unique presence is unmistakeable and intoxicating. Now their exquisite body is next to you, so close that you can feel the warmth and sweetness of their breath. Caressing your lips with a jeweled finger, into your ear they whisper, "How may I bring you sensual joy?"

Now ask your dream lover to rub your back. Feel their soft, soothing expert strokes up and down your body. You are feeling more and more relaxed. You feel very close to them, very intimate.

Now ask your dream lover to massage the front of your body, your face, chest, belly and genitals. The connection between you is getting deeper and deeper. You are one with them, and they with you.

Proceed with your fantasy, whatever it may be. Know that you deserve pleasure and set no limits to your enjoyment or that of your dream lover. Thank your dream lover when you are done.

Allow yourself an hour or two for a session in the beginning. At first you may feel a bit self-conscious, as our society does not encourage us to dream. But quickly you will become adept. This is your world, your dream lover, your fantasy, and you can do, have and be anything you damn well please!

Reverie, the state of mind where you are in between waking and sleeping, is excellent for this kind of play. So is hypnosis. These states are, in essence, waking dreams.

The benefits of creative visualization are many. Do not be surprised if creating a dream lover opens up new vistas in other areas of your life.

EDUCE EACH OTHER

Educe means "to draw out." Eduction is the act of drawing out. Eduction and seduction are not the same. Seduction is a maneuver. Eduction is a giving.

You want to find the deep rich valley of the sensory present when you make love. You want to stay in it as long you can. You want to be there together. Learn the fine art of eduction. Educe each other.

The Bridge Of Tenderness

Create a transition from the day-to-day struggle to survive to the love of lovemaking. The transition is a bridge. Rely mainly on non-verbal means—food, drink, herbs, massage, tender gestures, cuddling, games—to cross that precious bridge. Words may work, but touch, a universal language, is more reliable and direct.

Transition is necessary. This is why lovemaking can be so much better on a vacation. You are both relaxed.

Allow the desire for sexual union to flower spontaneously. But first create the atmosphere of peace and relaxation. Enjoy the shape of your togetherness as it is in that moment. How would you describe the shape of your togetherness? Its color? Its texture? If it was music, what would that music be?

If lovemaking arises, fine. If not, fine. This is the attitude that works best of all. This attitude keeps you in the here and now with your consort. You are eager for love and peace.

There will be times, though, that talking first thing is necessary. Do this in the very beginning. Later on, though, as you both relax, as you both begin melting in your mutual touching, you may have something you need to say. Say it. Don't suppress it. Talking is a way of touching another person using sound vibrations. Sexual intercourse is a touching of very sensitive organs.

If you don't force the format, everything will work out beautifully. Simply being together is itself the total fulfillment. You are already fulfilled. Everything that follows after your first meeting is discoveries of that fulfillment. But you will never be more fulfilled together than you are right now.

You may feel that your desire is spontaneous and completely natural. But this society teaches the forcing of sex. To be truly spontaneous in your lovemaking, avoid programming the experience. Free and easy, you share the joy of being surprised by the unknown in each new moment.

We seduce in order to guarantee our pleasure and have it our way. We educe in order to be amazed by the ordinary miracles which we usually neglect. A simple kiss, even a crystallized instant of fiery eye contact, contain all the sweet universes of pleasure.

Try the herbal tub soak, popular at top health spas and guaranteed to relax. Add Epson salts, bubble bath, and/or Kneipp® herbal bath essences. Scrub your lover's body with a loofa or sponge using circular movements. Dr. Bronner's almond, lavender or peppermint liquid soap, diluted half and half with water, is what we like to use with the loofa. A pumice stone is good on the calloused areas of the feet.

Relax, release, relish. It is good, so good, to just hold hands. It is glorious to be free to just breathe your consort's scent, to laugh and accomplish nothing whatsoever. To not have to do or prove or be anything, to be a carefree explorer of the mystery instead. The best way to guarantee that your lovemaking will be special is to share some relaxation and peace together first.

Remember, too, there is an art to receiving touch. Often it is the natural givers who must develop this.

Role Calls— Masculine And Feminine

The woman can assume the soft role of peacemaker, if she likes. This puts the power of the feminine, of the nurturing mother, to work. Like a knight returning from the battlefield, the man willingly surrenders to the peaceful balm of her gentle touch, of the bath she has prepared, of the bed in her boudoir. Not a word is needed. This sounds so archaic. For many couples, it is exactly what is needed.

In other couples, the man is the peacemaker. He is more able to express that peace than her. She is the warrior seeking refuge.

Women work in a battlefield, too. Now women tend to become hard in their struggle to survive and win as well. Neither man nor woman may have softness in reserve. But softness, roundness, is simply essential. Love makes the world round. Two hardnesses, two angularities, wound each other, they collide and crash. If yielding is not known, if only penetration is known, then lovers cannot melt and the other is not discovered.

When there is this yielding, the elixir of lovemaking is released. But demanding that the other yield is ineffective as well as inappropriate. It takes time. It takes trust. It takes a bridge from the world outside, where we struggle, to the world of making love and being in love, where we play.

Perhaps you can make this bridge for each other. But understand what you are doing. You are not just massaging, you are not just serving dinner. You are enabling the critical transition from fighting to loving. If the transition is not made, then lovemaking tends to be the same daily struggle to survive in another form. Lovers win or lose; score or fail to score orgasms.

Talking about peace and security can be the least effective approach. Caring deeply can be shown without using words. In an atmosphere of peace and caring, anyone will melt. There will be no conflict because nothing is being demanded. Then, as your consort falls into the sensuous valley of deep relaxation, you will be regarded very positively because you are giving what is really wanted.

Don't do this just as a strategy or it will backfire. Nobody really wants to be manipulated. You may have to be very patient. When the two of you find the place where just being together is enough, you have opened the door. Give and do not expect or demand anything in return. The results may astound you.

Prepare yourself for this role by taking the time to find more relaxation and peace in your own life. You cannot give to another what you do not have yourself. Take time out just before making the transition from fighting to loving. Take time out in your daily life for your own happiness.

Bring Him To His Senses

Women often ask us what they can do to bring out the gentler, more sensitive side of their man in bed. Realize, first of all, that he is different from you. He looks at life differently. He probably views himself as a warrior, even if he is an accountant or a gas station attendant. To him, life is war, and he wants to emerge the victor.

Men's bodies are different. They are harder and tougher. A man tends to relate to his body as if it were a suit of medieval armor. He wants a tough, strong, durable body that can handle any kind of punishment. This relationship to the physical body may be helpful in the business world, but it is a hindrance in the lovemaking world.

It is very likely that he himself does not know how to let out his sensitive side and take off his suit of armor. Therefore, you must give him a little push in that direction. He may not know where to start. He probably lacks experience in this. His training as a child and young man emphasized other things.

Assert yourself sensuously. Be sensually inventive. Make creative use of the sense of touch. If you would like to have him stroke your face, stroke his face first. Then gently bring his hands to your face. If you want to use words, use them to reinforce your sensuous message. Tell him how good it feels with your eyes, your body, verbally, too. One of our students, Margritte, a fully sensuous woman and hair stylist, claims this approach works like magic nearly every time.

"I give my men an exotic bath. I rub their backs as we watch TV. I show them how much fun it is to be sensual with me. I don't put the responsibility for being sensual on them. I am the woman. I lead them into the delights of love. After all, where can they learn about this? Who is there to teach them? So I assume they don't know anything about playful sensuous lovemaking but are eager to learn and they absolutely love me for it.

"It's very stressful being a man and having all those performance expectations on your head. I make it clear I don't care about orgasms. What do orgasms matter when you're having so much fun? Of course, this defuses the situation so that orgasms are more likely for both of us. The mere act of one human being touching another is a miracle that by itself just overwhelms me. They are grateful to me for taking an active role."

So relax first. The joy will soon follow.

PLAYMATES *opposite*
Where does a man learn how to play sensually and be a lover? From a woman like you.

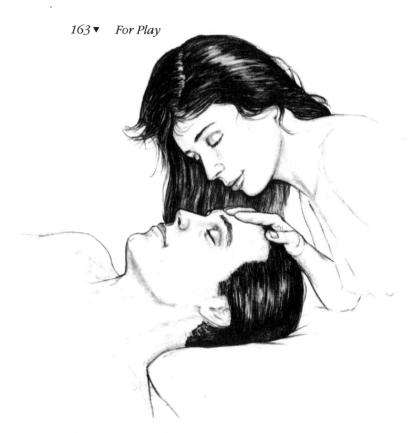

ENERGIZE YOUR HANDS   The most powerful life energy center in the hands is right in the center of the palms. To energize the hands, Bernard Gunther suggests that you clap them for about 30 seconds and then rest them (palms skyward) on your knees. You can also play an energetic game of "patty cake" with your consort and then rest your palms on their knees.

Another way to energize the hands is to pack an imaginary snowball between your palms, moving your hands slowly together and then apart. A sensation of heat or energy density or tingling may occur. You can start this off by rubbing your palms fiercely together for a few seconds.

Breathe deeply as you do this. Imagine a glowing ball of warm light instead if that gives you more energy.

Once you have the sensation going, you can move your hands more creatively while still playing against the feeling of density that is building up.

EROTIC MASSAGE   The sensual lover's erotic massage will include many areas that are not usually considered erotic zones. To begin with, all human skin is erotic. Wherever there are nerve receptors, erotic feeling is possible (see *Aculoving, Oriental Arousal*).

Besides the primary erogenous zone of the genitals, the list of sensitive and highly erotic body places includes lips, the nipples (of both sexes), in and near the ears, the nape of the neck, the middle of the palm, the side of the little finger, the inner arm, the hollows of the elbows and knees, the stomach and navel, the hollows of the buttocks, the base of the spine, the inner thigh, the crease where the groin and thighs meet, and the feet.

Have your basic massage tools on hand, including towel, oil and perhaps soft bristle brush, feather and silk scarf. Make sure the room temperature is on the warm side. The recipient is naked, while you can start in your robe.

If your partner needs help relaxing, we suggest that you start with the back. The back will feel more neutral to both of you. After making contact there, you can progress to more intimate strokes.

When you finish with the back, you may gently knead the base of the skull, a major tension stash spot many people ignore. Basic techniques for working on these areas can be learned in a few minutes. After you are done with their back, ask your partner to turn over.

A truly sensual erotic massage does not begin at or even close to the genitals. The touch is very light, much more so than regular massage. Always be slow and gentle. After tantalizing an area of their body with your sensuous touch, try breathing on the area, then titillating it with your tongue.

Try this sequence. After you do their back—make sure their legs are wide but comfortable—slowly move up the legs and the insides of the thighs. Use the palms on the inner thighs. Now attend to the moons of the buttocks. The heel of the palm is good here. Go tenderly around and between the buttocks on up to the waist as well.

Now have your partner turn over. Starting with the head, move down the face, to the ears and neck, the arms and hands, the navel and the feet. Do not neglect the perineum. After attending to this delicate area, your lover, now warm and melting like a pad of butter left in the hot sun, will be eager to make love to you. At last, you stimulate their genitals as you—and they—please.

These natural hot spots have their own ways of being stimulated so that a sexual type of feeling is experienced. The lips enjoy a light brushing caress with the tips of the fingers or a feather or silk, especially if the eyes are closed.

The ears respond to your warm breath as well as the proverbial rotating tongue. Some like to have their earlobes licked, nibbled and sucked on.

The nape of the neck, of women especially, is an erotic zone. It responds to licking, kissing and blowing.

The middle of the palm responds when a middle finger is pressed into it and rotated in little circles. The outer edge of the little finger tingles with sucking, licking or caressing.

There are many ways to stimulate the nipples, including nibbling and licking. Another approach is to caress the nipple with the thumb while the nipple is held between the first two fingers. Tender tugging is usually appealing.

Many enjoy being rubbed on their stomach. Moving the fingers in a clockwise circle is best. The navel responds to a tongue inside, going in small circles.

The base of the spine enjoys being warmed by the hand rubbing in circles.

The buttocks, thighs, groin and feet respond to a variety of massage techniques as well as tickling and rubbing. And don't forget Big Toe Fellatio, which all by itself has been known to take some lovers to orgasm.

EXTENDED FOR PLAY

Your biggest and most important sex organ is your brain. Lovemaking usually begins in your mind long before the clothes come off and the physical act takes place. Your imagination plays a major role in creating what you will experience. The physical act is partly a performance of the movies that play in your mind. This is why people can become so aroused via fantasy. The mind is a powerful tool that can work for you or against you.

The very meaning of "foreplay" can be redefined and expanded. Your pattern may be to go out for dinner or a movie, return home and eventually get into bed. Reframe this entire experience and call the entire time you spend together your foreplay. How you touch his or her hand, the tone of your voice, your choice of food, are now seen as forms of "foreplay," that is, play before intercourse.

You may find that you can, even in social situations, build a bridge of affection and intimacy between you by touching each other more often and more sensitively. When touch is intentional, as a chosen expression of positive warm regard or similar expansive feelings, its power is greatly increased. The effect on the recipient is not only obvious but beautiful.

Indeed, scientific claims have been made for the healing power of touch. While the power of touch has been used by Don Juans and femme fatales to manipulate others, these tragic travesties of genuine erotic love only prove the lasting value of skillful tactile communication.

By reframing and expanding your concept of foreplay, you will make better use of your "social intercourse," which relies heavily on words, as a preparation for sexual intercourse, which is chiefly non-verbal. As your understanding of foreplay/for play is expanded and refined, you may arrive at the conclusion that even one brief thought about your consort is a kind of foreplay or afterplay.

This fact can be put to advantage. One way to virtually guarantee a memorable lovemaking session is to delay satisfaction and build up anticipation. Elevate the natural strategy of teasing and tantalization to a new level of effectiveness. Spend one to seven days flirting with each other but don't allow sexual orgasmic release. Then, at the day and time you chose in advance, make love with wild abandon. Set aside plenty of time. Add to the special flavor of the occasion by enhancing your boudoir in new ways.

You can also build up anticipation by spending a few minutes each day visualizing your successful union. You may want to have romantic dinners, give gifts or dance together for the purpose of blending your energies in a graceful way. The more you put into it, the more you will probably get out of it.

The totality of foreplay as it usually occurs breaks down like this. Imagine in your mind that you are going to be meeting your consort after an absence. This might be after being at work, the first date, whatever appeals to you. First, you think about them and about making love to them. Then you see and/or hear them. You make eye and verbal contact. You may touch or smell each other, i.e., shake hands or hug or smell their cologne or perfume. If you begin kissing them, you taste them. Eventually, your encounter may lead to a full embrace. Your encounter may conclude with lovemaking.

This sequence can be observed in an experiment. Set up a time for a meeting at your home. At the chosen time, the consort at home is already in a separate room. They cannot be seen. When the other consort arrives, both remain quiet.

Spend a few minutes in silence, observing your thoughts of anticipation. Now you both make some sounds. Then, a little later, one of you enters the living room. You look at each other from a distance but say nothing. You experience this for a few minutes.

Eventually, you make eye contact, and experience this fully also. Then you make verbal contact, tactile contact and so on, pausing after each step in order to fully experience each stage of increased physical intimacy. Make an effort not only to stay in the present but to focus on that sense alone.

Concluding the experiment in sexual intercourse is optional. You may find that you no longer want to skim over the early stages, for now they satisfy. Perhaps you delay intercourse for another time.

You can use your psychic ability as well. Instead of focusing on the five senses, rely on your sixth sense to feel and perceive your consort's vitality level, the colors and shape of their energy field, their current mood and basic character.

Stand or sit in the same room about 20 feet from each other. Relax and open up to your partner. Stretch your sensitivity out to them, as if you are touching them with your mind or energy field. After doing this for several minutes, move in closer so that you are 10 feet away.

Continue to move progressively closer, stopping each time to tune in, until you are actually making physical contact. For some couples, this is a very powerful process and leads to a deep sense of connectedness and gratitude.

GOOD TIMES The best time to make love is when you are feeling calm, relaxed and full of energy. Be in neutral gear emotionally. This contradicts what today's romantic novels, movies and songs tell us. But you will notice that the supersexed heros and heroines depicted in these products argue violently, seesaw from one emotional extreme to another and live in a world of deception, anger, confusion and unhappiness. Such characters, real or imagined, are too preoccupied with their personal dramas to understand the subtleties and benefits of good sexual timing.

People think long and hard about when to buy a house, get married, change jobs or even go to the store. Surely it makes sense to consider when to make love as well.

Some couples are in the habit of arguing bitterly, then making up by making love. This is not a good idea. Wait until your system is completely calmed down before making love after an argument. Otherwise, you will only feed the negative cycle you have fallen into. According to ancient Chinese medicine, you may damage your heart, kidneys or liver by doing this repeatedly.

In fact, the Taoist sex experts advised against making love when either of you are extremely happy, depressed, angry or tired. Extremes of emotion were simply not thought to be healthy. Balance should be achieved as quickly as possible. Then, with the mind clear, a smart decision is easily made as to whether or not this is a good time to make love.

The Taoist sex experts believed that times of natural disturbance were bad times for lovemaking. This includes eclipses, heavy sunspots, earthquakes, tornadoes and fierce thunderstorms. Since it is now known that the electromagnetic field of the earth can be disturbed at such times, this theory may have some scientific foundation.

Matching biorhythms is a useful strategy. You may find that you are more responsive when the emotional (sensitivity) biorhythm cycle is at a peak or valley. The less frequent double and triple peaks and valleys may point to special times of even deeper response.

Astrological timing is also a valuable tool. The simplest guideline is to make love on the day or night of the full moon. Astrologically speaking, a solar or lunar eclipse is a powerful energy moment and may represent a good time for ritual lovemaking or some other sexual power awakening event. The summer and winter solstice (June 22 and December 22) are recommended because of the huge influxes of energy that occur at these times.

With very little effort, you can learn enough astrology to take advantage of many other heavenly opportunities. These include the moving Jupiter or Venus in the sky conjunct your natal Moon, Venus or Mars. A contact from one of these benefics usually results in a beautiful, uplifting experience. Square aspects release lots of energy and generally stimulate action, but they are harder to work with.

Contacts of the slower moving outer planets tend to last longer, whereas Sun and Mars contacts will be more short-term. Briefest of all are the aspects from the Moon, which can be timed to the minute. The advantage here is that the Moon offers special sexual timing opportunities almost daily because it goes around your entire chart in about two and a half days.

According to ancient Hindu sexual traditions, the best times are between 7 p.m. and 12 midnight, and again between 12 midnight and 2 a.m. The fifth or eighth day after her menstrual period ends is recommended. The eighth or fourteenth days of the dark of the moon are also suggested.

Another good time is when she is menstruating. She will be more sensitive and sexual activity, especially with genital orgasm, may help relieve menstrual tensions. Use woman above postures so that the blood is able to continue flowing freely.

ORIENTAL Although no part of the world has a monopoly on subtle
AROUSAL arousal techniques, the Oriental sexologists suggest unusual
points and ways of stimulation based on acupressure insights. Some of these points are not effective until after your
lover is aroused. Other points require sensitive methodical
stimulation for a much longer time than the rapid pace of
strictly genital-oriented sex allows.

Actually, the entire bodymind from toe to top is one
unified erotic zone. This is the undeniable feeling when
erotic arousal is experienced directly without the usual cul-
tural programming and limiting preconceptions. Erotic zone
boundaries exist mainly in the mind.

On the other hand, this is not a standard of arousability
against which you need to measure yourself. Everybody has
a different pattern of physical sensitivity. What is very arousing for you may do nothing for someone else and vice versa.

Have a good time discovering the individualized hot
spots of your bodyminds. Whole-body massage, erotic or
relaxing, is a great way to find these spots.

Oriental sexology stresses the value of personal cleanliness. The anus, for example, is a fabulously erotic locale—
but only when it is completely hygienic. In the Oriental ideal,
a consort should be able to probe, lick, squeeze and rub
every square inch of their companion's flesh without the
slightest concern. The thought that you cannot explore your
consort entirely for hygienic reasons inhibits lovemaking
before it even starts (see *Pleasure, Health And The Anus*).

According to Oriental erotology, the upper and lower
lips are connected differently in the man and woman. The
upper lip of the female is linked with her clitoris. The lower
lip of the male is linked with his penis. Keep this in mind the
next time you kiss.

On at least one occasion take two hours to explore these
secondary erotic areas before connecting genitals. You will
probably discover that you are naturally a great sexual artist.

These areas described below can be stimulated during
"for play" or while giving a massage. You will find them
illustrated in *Aculoving*.

If no specific instructions are given for an area, then we
suggest this subtle yet sensational sequence taken from the
Tantric repertoire: kiss, lick, blow, caress, nibble.

○ *Ankles:* caress and nibble
○ *Anus:* penetrate with finger at peak of genital orgasm
○ *Armpits:* gently bite or insert penis here
○ *Breasts (valley between)*

o   *Buttocks (including valley):* probe deeply
o   *Earlobes:* tug, bite, chew or suck
o   *Elbows (hollow behind)*
o   *Eyelids:* gently brush with fingertips or tongue
o   *Finger tips*
o   *Forearms (hollow behind)*
o   *Forehead (between eyebrows):* gently rub or lick
o   *Head:* rub scalp vigorously, hands curled into claws, with tips of fingers
o   *Hindu sequence:* repeated stimulation of female nose tip, armpits and navel in order before moving to genitals
o   *Incense heater:* move stick of lit incense up centerline of front of body two fingers width distance away
o   *Kidneys:* rub area vigorously with palms of hands, move palms all the way of spine on both sides and repeat several times
o   *Knees (hollow behind)*
o   *Lip (just under lower):* press hard for count of three to increase lip sensitivity
o   *Lips (both):* he gently chews her upper lip as she chews his lower lip
o   *Nasal kiss:* faces close, inhale each other's exhalation through nose (rub noses for extra thrill)
o   *Navel:* circle around navel with flat of palm
o   *Neck (back of):* long deep sniffs or breathe on from deep in throat
o   *Nipple tips:* freely stimulate tips manually and orally, including breathing on them, without any stimulation to rest of breasts
o   *Nose tips:* nibble and bite gently or rub noses together
o   *Palms (center and mound):* rotate and circle middle finger
o   *Penis tip:* man squeezes just before going in vagina to delay ejaculation
o   *Perineum*
o   *Pubis (mound, hair line and just above)*
o   *Roof of the mouth (hard palate):* use tip of tongue
o   *Sacrum*
o   *Shoulders (at bony part where arms are joined):* bite
o   *Soles of the feet*
o   *Spine (along either side):* rub and knead
o   *Tailbone (coccyx):* rub gently and repeat until warm
o   *Thumbs and little fingers:* alternate biting tips or otherwise stimulate together
o   *Thighs (upper inner)*
o   *Toes (big and little)*

SOLAR PLEXUS PEACE
opposite

PAIR BONDING AND TUNING

Each of us has his or her own unique and very personalized vibration. Every one of us "feels" different from every other person.

This vibration is often felt without even trying. You may not realize this is what you are tuning into. It may all be subconscious. Yet think about how often you make important decisions about other people based on these "feelings."

This vibrational factor takes on real importance when choosing a consort to make love to or live with. Can you tune into someone else and get behind their personality mask? Can you harmonize and strengthen your bond when it seems to be weakening? Can you deepen your bond when it is already secure?

Yes, you can do all this and much more, with little effort.

We have tried many techniques for tuning into each other's vibrations. Those included here worked the best for us. They do not rely on some far out theory to be effective. They directly enhance the feeling of being bonded and being in harmony with each other. They are very powerful.

These can be done with clothes on or off. Do them apart from lovemaking as well as just before making love. Some people refuse to do them because the reward seems too subtle, at least at first. This is understandable, but love can be rather subtle. Perhaps it is in the willingness itself to share little celebrations of closeness such as these that "true love" distinguishes itself. Nevertheless, couples in our workshops have reported remarkable results with these same simple techniques.

The state of "being in love" is glorified and imitated in

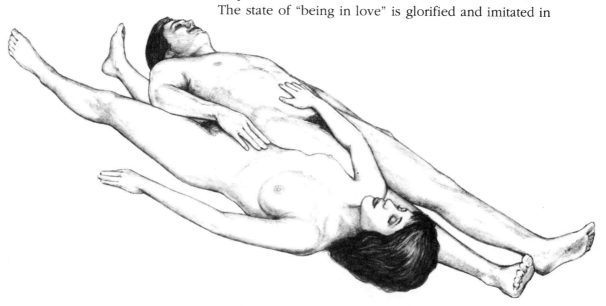

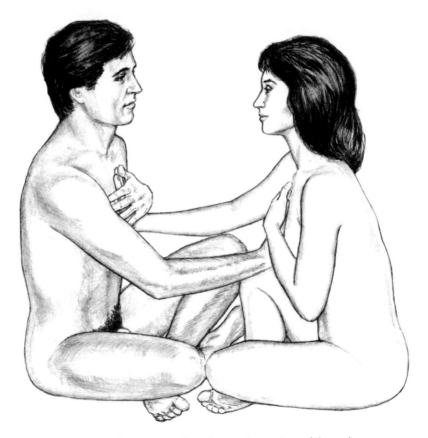

our society. The pop and rock music stations blare the message that "being in love" is the most exhilarating state of mind possible. With these techniques you can create and share this state of mind whenever you want to.

When "in love," it is natural to gaze deeply into each other's eyes, to hold hands as if never to let go, to hold each other close for hours, to sit together in silence, content just with the feeling of closeness. Yet for every couple, apparently, the initial magnetic merger of bodies and minds that is a natural high comes to an end, for some much more quickly than for others.

By gazing and holding and adoring any object, you can fall in love with it again and again. You are focusing your emotional energy. You are creating a powerful bond. You can do this with animals, seashells, flowers, rocks (remember "the Pet Rock"?) and, of course, people.

Triple Tuner   The Triple Tuner consists of the Solar Plexus Peace, Heart To Pulse (or Heart To Heart) and One Eye Love. This is the preferred order in which to do them. Performed in this order,

HEART TO HEART
opposite

ONE EYE LOVE
below

these exercises naturally and gently bring the energy up. In other words, you will first enjoy instinctive feeling (the solar plexus), then emotional feeling (the heart) and finally inspirational feeling (the head).

Allow at least 20 minutes for the Triple Tuner series. For some people, it is a good idea to bring the energy back down to the belly after an exercise like this (see *Ground And Store Energy* and *Hara*). For others, feeling the energy rise in this easy way will be a novel pleasure they want to stay with for awhile.

Solar Plexus Peace is as easy as it looks. As you relax, use your hand to tune into your consort's breathing. Feel their abdomen rise and fall. You may find that your breathing patterns naturally entrain.

This process is an easy way to sense the energy in your consort's body. You may also become aware of stress that they are holding. The chief benefit, though, is that you naturally and effortlessly become relaxed and aligned with each other. As simple as it seems, five to ten minutes of Solar Plexus Peace can transport you into the frame of mind ideal

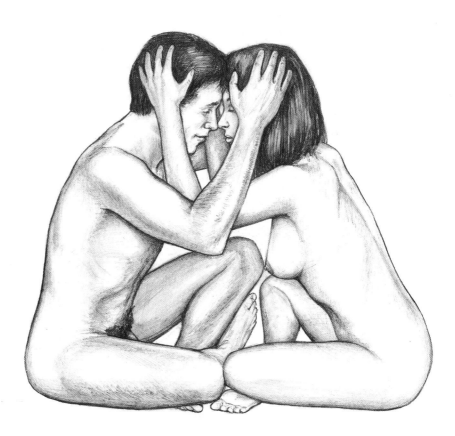

for lovemaking and just plain having fun together. Harmony is a natural by-product of this exercise.

In the Heart To Heart exercise you sit across from each other. To do the Heart To Heart, extend your right arm and place your right palm on the *Love Spot* of your consort. Place your left palm over the back of their right hand which is gently resting on your chest.

In the Heart To Pulse version, place your left hand over your own *Love Spot* and your right hand on the side of their neck where you can feel their pulse. Some couples like to start with this variation first, as you have the physical pulse to work with, and then go on to the more subtle Heart To Heart.

You can breathe together, make sounds of harmony together or just look into each other's eyes. Strive to feel the other person from your heart. The longer you do one of these exercises, the more you will get out of it.

One Eye Love is ideal for developing telepathic attunement. The forehead, of course, is the location of the third eye. Moisten your finger and apply a small amount of saliva to your consort's forehead. Or you can kiss or lick that area.

Join foreheads gently and close your eyes, seeking a deep rapport with your mind. Alternate co-breathing so that you send energy through the third eye as you breathe out and receive energy there from your consort as you breathe in is a more active possibility.

A fascinating variation, which some will find a bit straining to the eye, is to keep the eyes open and focus at the point between your consort's eyebrows. There, as the images of the two eyes converge into one, you will see the One Eye Love. If this is comfortable for you, it is an extraordinary meditation.

The metaphysical implications are many, should you choose to pursue them. This is a classic sex meditation technique in Tantric sex yoga, performed with the couple locked in the YabYum embrace. In this discipline, One Eye Love may literally be practiced for hours in order to achieve a transcendental state (see *Tantric Ritual Sex*).

Spine Wine   We also recommend doing Spine Wine, so called because of the intoxicating effect it can have. Sit back to back. To make your contact more sensual, try interlocking elbows. The Spine Wine exercise can build up lots of heat energy, which you may feel even when your bodies are separated.

This is a good one for energizing the two of you. You can try it when you both need something to pep you up. Some

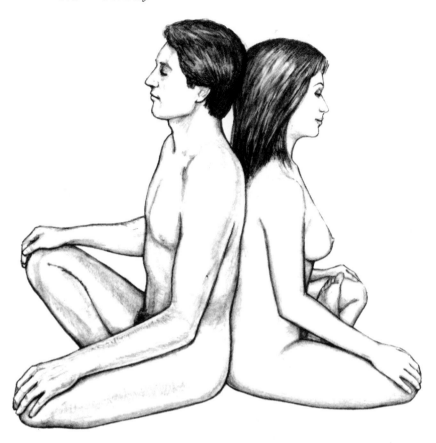

consorts meditate together this way. A good follow-up to the Triple Tuner, it has a grounding effect.

Trespasso   Trespasso is a very old exercise which gets its name from the fact that sustained eye contact is a trespass into the other person's identity. Take off any glasses or take out contact lenses. Take a few minutes to relax first. Imagine that your eyes are becoming soft like jelly.

Then, sitting across from one another gently stare into each other's eyes or at the center of your consort's forehead for at least five or ten minutes. Some report that looking in the partner's left eye deepens the opening and makes the exercise easier. To experience the full impact of this powerful technique, gaze into each other's eyes for a full half hour before making love.

Fingertip Om   An easy variation of Trespasso that most people in our workshops find more entertaining—and less threatening—is Fingertip Om. Sitting so that your fingers just touch, gaze into each other's left eye and chant "Om" (or another opening sound such as "Yum"). Focus on the delicate sensations at your fingertips as well as gazing into your partner's eye. You will find this increases your awareness of subtle body sensations, making you more sensitive to the subtle energies that surround and flow between you.

Making Love With Energy

Sometimes it is very difficult trying to make heart-felt contact during sexual intercourse. You may feel like you are groping for a handle, a contact but everything slips out of your hands.

One of the chief advantages of these techniques is that they are actually diluted intercourse, sex without the genital bonding. Sexual intercourse is a matter of degree and of physical convenience. Naked with genitals united isn't the only way to make love.

David made love in energy fashion to a woman friend while standing fully clothed on a quiet moonlit street corner. They never did kiss or fondle an erotic zone. The energy of their polarity was enough to lift them into ecstasy. Genital intercourse would have been a letdown compared to the blissful energy climax they shared, lasting into the next day.

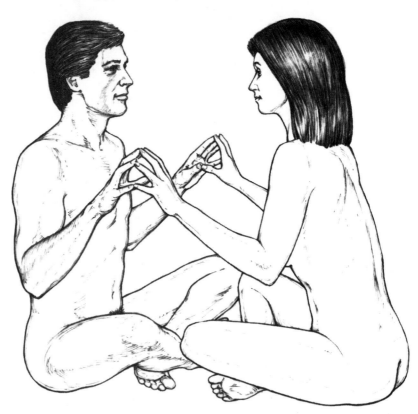

We would like to thank California psychic Betty Bethards for the solar plexus exercise. The heart and head exercises are taught in the Sufi spiritual tradition. *Tantric Sex* by E.J. Gold and Cybele Gold offers many other fine couple attunement techniques.

PLEASURING THE LINGAM

Lingam is Sanskrit for penis. We like to use this more exotic and sensitive sounding word here to emphasize the noble mystery that surrounds this sacred jewel of love. In India, the firmly enlightened consciousness of Shiva, the god of Tantra, is symbolized by ancient, sacred, abstractly phallic stones called *Shiva Lingams*.

If AIDS is a concern, we recommend that you study the books listed in *Safer Sex* and call the information numbers in the *Appendix*. New information is always becoming available. Please do your research.

Giving A Man Pleasure

There is, perhaps, no greater thrill for the man than to see his consort loving and adoring his lingam with enthusiasm. An innocent, bright-eyed, worshipful yet playful attitude can make up for any lack of technique. The truth, plain and simple, is that men don't just want their lingam sucked on, they want it worshipped! This psychic blending of love, devotion and ecstasy is perhaps the greatest aphrodisiac of all for a man.

A major complaint of men in a recent study was that women didn't perform fellatio often enough. Other surveys revealed that fellatio is what men most often say is lacking in the sex lives with their wives. It is the most popular service performed by prostitutes.

In spite of its mystique, the "69" position is not optimal for stimulating the male. The angle of the lingam is wrong for her mouth and the most sensitive areas are facing away. Neither partner is free to focus on just giving or receiving.

Whether he is sitting or lying down, it is optimal for you to be face to face with him. Then the most sensitive areas of the lingam, the tip, the frenulum, the crown or glans, and the corona, the ring around the crown and the notch beneath it, are all presented to you (see illustration on page 181).

A reliable position is facing your man in the classic "jade flute" position, your fingers poised around his shaft as if to play it like a musical instrument. However, as we play the flute horizontally, the position should perhaps be renamed the "jade recorder."

FINGERTIP OM
opposite

A widespread observation is that women are too delicate in their approach. As women generally prefer a much lighter touch on their own genitals, they are perhaps stimulating the man the way they would like it.

Washing the lingam before oral sex can be performed by you as a sensual act. Mildly scented liquid soap, such as Dr. Bronner's, works nicely for this. Or he can take a shower first, favoring the genital and anal areas. We love taking showers or baths together and washing each other which can, but certainly doesn't have to, invite erotic play.

Do everything very slowly. Generally, anything when done with rhythm feels better. Lick your lips to moisten them before you begin.

Depending on the natural fullness of your lips, you may need to tighten the lips around your teeth so you don't accidentally bite him in the wrong place. While men generally like their lingam pleasured quite firmly, it is possible to cause him serious pain by biting his corona hard when he is erect.

Main Course

Position yourself so that you are facing him. Start by massaging his inner thighs. Stroke up his inner thigh through the crease of the thighs and then down the top of his thighs. You can reverse the direction of your hands, too. Kiss and lick the upper thighs.

Pull on the scrotum, putting his balls in your mouth. Pull down with the mouth, as you did with your hand. When you pull the balls down, be gentle. Avoid pulling on pubic hairs. Kiss all around the genital area.

Begin stroking the lingam from the head down to the base. Men generally like downward strokes. A good way to make first contact with the lingam is to take your tongue and roll it around the corona. Look up at his face to see how he is enjoying it.

Some men will want lubrication. A little saliva on your index finger may be enough. If you are mixing oral and manual stimulation, use the sensual jojoba oil or a vegetable oil, something you won't mind tasting in your mouth. For a long session, the Brauers' recommend unscented Albolene, an oil-based makeup cleanser available at your drugstore or a cosmetic supply house.

Circle the lubricated finger around the corona, then follow with the tongue. Now work your tongue gently down his shaft, gently licking with the tip. Gently breath out to tantilize him and work your tongue down from the top, down the shaft and back up. Tenderly flick your tongue in and around the corona and top as if you are quickly licking the edge of an ice cream cone. This usually brings him a tantalizing thrill.

Now you can do a series of fast licks starting at the corona and going up, again like licking an ice cream cone. Tease and blow some more.

Take a break from stimulating the corona and play the flute or piano keys on the shaft. Place one or both hands below the corona—they must stay down below the corona— and do quick little squeezes down with one hand. Alternate with a sliding squeeze that finishes with pulling his balls down a little.

Intersperse massaging the balls and pulling them down a little. Return to feather strokes with the hands on the shaft, only do them more quickly, while your tongue twirls around the corona. This feather stroke can continue on down over and past his balls, flowing onto his thighs. Do an occasional hard suck from the corona up.

Another tactic is to twirl your tongue around his corona, then firmly surround the corona with your lips and work your tongue up in a spiral. Your tongue moves with plenty of force along the side and up and down, perhaps twirling around the entire head of the lingam.

Now for the deep suck made famous by the movie *Deep Throat*. Go very gradually, teasingly. Take at least a minute to take him all the way down in. Move your tongue around while you go down if you can, although this usually takes some practice. When you get him all the way down, create suction by sucking in the side of your cheeks. Relax the back of your throat as much as possible. Give the lingam several good hard sucks. To release the suction, open your mouth.

At this point, he is probably very hard and aroused. Just stay there, your mouth encompassing his lingam. The warm wetness of your mouth is very pleasant to him. However, if he is in so deep that it is uncomfortable for you, release the lingam a bit, leaving some of it still in your mouth.

Now go below the corona (remember, never bite the corona!) and gently nibble your way down the shaft. Your lips should be pulled away from your teeth. All these move-ments are from the corona going down the shift. If you are coordinated enough, you can tease with the tongue at the same time. Otherwise, just keep the tongue flat against the lingam. He may also enjoy the pressure of the roof of your mouth against the crown.

When he is very erect and in deep, you will need to relax the muscles at the back of the throat. You can practice on a dildo or a thick, room temperature cucumber. A good trick

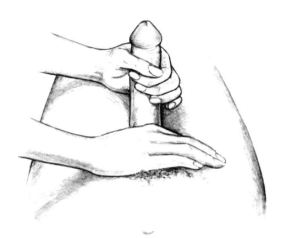

when he is not in too deep is to keep on swallowing. He will find this arousing and you will be able to keep him deep.

While the head quickly bobbing up and down mechanically is not usually preferred—to each man his own—a slow, sucking movement is. Using your mouth like a vacuum cleaner, suck his lingam in about halfway. Then gradually let it slip out of your mouth, strongly sucking as you go up. This is a good way to give him a firmer erection.

Here are some hand movements you can do once he's aroused. They do require oil, preferably of the edible kind. Keep the fingers together and using the palms and back of the fingers, try a twisting or rolling movement. Using both hands, create a rhythmic pressure that twists or rolls the lingam just slightly, then release.

Another stroke to use with oil is to make OK signs with your fingers. Starting at the top, pull the circle down over the corona down to the base, followed by the other hand.

Play the flute with the pads of your fingers. Only this time, roll your fingers at the base in a rhythm (almost like drumming fingers on table) from index finger to little finger.

When his lingam is completely aroused, he will usually prefer full strokes down, like the OK stroke, rather than teasing. In fact, at that point it will probably be pleasurable for him if you just put both hands around his lingam and hold on firmly for awhile. Look at his eyes and facial expression as men vary in how firm they want it and women tend not to be firm enough.

When he is ejaculating, a man seems to prefer that you have him as deep in your mouth as possible, since he is shrinking as he is ejaculating. Flick your tongue back and forth at the tip to make it more arousing. If your hand is well

THE OK STROKE *above*
The tendency to play with his lingam like a toy is almost irresistible.

MOUTH MAGIC *opposite*
Enthusiasm is the most effective aphrodisiac.

lubricated, he may like for you to rub on the shaft as he comes. Friction on his frenulum during orgasm may also appeal to him.

A point for him to remember is to not move his lingam around vigorously when he is in your mouth. This only makes your task more difficult and could cause pain to either or both of you. Medium and hard thrusting is best reserved for intercourse.

The taste of his semen varies with his diet. Many women report that if a man drinks alcohol or coffee, they can taste it. The semen of a vegetarian is said to taste the sweetest. If she can keep the back of her mouth open, she doesn't have to taste it as then it will not go over the tongue. However, since ejaculate is 70 to 100 calories, you may not want to swallow it if you are on a diet!

If you choose not to swallow the ejaculate, we recommend keeping a towel or tissues handy. Be subtle about it, as your partner may take this personally. If your man is very sensitive about this, Xaviera Hollander suggests hiding a towel in or near the bed.

The more aroused a man is, the slower these movements

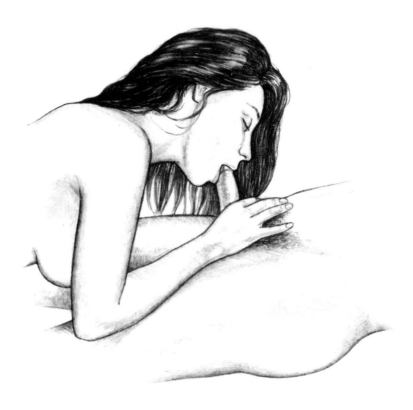

should be performed if ejaculation orgasm is to be delayed. Since the corona or glans is the most sensitive part, when he is very aroused you can do more on the shaft, pull on the balls and so on. It is usually pleasant and relaxing for a man to be stimulated in the area around his lingam, scrotum and perineum.

Gently pulling down (but not squeezing) on the scrotum once the man is fully aroused feels good and delays orgasm as well. A vibrator can also be quite thrilling behind the scrotum on the perineal area.

Other games to play with his lingam include giving it a name, wrapping your hair around it, and playing guess the caress, where you use different stimuli (fake fur mittens, silk, feather, oil) while he, eyes closed, tries to guess what you're doing. It may be easy for him to figure out what you are using but the game puts him more in touch with his sensations. Whipped cream and honey a la lingam makes for a pleasant mutual treat. Our *Spreading* technique also works nicely.

A successful strategy for safer sex is to add a drop or two of water-based lubricant to the lingam and slip a condom over it. Then stimulate his lingam by moving the condom up, down and around. Since lubricant inside the condom clearly makes for a slippery situation, discard that condom and dry the lingam off if you want to shift to intercourse. Start intercourse with a new condom lubricated on the outside (see *Safer Sex*).

Pleasuring His Prostate   The prostate is the equivalent of the woman's G spot. It can be approached indirectly by pressing on the Prostate Point in the middle of the perineum between the scrotum and the anus. Or, it can be approached directly through the anus.

Once he is aroused, tell him you want to locate his Prostate Point. Press at different points near the middle of the area between the scrotum and anus and ask him how it feels. Also ask him how different degrees of pressure feel. You may find that there is a certain spot that is just right. Make a mental note of this point.

If he is very aroused, you may be surprised at how hard you can push on this point and still have him tell you to push even harder for his enjoyment. Press firmly with the tips of your fingers or thumb. Your fingernails will need to be short for this technique.

Genital and anal cleanliness become especially important when you want to stimulate the prostate gland. If you are going to stimulate him through the anus, it is important

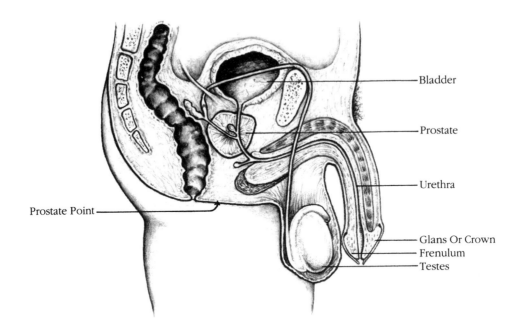

Bladder

Prostate

Urethra

Prostate Point

Glans Or Crown
Frenulum
Testes

that you use a latex surgical glove or finger. A light enema just before is not an unreasonable request. Use plenty of water-based lubricant, such as Astroglide®, and go very slowly (see *Pleasure, Health And The Anus*).

Whether or not stimulation of the prostate gland leads to an exceptional orgasm, as some report, a rhythmic, pulsing pressure applied every now and then through the perineum or directly through the anal canal is not only pleasurable but a reliable way to prolong arousal and delay ejaculation. The relief is quite tangible as the prostate, behaving not too different from a balloon filled with air, relaxes as some of its pent-up fluid is released (see *Voluntary Orgasm For Men*).

The prostate can be stimulated as you stimulate the lingam. Rhythmic pressure on the prostate or external point just before orgasm is reached can lead to the ability to stay on the verge *(OTV)* for many minutes. The Prostate Point can also be stimulated during orgasm to extend it.

A rapid, almost musical rhythmic alternation of prostate and lingam stimulation can lead to a considerable prolongation of orgasm. This is an art form, perhaps, that takes time and practice to develop. His sensitivity to the subtle stages of arousal up to and into climax greatly increases.

The man grows more and more comfortable with the

MALE ANATOMY LESSON
above
Press firmly on the perineum to stimulate the prostate indirectly. He will definitely feel a sensation there. It feels good.

practice when he does his own PC clenches, breathes completely and consciously relaxes his anus.

To facilitate simultaneous stimulation, try hooking the thumb or index finger of one hand around the lingam. Press on the Prostate Point with the free finger(s) or free thumb of that hand while performing a stimulating stroke with the other hand. While we can't predict your man's response, combining prostate and lingam stimulation should lead to some new orgasm experiences for him.

PLEASURING THE YONI

Yoni is Sanskrit for vagina. We prefer to use this more exotic and sensitive sounding word here to emphasize the extraordinary beauty of this sacred flower, symbolized by the rose in the West and the lotus in the East. Yoni not only sounds less clinical, its mellifluous sound adds a touch of poetry to lovemaking.

If AIDS is a concern, we recommend that you study the books listed in *Safer Sex* and call the information numbers in the *Appendix*. New information is always becoming available. Please do your research.

Here is a delightful approach to making oral love to a woman that we learned from the Hindu erotologist Godfrey Anderiesz. It takes into account the Tantric knowledge of a woman's secondary and tertiary erotic zones.

Giving A Woman Pleasure

Eastern erotic mythology compares orally loving a woman, or cunnilingus, to the relationship between the bee and the lotus flower. Due to the exciting provocation of the bee's activities deep in the lotus, the flower eventually climaxes, secreting nectar-like substances of great beauty and nourishing sweetness.

While it is true that cunnilingus seems to consist of kissing, licking, sucking and so forth, there is a logic to the female body as a whole that must be honored. Though a woman generally cannot go wrong with men if she starts at their center of sex stimulation—in other words, if she leaps on his lingam like a hungry tigress—the opposite is true for the woman. To properly arouse most women, it is best to start at the periphery and gradually move in towards the center of the body, leaving the clitoris for last.

For the man, the circle of arousal naturally expands from the center outwards. For the woman, the movement is from the perimeter to the center.

In Taoist sexology, the woman is first aroused by rubbing

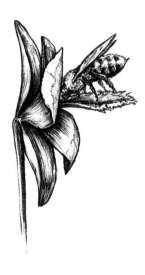

her hands and feet, then gradually massaging her body up her legs and down her arms to her belly and, eventually, her genitals. *Tao Of Sex* masters use their intimate knowledge of acupressure meridians to further intensify foreplay effects.

Our Hindu technique starts with nibbling the tip of her nose. This is based on the ancient yoga teaching of a connection between the tip of the nose and the root chakra at the base of the spine where the life force energy (Kundalini), responsible for sexual ecstasy, resides. The rest of the approach can likewise be traced to other energy-oriented observations, little-known outside of Eastern erotic lore.

One other point is worth mentioning. In the Hindu way of thinking, the fluids that the woman secretes as she becomes aroused and, especially, as she orgasms, are considered the nectar of the Goddess. These fluids, imbibed orally or absorbed via osmosis through the lingam during intercourse immediately after oral love, are considered highly beneficial to male well-being. The Taoists enthusiastically concur on this point.

For this reason alone, it is advised that you bring her to orgasm as many times as she wishes first. Then she can orally love your lingam or, if you prefer, intercourse can begin immediately. Remember, she may be capable of many more orgasms in your love session than you.

This approach acknowledges the difficulty many women have achieving orgasm during intercourse. Not only is she likely to achieve orgasm through oral love, the chances will then be greater for her to achieve orgasm during intercourse as she is already aroused.

Men like techniques. The male Hindu erotologists also delighted in detailed, step-by-step instructions, as the *Kama Sutra* aptly demonstrates. We encourage you to thoroughly master our system of arousing your woman to ecstasy. Then, after you have seen its value in practice, go on to improvise, allowing the love artist within you to confidently emerge.

While a man can familiarize himself intimately with her anatomy and learn the techniques, it is vital that she still be willing to verbalize her wants. Naturally, there are non-verbal cues, such as when she shifts her position to increase stimulation to an area. Still, she is encouraged to speak freely. It is understood that he is ready to do whatever she asks.

According to Hindu erotology, the approach to a woman should not be random. A random approach leads to a random response. Rhythmic, almost musical stimulation, combined with a gradual build-up, is optimal.

In this Eastern way of oral love, a cyclical current of energy is set up by going from the nose tip to the armpits and breasts to the genitals and back to the tip of the nose. A typical response is a thrilling, tingling sensation, not unlike tickling, that may start her writhing about. Areas that show a marked response can be given more attention next time.

Hindu erotology teaches that her breasts crave stimulation. Only after her breasts have filled with energy and warmed her heart will her lower gateway be fully ready. Then she will not only be warm and wet. Much energy will have gathered there and your union will be deeply fulfilling, not only for her but for you as well. The vibrant overflow of sweet energy from her nectar-filled yoni and lush, melting body then satisfies you to your depths.

To begin with, the genital and anal areas should be clean. The *Koka Shastra,* for example, suggests washing, perfuming and placing honey in the yoni. For this technique, special attention to washing the armpits and anus is also suggested.

A reliable position is for the woman to sit at the edge of the bed, her thighs spread wide. The yoni is open, the clitoris partly exposed. The position is favored also because she can easily see what is happening, in itself a powerful aphrodisiac stimulus. In other positions, mirrors can be placed so that she can still see the action.

Main Course Here is the technique proper. Note that the yoni is the last area to be stimulated. Be gentle but feel free to nibble, suck, kiss, lick, titillate, tease, rub, roll, tug and otherwise arouse and tantalize. A gentle back or foot massage to start things off is usually a welcome way to transition to the relaxed state that is ideal for receiving pleasure.

Begin by nibbling and kissing the tip of her nose. Then move down her front of her body, pausing at her lips, and continue to her upper chest. The traditional advice here is to switch to her armpits, which you stimulate by nibbling and pulling on the hairs with your mouth. However, chances are she shaves there.

During this time, your hands concentrate on her nipples. Her breasts, however, are avoided. They are reserved for intercourse.

Now switch your mouth to her nipples and your hands to her navel. Move your hands in a circle around her navel until you reach her pubic hair.

When her nipples are fully aroused, move your mouth down between her breasts to her navel. As you play with her navel with your tongue, play with her pubic hair and venus mound with your hands. Now move your mouth slowly from her navel to her venus mound and your hands to her inner thighs.

Eventually, move your mouth to the groin area at the line of flesh between her pelvis and thighs. Then kiss and lick all the way down her left inner thigh to the soft hollow behind her knees. Repeat on her right thigh. While you do this, use a feathery touch up and down each leg. Then, when you move your mouth up her leg, take one hand and caress the perineum between anus and yoni.

When your lips are all the way back up the inside of her legs, place a firm, wet kiss suddenly on her whole yoni. This is called "the leap of the tiger." She may jump with excitement. Do not repeat this kiss yet.

Now, with the outer lips of her yoni create a roll of flesh between your fingers and place your mouth there. Your mouth, lips, teeth and tongue active, go from the bottom of her yoni up in the direction of her clitoris. Suck as you nibble.

Let her outer lips go and pat her anus firmly with a finger. Orally stimulate and suck on the lower area of her yoni, using your tongue. Gently chew her outer and inner lips, going back and forth between them. Remember, *never* blow into her yoni.

Her Clitoral Jewel   Now you are ready to worship her clitoral jewel. However, even now, you are not direct. She has been provoked and inflamed, ravished and titillated to this point, but even now you must be subtle.

Place your mouth on her venus mound just where the clitoris begins, gently nibbling there. Eventually, use your tongue or fingers to push the hood back. Pressure on both sides helps to lift her clitoris up and expose it further. Keep one hand in this position until she achieves orgasm.

The best direct stimulation of her clitoris is achieved by fixing the lips around the clitoris as you suck and loll the tongue there. Your other hand excites the vagina, buttocks and inner thighs.

Here is an important point. Once you have planted your mouth firmly, do not move. Stay in place but gradually increase the rate of stimulation.

Pay attention to any action she suggests with her body language and help her intensify the sensations there. According to the *Kama Sutra,* her eyes will shift around to show the next area she wants stimulated in order to take her to orgasm.

Now when she actually begins climaxing, make your oral loving very forceful. You may have to stimulate her clitoris much harder than before.

Now, thrust one hand in her vagina. The erotic sages suggest simultaneously plunging a finger of the other hand in her anus. Obviously, this is a matter of personal taste and hygiene as well as of lubrication.

Even though her orgasm may seem complete, here is an extra treat for her. Continue to orally caress the area from her anus to her yoni up to her venus mound. Many women find this last step one of the most satisfying.

When her yoni is back to its usual size and its mouth closed, then she is ready for your lingam. Timed properly, this leads to yet another orgasm for the woman as her yoni eagerly consumes your lingam.

In general, be sure to stimulate around her clitoris, using the indirect movement of the skin and lips near the clitoris. Once you have assessed her sensitivity, you can pounce on her clitoris with a big, juicy kiss. When selfloving, many women stimulate around and on the clitoris only.

Slowly and gently survey her yoni with your eyes, lips, tongue and fingers. Many women are very, very sensitive in and around the clitoral area as well as the labia and opening of the yoni.

Some women may like a commercial lubricant such as Astroglide®. Others will prefer a dry but clean hand and the natural lubrication from inside their yoni. Most women will want plenty of lubrication. It is better to go overboard with lubrication than to not have enough.

If you are mixing oral and manual stimulation, use sensual jojoba oil or a vegetable oil, something you won't mind tasting in your mouth. For longer sessions, the Brauers' recommend using unscented Albolene, an oil-based makeup cleanser available at your drugstore or a cosmetic supply house.

Many women will feel more comfortable if they have washed themselves just beforehand, although they may like it when you wash them. Use only a mild soap and warm water and a soft sponge or washcloth. Make sure your hands are clean as well.

Manual stimulation is a separate art in itself, and some women, depending on their sensitivity at the time, may find the touch of your hand too heavy. Don't be discouraged.

ORAL WORSHIP *opposite*
Taoist sages praised oral love, claiming her "tide of yin" (orgasm) is good for the man.

Remember, when she stimulates herself her hand is coming from a different direction than yours (unless she uses a vibrator). Since most women prefer a soft touch with move-

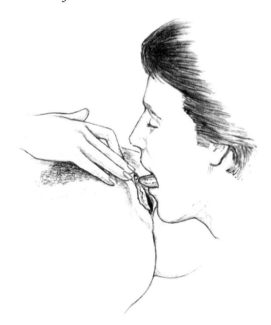

ment from the wrist rather than the finger, you will probably find it necessary to rest your arm on a pillow so that you can both relax.

If you have any difficulty in locating her clitoral bud, go ahead and ask. She will be glad you did. You won't be the first man who had trouble finding a woman's clitoris.

One approach is to recline beside her and rest your arm so that it is very relaxed. Use only the pad of your middle finger, not the fingertip. Let the movement come from your wrist rather than your finger. A soft but firm vibrating motion side to side is usually preferred.

As she becomes more aroused, you can usually feel the bud expand. An even stronger vibration that ranges further to each side may then be preferred.

An alternative is to place your hand so that your thumb is at the root of her clitoris and your fingers are free to rhythmically stroke her clitoral bud. Your other hand is free to play with her yoni and stimulate her G spot. Soft blowing near (but definitely not into the opening of her yoni!) is often pleasurable, especially near her clitoral bud.

Her G Spot   Once she has orgasmed via her clitoris, you can now enter with your hand to stimulate her G spot. You will find it a few inches inside her yoni towards the front. Press down gently with one hand on her pelvis while you stimulate her G spot with the other. This is optimal timing, as the consensus

FEMALE ANATOMY LESSON
opposite
Her clitoris and G spot are
both easy to reach. The
G spot may be easier to
find when she is aroused.

SHE DISPLAYS HER YONI
below
Unique, beautiful and
mysterious, her yoni is
worthy of your adoration.

seems to be that for G spot stimulation to bring deep satisfaction she must be either fully aroused or just have had an
orgasm. Nonetheless, women with sensitive G spots may
prefer direct stimulation with no clitoral prelude.

The G spot is hardly a new discovery. The *Koka Shastra*
calls it *purnachandra,* or "full moon." According to the
Ananga Ranga, it is called *saspanda.* It is described as a
rough area in the yoni inside and towards the navel which,
when stimulated, causes the *kama salila,* or "juice of love,"
to flow abundantly. Friction to this area, the author notes,
leads to an intense orgasm characterized by convulsions.

To easily locate her G spot, place your middle finger
inside her yoni palm towards you, facing front. Slowly move
the tip of your finger to and fro, towards and away from
yourself. Her G spot will feel a little rougher than the surrounding flesh. Once it is stimulated, it may feel to her like
she has to urinate. This is perfectly natural.

Probably the best stroke is a soft, smooth, rhythmic
motion. Steadily move your index and middle fingers up and
back as well as in and out. Do this for at least five minutes or
until she experiences the deeper, stronger G spot orgasm.

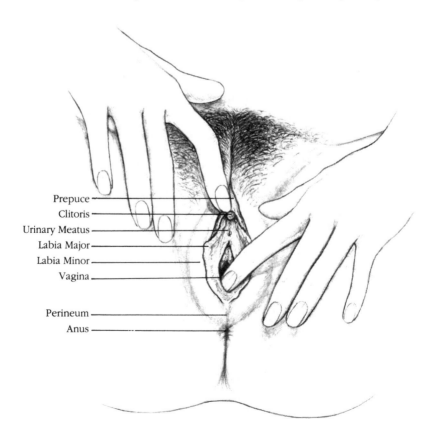

Prepuce
Clitoris
Urinary Meatus
Labia Major
Labia Minor
Vagina

Perineum
Anus

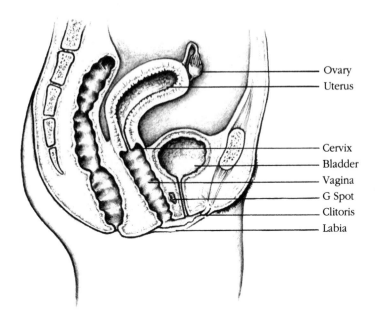

Ovary
Uterus

Cervix
Bladder
Vagina
G Spot
Clitoris
Labia

The *Kama Sutra* suggests stimulating the G spot with the middle and third fingers (the index finger being considered too heavy), moving them in and out of the yoni "like the trunk of an elephant."

According to Native American teacher Harley Swiftdeer Reagan, all orgasms are clitoral. But in the G spot or so-called "vaginal" orgasm, the sexual "serpent" (which has as its head the clitoris) reaches back and bites its own tail, the G spot. Then a more intense, longer lasting "fire" orgasm occurs. This kind of orgasm is said to awaken Kundalini.

Certain dildos and vibrators are shaped and curved to touch this spot. Some are even designed for simultaneous clitoral stimulation. Far from being a threat to sexual intimacy, these devices begin to make a lot of sense after several long manual sessions. Let technology lend a hand—literally.

Some women find that a rhythmic, musical stimulation going back and forth between clitoral bud and G spot extends orgasm, either in the form of a lasting plateau of pleasure or multiple climaxes. At any rate, do experiment and encourage her to tell you exactly what she likes.

Teasing Teasing is not a technique per se, for it is natural to erotic play. Nonetheless, you as a man need to know that when she says she wants you inside her, she still may not be *really* ready for you.

There is an important difference between a yoni that is wet enough or open enough to allow a lingam inside and a yoni that is on fire with the desire to consume your lingam. That difference may lead to a satisfied woman who is eager to pleasure you back or . . . ?

Make sure her oven is warm enough before you serve the main course to her. Like most worthwhile things in life, this takes time.

A typical scenario might go like this. You have been stimulating her clitoris for awhile. "Please come inside me," she says. "I want you." Don't you believe it!

Keep on stimulating. Seconds or minutes later, you hear "Oh, honey, what are you waiting for? I want you. Why are you teasing me like this?" Not yet.

Sooner or later, though, her tone changes. Desire has now taken her over completely. "Oh God, I want you! Now! Why are you torturing me?"

She may start pushing your hand away from her clitoris. Grabbing wildly for your eager lingam, half-blinded by bliss, moaning like a monsoon, she is now a woman who is *ready*. Now is the time to place the holy jewel in the sacred lotus.

Of course, every woman is different. Maybe she is a non-stop talker. Maybe she is very quiet and lies in bed like a sleeping princess, gentle quivers the only sign of her tumultuous inner pleasures. Or maybe she screams and bites if you delay her pleasure too long!

Gently tease your woman to her outer limit. Learn to read her signs. Be able to know for certain when she is *really* ready.

It is a great joy to open the door of ecstasy for her. Who said chivalry is dead?

If she wants to orgasm on her own first, that is good, too. Unlike a man, her orgasm capacity is virtually unlimited. She can rise to higher and higher planes of ecstasy as orgasms pile up like so many silky clouds in a sky of rainbows. If she is a "big bang" woman, then her one orgasmic blast will usually be enough.

Tease her into ecstatic madness. She will return the favor. Then you will see what sort of stuff you are made of. How much ecstasy can *you* take?

If He Needs Her Help   The man may be uncomfortable with orally loving her yoni because he tried it with a woman who had a strong smell and hadn't washed and cleaned, if not perfumed, her yoni in advance. But he may have difficulty expressing this concern about hygiene as it seems unmanly.

Another common issue is that the man may feel inadequate. After all, where does a man learn about this? Who will teach him?

As much as he wants to please and pleasure her, he does not want to fail. If he has doubts about his ability, he will probably tend to avoid cunnilingus even though, secretly, he would be thrilled to pleasure his woman that way.

Here is where she can take the initiative. Most likely it is not a personal thing. It is hard for a woman to understand just how important it is to a man to be a success, to be an expert in lovemaking.

The only way to get good at anything is to practice. Reduce the performance stress by approaching it as play. Let go of the orgasm as goal orientation and approach it as a shared adventure (see *Educe Each Other*).

Orgasm Bond   Modern research confirms that many women don't orgasm during intercourse. When the man has learned to pleasure the woman to orgasm orally and manually, he can arouse her in advance, increasing the likelihood.

If she doesn't orgasm, then he can satisfy her afterwards. He will feel more confident because he knows he has many ways to satiate her and be her special lover.

A great way to develop direct, open communication is to watch each other selfloving. Try this one at a time. Close your eyes while you stimulate yourself, at least at first, as this may help you relax.

The first time you demonstrate we recommend that your partner watch silently. Later you can have sessions where your partner asks specific questions about what you find pleasurable and arousing, including what you are seeing in your mind's eye, what you may be saying to yourself and the feelings you are having in your body (see *Total Orgasm*). Naturally, you can do mutual selfloving, too.

SPREADING   Spreading is a technique that Ellen developed to help spread energy from the genitals to the rest of the body. It is a fun way to relax and get energized at the same time. It is also good training for all the Sexual Energy Ecstasy lovestyles (see *Nights Of Tantra*). Spreading practice helps you hold bigger and better sexual energy charges, enhancing your lovemaking in any style, hard or soft.

The main advantage of Spreading is that you are free to focus completely on spreading your sexual energy and feel-

SPREADING *below*
More than massage, it is the basic training for discovering how to relax and stay with high intensity ecstasy.

ing the enlivening arousal throughout your entire body. You don't have to perform or exert effort or succeed. For some consorts, this experience of total yet relaxed arousal is felt as an ecstatic expansion of the energy field around the body.

If you are the physically passive partner, you are internally active. Sense, feel, breathe, direct, imagine, send the sex energy. Gently encourage it to move from the genital locale to other parts of your body.

It is especially easy to work with your *Energy Centers* in this way. Spread the energy to the solar plexus, heart, throat, third eye and crown of your head. Then, eventually, the energy is brought down in reverse order and grounded in the center deep in the body below the navel or out the soles of the feet (see *Hara, Ground And Store Energy*).

Remember to breathe deeply and completely throughout the exercise. Unconscious breath holding is very common and the active partner can point this out when it happens. Gently return to your complete breathing.

In fact, if a certain part of your body is in need of healing or is starving for energy, direct some surplus to that area. Naturally, this very same skill can be applied during inter-

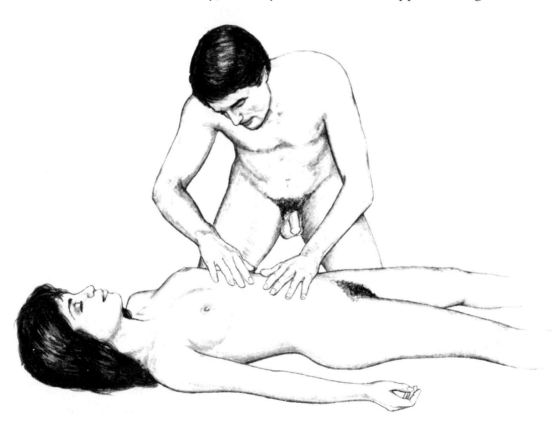

course for personal and interpersonal healing. The results may surprise you.

Going Both Ways   Partner A is active. Partner B is passive. B lies down with his or her back on the bed, genitals exposed.

Motionless, B relaxes as much as possible. To insure maximum relaxation, B's hands are palms up. The arms are at about a 45-degree angle to the trunk. The feet are slightly apart. The toes naturally fall outward. Relax the jaw so that the teeth are separated slightly. This position may be familiar to you from hatha yoga class. It is the *Shavasana* pose for the "final relaxation" (see *Deep Relaxation*).

A stands or kneels on the side of B and smoothly strokes B's body all over. The touch is always gentle. When A's hands leave B's body at the end of the stroke, it is done with a gradual lessening of pressure. This "helicopter" stroke is continued throughout the spreading. The "helicopter" stroke moves the hands half an inch to two inches above the passive partner's body.

A stimulates B's genitals until he or she is clearly aroused, then "spreads" the arousal to the rest of B's body. Concentrate on the genitals for only a minute or so, or even for just a few seconds. The emphasis is on Spreading.

Once B is aroused, A slowly sweeps the hands three to five times down B's legs ending near their feet. A uses a feathery touch and gradually lessens the pressure before leaving B's body briefly but completely.

Next A repeats the spreading stroke, moving up the body from the genitals three to five times.

Do this for 10 to 15 minutes, then switch roles. However, even a few minutes for each partner is valuable.

Once you get the hang of this simple exercise modify it to suit your individual needs. Be sure to include the "helicopter" stroke as you taper off each caress.

Practice Pointers   Sexual activity, especially of the non-orgasm variety, may leave a residue of tension. A similar technique passed on to us at our workshop by a sex surrogate training graduate is effective. Wipe tension off the body upward and downward from the abdomen. You can do this yourself or your consort can do it for you.

In working with the Spreading technique, Santa Barbara therapist Jonathan Robinson has found that some women prefer a different approach when being pleasured. Instead of starting with her genitals, her partner concentrates on stimulating and arousing the rest of her body first. Then the vagina and clitoris are aroused and the energy is spread up the body.

While the Spreading technique proper is based on classical massage, which accounts for some of its startling effectiveness, some couples may find this approach too formal. If so, you are encouraged to simply incorporate it into your lovemaking as a kind of foreplay, kissing, licking and touching to achieve arousal, then doing the Spreading. Even then, the formality of taking turns with partners assuming distinct passive and active roles is highly recommended. If you like, think of it as a game (see *Technology For Lovers*).

Many couples find an informal variation of Spreading quite useful. While stimulating your partner, reach out and touch another part of their body.

As you do this, talk about it, as this helps them focus on the sensations. "Okay, now I'm caressing your chest. Feel the warmth of my hand there. Okay, now my hand is slowly moving down to your belly. Feel the softness of my touch." Arousal can build and build leading to extended orgasms that push you into new frontiers of ecstasy.

The dialog can go the other way, too. For example, if the receiving partner is working to spread arousal up to the solar plexus or third eye, they can tell the active partner to start Spreading right to that spot. Your partner can also rest their hand there or caress or breathe on the target area.

Such intimate teamwork also has the effect of breaking down barriers to the total sharing of emotion and energy during lovemaking. You are learning the art of surrender through the rich poetry of fully sensual touching.

Consciousness raising massage practices like Spreading are a key practice of Tantra. By surrendering to the subtle, vibratory sensations as they occur at the tactile boundaries of the body, the usual sense of being confined to the body melts away (see *Meditation And Tantra*).

Relaxation is the beginning of allowing life to emerge in a natural way, moment by moment. But it is not the end. Hidden within is a blazing glory. When the outer layers of the body are completely pacified, Spreading arousal leads to an awakening of the primal energy of the body.

At whatever level you choose to approach it, Spreading is a delightful, effective way to greatly enhance your ability to receive, enjoy and sustain great amounts of ecstatic energy. It has the added benefit of bringing you close together emotionally. As you relax more and more, you discover what a great joy it is to be, to simply be. Indeed, you discover that the source of all joy is simply being.

Swept
Away

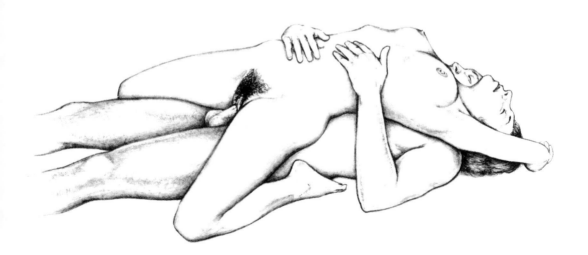

CONSCIOUS
CONFLICT

man and woman is a dream
in essence there is no difference between them
alike they are in fact

still, fire and water
the difference is necessary
to keep the world spinning

conscious conflict
created out of love
in a context of peace
is the secret

of everlasting love
be it for a night
a year
a life

for in all life
variety
is inevitable
and necessary
uninvited
conflict destroys
invited
conflict invigorates

the conflict of fire and water
is a delicious play
that boils away fear, guilt and anger
in the bold honest
heroes of the heart

to open to the opposite
is the only possible path
you are already what you are
your transformation is complete
but you cannot see it
from where you stand

your opposite has eyes
where you have doubts

THE ART OF
EROTIC
AWAKENING

You arouse your consort; you awaken him or her. You rouse their senses from the deep dullness fostered by daily living into vivid expanded vibrating aliveness. You penetrate self-protective layers with your caring life-giving touch. Now he or she is in the present. Now he or she is more able to appreciate and celebrate the gift of life.

Go beyond the conventional notions of "foreplay" and "arousal" completely. Act as if giving the awakening touch is the climax, that genital union does not exist at all. Maximum fulfillment during genital intercourse will result.

Consorts who are gifted in awakening may take hours worshipping and adoring their flesh cosmos. Transported to an ecstatic plane long before genitals are joined, mutual ecstasy during genital intercourse is virtually assured.

Quite a variety of skills are described in this section. You may find some of them very useful. Even so, the most valuable and most authentic lovemaking skill is to feel. This skill, like any other, can be developed.

When the human heart aspires to total wholeness and consumes the entire bodymind, so that the whole bodymind is given over to living love now, even for but a moment, then a touch or glance conveys the entire potency of the erotic promise. In order to make love and not merely to have sex, tender heart-felt caring, identity with the consort or other self-forgetful moods are sustained while moving through the physical act. This can be achieved with practice.

Without deep feeling, without the participation of the heart, the thousand and one techniques of the ancient and modern lovecraft will never lead to total satisfaction. Total satisfaction requires total participation.

Love, or maximum feeling response ability, is the only method. But love is not a method. In order to feel with your whole being, the whole mind, the whole heart, the whole bodymind must be awakened. These skills will help you do just that while you enjoy lighthearted pleasures.

To understand and expand sexual awakening, try this. At a time when you feel sexual desire or arousal and the situation is convenient for contemplation, take 20 minutes to explore the sensations. Place all of your attention in your bodymind there. Then penetrate it, become it, allow it to unfurl like a rose. Contemplate how this emanation of energy is part of the life energy that sustains you and the rest of the universe every day.

If you continue the contemplation long enough, the usual feelings of arousal change. You will feel a tingling and a brightness that spreads through your whole bodymind.

Ironically, one of the best ways to prepare for a profound lovemaking experience is to contemplate or meditate upon the reality of change in general and of physical death in particular. Do this for half an hour or so privately. You will awaken to the preciousness of this moment and of your consort. Making love in the here and now, you may experience a sense of beauty and wonder that can only be described as miraculous.

CO-INSPIRATION   Inspiration is a beautiful word that means both the act of breathing in and the act of enlivening and uplifting. Co-inspiration is the act of enlivening and uplifting each other by breathing in each other's vitality and personality, as well as relaxing and energizing your own bodymind in the process.

Have you tried breathing together during lovemaking? It may happen to you spontaneously. Rhythmic deep breathing together as you are approaching climax can help create a truly mind-blowing experience. Rhythmic deep breathing together at any stage of intercourse will intensify the feelings and energy level.

You do not have to be in motion, though. During a *Full Stop* you can co-inspire each other.

Breathing is a beautiful way to communicate nonverbally. Breathing together is an adventure in itself. Generally speaking, fast breathing is associated with excitedness and slow breathing is associated with calmness. Breathe according to the effect you want to have on each other.

People talk about flowing together or being in rhythm. There is no better way to do this than with the breath. However, this does not have to be a rigid one-two one-two. By giving yourselves an opportunity to fall into a rhythm, it can happen automatically.

Logically, two people can breathe together in two ways. Consorts can breathe in and out as one, or they can alternate like two pistons, with one breathing in as the other breathes out and vice versa.

Kegel contractions can be combined with your in or out breaths when genitally united. Concentrate on pulling the anus up and in when you do this. You may want to intentionally hold your inhalations or exhalations together, perhaps in time with music. When you maintain eye contact while breathing together, the effect is intensified.

Facing each other sitting up or lying on your sides you can place yourselves so that your nostrils are side by side. Or you can hold a passionate kiss on the mouth as you breathe in and out the nose together or alternately. Face to face, you feel your consort's warm breath on your skin and you hear them breathe. You are giving each other life energy when you breathe together in this way.

A tranquil alternative is "spoon breathing." Lie on your sides, belly to back.

During a *Full Stop* while making love, hold each other close. Draw the energy up to your crowns and hold for a few seconds. Rolling your eyes up may help. Then release the energy with your exhalation as a gift to your consort.

Knowing something about the subtleties of the breath in lovemaking may come in handy when making love to a new consort. Breath harmonization leads quickly to interpersonal harmony.

You set the breathing pace. If your consort is new to soft style lovemaking, they will pick up your lead without realizing it and soon be comfortable with this approach. If they are breathing too quickly, first match breathing patterns with them. Once you are on their wavelength, you can begin to slow down your breathing rate. They will then follow you into your more serene rhythm.

Just simply being aware of the drama of breathing as it unfolds in your world of two can be quite a treat in itself. Be aware of your breathing as it is for at least several minutes and then go where that takes you. In this way, you will experience the effects of breathing variations firsthand and develop your own ways to co-inspire each other (see *Inspire Yourself, Fusion Breath Sex*).

Tantric Breathing   David recounts one of his Tantric sexual experiences in a chapter he wrote for the book *Enlightened Sexuality*. His yogini teacher used the power of her breath to initiate him into conscious, caring spiritual sexual intercourse in which the Tantric orgasm is achieved.

"My first Tantric teaching transmission where I had some sense of what was going on occurred after I dropped out of college to join an educational commune experiment near Mendocino, California. It was a great place to consider the direction of my life and meet interesting, even wise, people while enjoying nature.

"I arrived in the winter. That spring I met the Bird Lady of Mendocino. I don't remember her name. We saved ten seagulls from an oil spill that day. To show her appreciation for my help, I suppose, she made lunch for me. I watched in amazement as she skipped around the lush backyard of her friend's house where she was staying—she was a wanderer, essentially—picking flowers, weeds, leaves and herbs. The lunch was excellent.

"She was also a gifted yogini, for she slid effortlessly into advanced poses. She must have seen something in me because it was that night or the next that we ended up in bed.

"I had a cabin, a shack really, that overlooked the juncture of three rivers. It had no windows and the wood was rough. But the bed was quite good.

"The sun was going down, filling the cabin with a brilliant orange-bronze radiance. I remember sliding inside her and feeling the taut muscularity of her slick vagina. She raised her legs somewhere over her head for maximum penetration. There was a magical impersonality about the moment, a lack of conventional passion and urgency that somehow made the occasion fascinating, as if by being more distant in this manner, we were, in fact, much closer.

"Then, I can't explain exactly how, the breathing started. It was not like any ordinary breathing. It was a breathing that seemed to surround me, that I could hear with my skin.

"Slim yet strong and wiry, she had a feeling of enormous energy around her. When she began to breathe in this deep, forceful, rhythmic manner, she seemed to create a gap in space, a vacuum into which I was irresistibly drawn. This vacuum appeared to take the shape of a tunnel, at the end of which glowed a brilliant white light.

"It felt quite literally as if she was breathing me. The breath was like a tangible bond, a solid, tactile glue that tied us together far more deeply than the ordinary union of sex organs. It felt as if, through the breath, she had actually gained access to the inside of my body, the inner, vibrant, soft, pulsing core of energy that sustains my flesh.

"She initiated and controlled this potent co-inspiration experience. My job was simply to surrender, to respond openly, which I apparently did well enough.

"The whole relationship had not been ordinary. I had had the sense pretty much from the beginning that she was superior to me, wiser than I. I felt fortunate to be with her. She was going to teach me something, something about love or truth or happiness—that much I knew. Following some unspoken protocol, I had meekly followed her lead from the moment we met.

"Somehow, then, through her power, this special breathing began. It was like a slow steady pulse that filled our bodies and the space around us. It expanded and contracted with its own rhythm and we moved to it. I moved in and out with it. We breathed together with it. The pulse became slower and slower, the breathing deeper, the pauses between breaths longer. Soon it felt as if we were literally breathing each other. A moment arrived when I could not tell who was who.

"There was no movement, no sound, no separation, just a primal dreamlike fusion that melted my mind into an endless glowing void. At this time, too, came the open-eyed vision of a colossal red pyramid pulsating with elemental power. I don't remember having a conventional orgasm. The notion of coming or not had been totally eclipsed.

"We had sex just this once. But the experience was, without the slightest exaggeration, absolutely unforgettable. After this I knew for certain that love and sex, sexuality and spirituality, did not have to be in conflict, that, in fact, their integration can take us to new heights of consciousness."

COMPLETE CIRCUITS There are biomagnetic circuits within the bodymind and there are biomagnetic circuits that can be created between two bodyminds. These circuits correspond to acupuncture energy flows. When completing biomagnetic circuits with your consort, think of it as completing circuits within one whole bigger bodymind.

Completing your biomagnetic circuits brings you closer together emotionally. You may share moments of bliss as your energies joyfully merge into oneness. You may improve your health and sense of well-being. You don't have to know that you are completing biomagnetic circuits during your lovemaking to enjoy the benefit. Just the act of the penis entering and resting in the vagina completes many biomagnetic circuits.

Biomagnetic circuit closure can be solo or duo, simple or fancy, in any comfortable position. One simple solo way is to put the palms together in a prayer position or make a cup out of them and interlock the feet at the ankles or press the soles of the feet together.

Fancier solo methods include the Ring Of Calm *(Gyana Mudra)* and the Tongue Press *(Kechari Mudra)*. To do the Ring Of Calm, press the thumb and index finger, middle finger or little finger of either hand or both hands together in an "OK" sign. This gesture helps circulate sexual energy.

The Tongue Press seems more unnatural, but it may be the most powerful biomagnetic closure technique that a person can do solo. Among other things, it is said to balance

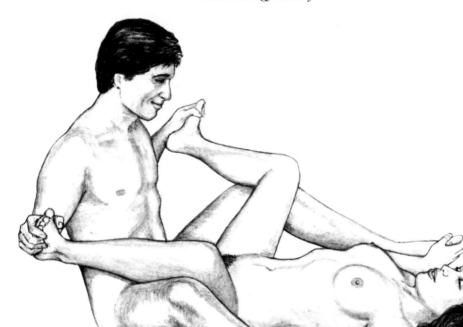

the activity of the brain hemispheres, complete the major energy circuit in the body (up the back and down the front) and increase the flow of saliva (increasing saliva may have cooling, calming, healing benefit). It is also said to directly stimulate the pituitary gland. The Ring Of Calm and the Tongue Press can be performed during intercourse, then dropped at orgasm to increase release.

Place the tip of your tongue against the soft palate in the back of the roof of the mouth. If this is too uncomfortable, place the tongue just behind the first ridge of the gum in the indentation where your palate has a soft spot. The rough area of the hard palate is not recommended as this tends to dry out the mouth. Keep your jaw loose and relaxed.

If either of these approaches is uncomfortable, just keep the tip of the tongue behind the two front teeth where the gum begins, your upper and lower teeth slightly apart. When the mouth and jaw are relaxed, this alignment happens automatically. A tight or clenched jaw is often a sign of pelvic or genital tension, which is reduced by releasing the jaw in a big pretend yawn.

COMPLETE CIRCUITS
above

TONGUE PRESS
opposite

Perhaps the ideal time to experience solo circuit closure is when you are in a passive, receiving role during your lovemaking (see *Stairway To Heaven*). In this role you are free to go within and feel the subtleties of your experience.

A unique combination of effects is achieved by performing the Tongue Press as you cover the eyes with the fingers and the ears with the thumbs. This the "womb gesture" *(Yoni Mudra),* a Tantric strategy for internalizing erotic awareness.

You can stimulate a private phospheme light show by pressing firmly but gently on the eyeballs. Various breathing patterns can be used to further deepen the sensitivity these techniques foster. Try this as your consort takes you into orgasm.

During lovemaking a great amount of energy, which some call the Kundalini, builds up. While it is good to be able to shoot energy out through the crown (see *Elevate Energy*), containing this special energy is also important.

Here is a simple way to accomplish this. Place the palm

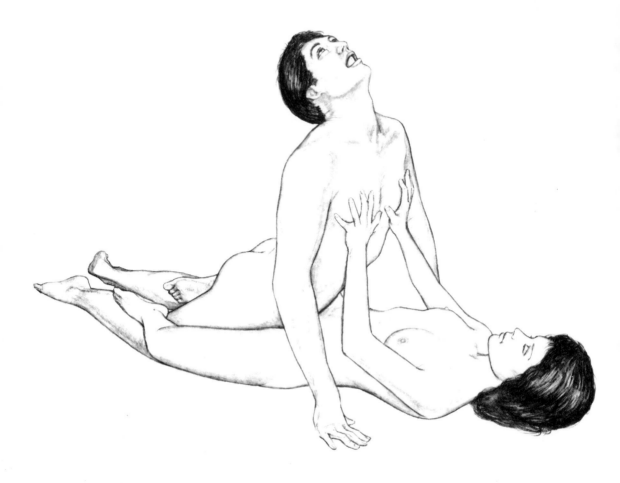

of your hand firmly on the top of your consort's head as you make love. Be sure to cover the indentation towards the back of the head as well as the center. Keep your hand on the top of their head. Allow the energy to build and build.

You may be surprised by the intense reaction, such as wild shaking, that may eventually follow. You have sealed off a major escape valve for the expanding energy. This containment effect is enhanced if they do the Tongue Press and PC clenches at the same time. If you are looking to accumulate energy for healing or restorative purposes, use this technique. Then do *Taoist Circle Of Gold* or a similar method to circulate the energy and store it in the *Hara*.

Biomagnetic closure between consorts can be as simple as matching same bodymind parts. This happens to some extent during lovemaking (including for play) but the effect can be enhanced by making this a chosen activity. You can match forehead to forehead, palm to palm, belly to belly, chest to chest, back to back, sole of foot to sole of foot and, of course, mouth to mouth and tongue to tongue.

Connections can also be made between different body parts. These connections include hands to feet, hands or feet to chest, and hands or feet to head. Other examples are mouth to hands or feet, and mouth or hands to genitals. Some positions, i.e., 69, make completing circuits feasible for both consorts at the same time, increasing the effect.

There is no right length of time for maintaining a connection. You will be able to feel the soothing effect of the life energy as it flows through a completed circuit. Disengage when this sensation goes away or you feel moved to create a new match between bodymind parts. You may find that you are performing a joyous biomagnetic dance as you hold one arrangement for awhile, then move on to the next.

If you find that your tendency is to hold configurations for only five or ten seconds, try holding a few for a minute or two each. You may be delighted by the new sensations you experience.

Howard John Zitko suggests a version of the classic Tantric ritual touching *(nyasa)* as a preparation for intercourse. Sitting naked facing each other, holding hands, the couple meditates together. After achieving a rapport, they begin to breathe in unison. To further develop the psychic rapport, they touch each other simultaneously. The male touches her body on the right side using his left hand; the female touches the male on his left side using her right hand. The touching, which is a kind of slow, deliberate healing caress, begins at the head and gradually continues on down to the legs. This practice is said to awaken the Kundalini by creating and closing a polarized energy circuit.

As breath from the nostrils or mouth also carries biomagnetism, just breathing on an area of your partner's body tends to create a circuit. While breathing on their body can be very sensual, you may find the experience is even more intense if you imagine or feel that your breath carries energy that soaks into their skin at that point.

According to the *Karezza* approach, the ideal is not only to invest your breath with energy, but to summon up the deepest feelings of love and affection that you have for your consort. This love saturated breath is then used to non-verbally communicate with them in a most subtle form of touch.

The eyes are also a powerful way of connecting. Looking in each other's eyes while making love can be challenging as well as inviting. A fascinating game is to maintain eye contact throughout the sex act (see *Pair Bonding And Tuning, Creative Climax*).

ELEVATE ENERGY

People in ecstasy are often depicted with their attention directed upward, sometimes with eyes rolled up or hands raised in jubilation. As the expressions "to be up" or "get high" show, ecstasy is somehow related to rising up, to ascension. Likewise, we are all too familiar with what it is like to be "down" or "low." In conventional religion, of course, heaven is above (see *Energy Centers*).

Kundalini Kegel, *Elevate Energy* and *Taoist Circle Of Gold* are applications of this same sex yoga principle, which you should feel free to adapt to your individual taste. After all, the real key is to find what helps you personally feel the movement of energy. For one person, it will be touching. For another, it is the breath. For others, it will be visualization or focusing on body sensation or making sounds or something else entirely different.

It is best to practice alone at first. This is a powerful opening practice and a way to awaken energy flows in your bodymind that leads to Tantric orgasm with or without the usual genital climax. You will find several related practices for couples in the *Nights Of Tantra* section.

Basic Version

First, the basic version of Elevate Energy. Inhale gently, hold your breath, clench your PC muscle and pull your anal muscles up and in. Close your eyes and direct your attention above your head. Don't strain. Just relax and float away.

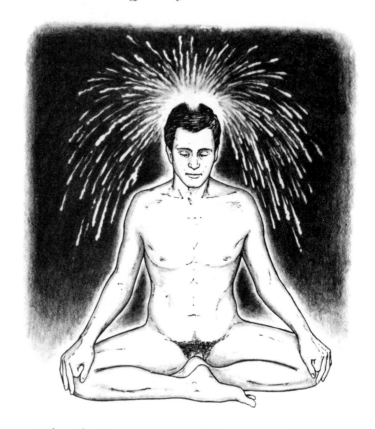

When the time comes to exhale, you may find it helpful to take in a little sniff of air. As you exhale, relax the PC and anal muscles.

Hold no more air than is completely comfortable for you, which will probably be about half capacity. The whole experience should feel very relaxed and bring a sense of relief.

There is plenty to work with even in this simplified form. Instead of directing energy to a point above the head, you can experiment with sending it to other points along the vertical channel, such as the solar plexus, heart, throat or third eye.

Advanced Version Now for the more elaborate version. Sit on a chair, in a meditation posture such as easy Burmese (see *Sexercises*) or lie on your back. If you sit on a chair, place your feet flat on the floor. Place your palms flat on your thighs.

Inhale through your nose deep into your belly, scraping the air deep against the back of your throat. You may even feel it touch your lower back or the base of your spine. As you do this, slowly roll your eyes upward and inward and gently tighten your PC and anal muscles.

Press your tongue against your soft palate, at the roof of your mouth towards the back. Or, you can rest your tongue behind your front teeth.

A very gentle tucking in with the neck so that the head bends just slightly forward and down may be helpful. This should feel more comfortable as you retain the air. A gentle abdominal lock, performed by pulling the lower belly in, completes the energizing posture.

As you inhale and hold, relax and melt away into a light, expanded experience of spaciousness and brightness at or above your head. Encourage any yearning for ecstasy or release that may arise. Take time to enjoy this natural high.

When you are ready, allow the eyes to roll down, following the descending flow of energy. However, if you find that you want to stay lost in an ecstatic space, and the eyes want to stay rolled up and back, by all means maintain the pose.

When you release by exhaling, your head may want to lean back slightly. As your head goes back, encourage some sort of vowel sound. This helps to open up the throat center so that the energy does not get stuck there. If you are lying on your back, it is enough to arch the back a little and let any sort of moan that wants to come out express itself.

An extended "Ahhh" or "Sahhh" is our favorite sound for this kind of opening. Feel the sound deep in your belly, as if you are pregnant with it (see *Sound Sex*).

However, at some point you should return the head to an upright position so that the energy has a free pathway to the top. As you become sensitive to the ascending currents of energy, you may find it feels more natural to keep the head erect or even tilted slightly forward, linking the *pai-hui* point just behind the center of the crown with the heaven energy.

If you are visually oriented, you can imagine that a stream of white or golden-white energy is rising up your spine or through the core of your bodymind into the center of your head or out the top of your head. If you like this option, you may find it helpful to talk yourself deeper into it: "I see a bright column of white light up my spine, blinding in its intensity. Now it is beginning to pulse. Waves of energy are going up to my head at a faster and faster rate."

The precise visualization of energy is not necessary, however. It is enough to just direct your attention to the center or top of your head. Work with getting a strong, clear feeling of going up or floating upward. As this sensation gets stronger with practice, melt into it more and more so that the whole experience takes on a delicious, blissful, almost liquid quality.

ELEVATE ENERGY
opposite
What goes up (yang, fire, the stars) must come down (yin, water, gravity). First, though, we focus on rising—rather than falling—in love.

In fact, Elevate Energy can become an intensely sensual, erotic experience that feels very much like you are making love to yourself. More accurately, perhaps, you will feel like you are savoring the subtle essence of the experience of making love.

Perhaps the best way to visualize in Elevate Energy is to have the *impression* of a light above the head. It is a common mistake to think that imagery must be detailed and vivid like a motion picture. While that is possible, for Elevate Energy it is quite enough to *feel* or *sense* that the light is there. Trying to generate hard, precise images can actually block the subtle, inner, tactile sensitivity that is the key to Elevate Energy.

You are going towards and into this light in a soft gesture of melting surrender. This has a very sensual quality to it, a feeling, perhaps, of touching your flesh from the inside out. You may feel like you are stepping out of bulky, awkward clothes into a luminous openness. You may become aware of the light within your body as you do this.

Allow your face, jaw, shoulders and so on to relax. Feel the pull of gravity and let the body sag. Just let it go. The more relaxed your body is, the easier it will be for you to feel your energy and sense its blissful, nourishing movement.

Remember, easefulness is the key to Elevate Energy. You are listening to, feeling and following the natural flow of ecstatic energy through your bodymind. Virtually no effort is required. This is selfloving of a very subtle kind that opens the inner pathways.

The point between the eyebrows is a trigger for the third eye. You may want to focus there instead of the top of the head or above. This point is often an easier place for intellectual persons to focus, while the center of the brain or the crown tends to feel more natural to intuitive types.

Fountain Of Light   After you have practiced Elevate Energy a little, it is good to work on opening the crown energy center. By bringing the energy all the way up to and through the crown, you connect with the center of light above the head. Even if you don't seem to feel anything at first, end with your attention concentrated at the top of or above the head with the sense that the top of your head has opened up (see *Energy Centers*).

Do not be concerned about the precise location of the crown center. If you can feel a little openness or tenderness at the top of your head, that is enough. Know that you are somehow connected with the universe there in a stream of clear bright white light. It may help to think of this stream of light as your umbilical cord to the cosmic Mother.

Now you are ready to emphasize breaking out through the top of the head as a fountain of clear bright white light, literally like an orgasm through the crown that fuses you with the blazing hearts of stars. Some people find the imagery of a volcano spewing lava, or even of a pulsating penis emitting semen during an orgasm, compelling and effective for getting this feeling of "jumping" through the crown.

An excellent way to strengthen your sensation of shooting out the crown of the head in a fountain or torrent of light is to take a slight inbreath in the upper chest just as you approach the end of your breath retention. Not only does this sniff of air make the subsequent exhalation easier to perform, it helps you get the feeling of "jumping" right out or pulling yourself up through the top.

You can also use your exhalation to pop out the top. Begin the exhalation from your concentration point within or at the top of the head and use the thrust from the exhalation. Try a long, tender exhalation, coordinated with rolling the eyes back a little more, that floats you higher and higher.

When the crown is felt to really open it has a grounding effect as well. You may feel as if you have connected, even merged with a source of energy or light that is unlimited and all around you. There may be a feeling of flying through space. If, instead, the third eye is concentrated upon, flashes of light and colorful imagery of various sorts tend to occur. This is excellent preparation for non-genital Tantric orgasm.

Waterfall Of Love

Grounding the energy will be a concern for some people. The symptoms of too much energy in the head include spaciness, headaches, or a feeling of not being connected with your body. To ground the energy follow the radiant fountain of light out the top of your head with the waterfall of love.

Allow the fountain to spill over and shower down upon you like a rain of unspeakable beauty and kindness, a peaceful, blissful waterfall that soaks you to the core with contentment. When you exhale, imagine that energy is pouring down in waves around and through your bodymind right down to and through the soles of your feet, reconnecting you with the earth.

Go deep into the feeling of this wonderful life-giving rain on your skin and allow it to sink deep in, saturating you completely. You may find it easier at first to feel it streaming down just the outside of your flesh, but eventually the experience of saturation to the core will occur.

Feel this waterfall of love relaxing and healing you. Feel

it go to the exact places in your bodymind where you tend to block or store tensions. Feel it gently and effortlessly soften, open and clear those spots, as if it has a dynamic, loving intelligence of its own.

Feel this saturation from the top of your head to the soles of your feet. Encourage the feeling of bliss to soak right into the ground beneath you, so that you are surrounded from every angle by bliss.

Get the feeling of bringing the energy to the feet, even if that means skipping some parts of the body on the way down at first. That way you can feel the connection between the soles of the feet and the top of the head.

If one breath does not last long enough at first for you to go from the top of your head to the bottom of your feet, you can pace the energy waves by exhaling and inhaling several times on the way down. For example, you can do one breath from the head to the chest, another from the chest to the abdomen and a third from the abdomen to the feet, ending on an exhalation as the wave flows down around your feet into the earth.

However, with practice you will be able to move the energy down in one long exhalation. Then you will feel a wave up the entire body with the inbreath and a wave down the entire body with the outbreath. This is a very pleasurable feeling and leads to a state of deep calm. Sitting in a chair with your feet flat on the floor is a good posture for this.

Then, from this natural peak, it is easy to feel the energy fall down all around you like a natural mountain stream being pulled below by the irresistible force of gravity. This blissful shower feeling is, in fact, a very effective grounding technique that puts you solidly in your body.

This is a purifying practice. Grounding culminates with recycling the psychic wastes that sometimes surface—seen, perhaps, as dark substance—down through the layers of the earth into its fiery core. There they are harmlessly consumed, fertilizing the soil and creating life. Thanks is then given to the Earth Mother for Her love and the fragile gift of life.

Practice Pointers   The Elevate Energy technique is thought to stimulate the pituitary and pineal glands for longer life, more vitality and personal growth. It may accomplish this by increasing the flow of cerebrospinal fluid which already circulates through the spine and the brain.

Because this technique involves holding the breath, it is not recommended for persons with high blood pressure. However, if this is a concern for you, Elevate Energy can be performed without breath retention. Performed with your easy, natural breath pattern it will still delight, heal and ground you.

As a final point, some sources recommend rising up the spine from the sacrum on the *exhalation* and drawing energy down with the *inhalation* (the exact opposite). An easy but reliable approach is to fill *Hara* on the inhalation and then shoot energy up the spine to the crown with the exhalation. The feeling is that the belly is acting like a bellows.

Ultimately, Elevate Energy is about being in love with yourself. Your bliss is not based on any outside source but arises from deep within you. Your external lover is the trigger or reminder who renews and reveals your connection with your own deepest center. A convenient time to do Elevate Energy while making love is during a *Full Stop.*

FOCUS   Your most valuable sex organ is between your ears, not your legs. The ability to concentrate, to focus the mind on what is happening in the body or on positive features in your experience, is universally agreed to be a key factor in success.

The power of concentration can enhance lovemaking to an extraordinary extent. The love elixir that many people are looking for is the ability to totally concentrate, to fully focus. This ability is acquired through practice.

A simple concentration training exercise is watching the second hand of a clock. An even more basic technique is to follow the breath in and out. If nothing else, trying these techniques quickly proves how easily our minds wander.

Just touching can be practiced as a training exercise or while actually making love. Just touching can be practiced by touching your own body, or oranges and apples, cloths of different textures and so on. Just touching for tactile sensitivity training can also take the form of very slow, barefoot walking.

You can practice being more in the sensory present. You will benefit your entire life as well as your love life. The Buddhist way of meditation called vipassana, insight or mindfulness meditation emphasizes this training.

There is another kind of focus which is rarely spoken of in the context of making love. This is, in the words

SEATED BODHISATTVA
right
Ch'ing dynasty.

of philosopher Franklin Merrell-Wolff, the state of "high indifference." This is not a heartless, cold state of mind. You feel a delightful detachment, a spacious ultra-involvement, that takes you out of your head and into the present.

Try making love at a time when you are a bit indifferent to sex, when you can take or leave the genital orgasm. This mood of detachment may lead to some of your best experiences. There is something about the tunnel vision that results from trying too hard or wanting something too much that seems to prevent the very sense of reward we seek.

FULL STOP   The Full Stop is taking the time to take stock, to just feel, to appreciate. You step off the elevator of arousal and explore the floor you have reached, be it the 9th or the 49th. You take this time to reestablish the reality that it is you two, and only you two, here now together.

Look into each other's eyes. Feel each other from deep in the belly and chest. Caress each other, breathe on each other. Acknowledge that the fact of your being together is itself a miracle. Take at least a minute or two for this. Take five minutes, fifteen minutes or more. If it ends in sleep, that's fine. You will feel completed afterwards, without any sense of frustration.

You may want to squeeze, really squeeze, each other to say "I really care." It is sometimes difficult to remember to do this as you rush past each other in pursuit of solitary crescendos. Stop and squeeze each other in an enthusiastic bear hug. Make it a long one.

Resist the temptation to pull back if deeper feelings come up. You are making love.

We like to full stop in YabYum. We will sit upright in each others arms, silently, and direct the attention within. These peaceful moments are some of the moments together we treasure the most. Seconds before we were a raging fire. Now we are a cool mountain breeze scented with pine. The contrast is not a problem, it is the source of delight. We also prefer the Seesaw for Full Stops (see *Peaceful Positions*).

A playful version of the Full Stop is the freeze or alarm clock game. There are two ways to go about it. The first is to set a timer, or several timers, in advance. The second is to assign one of the partners the role of alarm clock. Switch roles at some point, either halfway through that session or during an entirely separate lovemaking session.

When the timer goes off, both freeze. Stop completely.

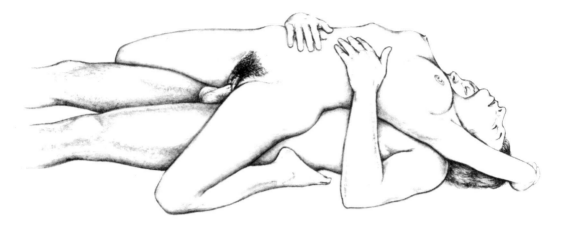

Do not move. Simply lie still and be aware of the continued motion of your sensations, thoughts and emotions. The main thing is to not move in the slightest. Do not move for at least one minute, if not longer.

What is the benefit of this game? Typically, we tend to make love with a driven, compulsive, edgy feeling. This exercise will give you some valuable distance from that compulsive feeling. It also adds that element of playfulness or surprise that so often is missing.

You may want to breathe in unison, very informally, as you tenderly return to the peak of passion. You can be like a two person steam engine, breathing slowly at first, then more and more quickly.

Without the valley, the peak is meaningless. Without the peak, the valley is fruitless. Take time to enjoy both.

The ups and downs of lovemaking are inevitable. Somehow when you make rising to the peaks of excitement and descending to the valleys of peace a choice, the cyclical, ebb and flow quality of ecstasy and intimacy in lovemaking is more acceptable. This is true of relationships on a day-to-day basis, too. Like surfers on the ocean, sooner or later you learn to ride the waves.

Since taking a break short-circuits male arousal, intercourse can be prolonged indefinitely in this way. Lovemaking with frequent Full Stops takes on a rhythmic, flowing dance-like quality (see *War And Peace*).

You may want to talk to your partner first about taking a Full Stop. Although it is not likely, without advance notice they could take your desire to stop as a rejection.

If they protest, be assertive. "What's the rush, honey? Making love with you is such a beautiful experience."

CRY OF THE EAGLE *above* In Sweden, they move from the snow to the sauna and back, again and again. The contrast creates an intensely delicious experience.

While making love, be gentle, of course. "Let's stop for a moment. I just want to hold you, to feel you, to feel all of you, to know that you are really here with me."

In the still, moonlit serenity of a moment of no motion, not only can such words be said, they can be heard. Swept away by a river of intimate, sensual joy, you taste a glory, a living presence, the precious, healing stream of unblocked, pure feeling, the brave, pulsing heart of life.

Above all, follow your own path. These are suggestions only. Surrender to the moment. Know through feeling.

Partners can use the time to *Elevate Energy*. It is also a convenient time for either partner to press on the man's perineum to relieve prostate pressure and delay ejaculation or to use other delaying techniques. Or the Full Stop can simply be used to give permission to each other to internalize and go deep within to claim and relish the waves of pleasure that lovemaking creates.

GOD AND GODDESS

Some cultures have developed the art of god and goddess visualization to an extraordinary degree. Perhaps this is an expression of their reservations about the sexual act in its natural form. However, the uninhibited erotic beauty of the Hindu temple at Konarak, even if merely symbolic, suggests instead a time of wonderful sexual freedom in which religion and sexual energy enjoyed a unique fusion. At any rate, the expressed purpose of visualizing yourself and your consort as a god or goddess is to elevate the sexual act to a higher plane (see *Make Love With Your Mind*).

Those of us raised in the Judeo-Christian atmosphere have not really been provided with an adequate archetype for this practice of melding with a symbol of God in sexual union, as Christ is depicted as celibate, if not asexual. Therefore, you may be surprised by an unexpected reluctance.

Eventually, though, if you persist, you will discover that this is a very effective method for experiencing the sacredness of sex, even the descent of the Shekhinah (Goddess Force). It is more that we tend to see it as a threat to spontaneity. Romance as worship is natural to us.

While plenty of energy certainly does become available during the sex act, this output is not easily managed. The deity visualizations are designed to provide a conduit for the energy to flow in a predetermined direction towards spiritual or psychological success. In the Western Occult tradition, this is called "Assuming the God Form."

Easy Beauty However, many of us would just rather enjoy our loving more and feel closer to each other when we are intimate. One very simple but very effective strategy is to smooth out your lover's physical imperfections with an imaginary paintbrush.

Let erotic imagination go wild. Give their skin a lush, unearthly golden glow. Set an open, vertical third eye like a jewel in their forehead. Make their hair shine like lightning, their eyes blaze like fire.

Go ahead and make their other features as perfect and idealized as you like. Remember, you can have anything you want. So why not create unearthly good looks?

Soft lighting, such as amber bulbs rather than white, or candlelight, a few glasses of wine, some incense and sensual music provides the physical setting (see *Boudoir Basics*). The dimmer lighting is important, for in the soft lyricism of twilight our imaginations are free.

Unusual, ethereal names such as "Devi" or "Maha" add to the exotic feeling. You may also want to use a little face paint to illumine your face and perhaps parts of your body that add to this ritualistic mood. A simple third eye painted vertically on the forehead provides strong reinforcement for your vision. *Tantric Sex* by Gold offers some excellent pointers for cosmic role playing.

Archetypal Love Affair This approach can be developed into a full-blown role playing as god and goddess. There are archetypal love affairs, such as Krishna and Radha, that resourceful lovers can explore. Mythology is a particularly rich and detailed source of such images and roles. For some couples, this is a very potent approach. Traditionally, this process can ultimately take the form of undying devotion to a holy form, the path of bhakti (devotional) yoga.

Do you have a clear mental image of your ideal lover's body? Perhaps you have seen a photograph or drawing of someone whose body seemed absolutely perfect to you. Practice recalling this image to mind. Make a mental note of the details. You will not need to have the photo or drawing anymore. If they were close to your ideal, you will have this image more or less burned in your mind anyway.

Now, when you make love, gently project this image

over your lover. Imagine that you are making love to your perfect archetype. Allow yourself to believe that you are with that perfect lover of your dreams.

You may be astonished by the vigor of your response. Often it is too much realism that kills the erotic thrill. In this setting you have so carefully arranged, allow fantasy to run wild, for illusion and love are not so far apart.

Making love with your archetypal perfect lover is also an excellent way to approach *Selfloving*. Develop the details of their body, face and appearance in advance. Try out your tryst as a *Selfloving* session, too, if you are uncomfortable relating to a fantasy persona while making love with another.

Real Fantasies   One note of caution here. Do not choose as your fantasy lover someone you know or actually want to have sex with.

Likewise, if there is an actor or actress that represents this fantasy character for you, it is preferable to use their appearance as a starting point only. Go on to create a magical, mythical person and give them a new name.

In traditional Tantra, where this kind of visualization has been developed into a profound art, after the image has been created and fusion with it has been enjoyed, it is dissolved. In one practice, the god or goddess is seen to arise from a point or *bindu* that itself originates out of a vast expanse of restful blue sky. After achieving mystical union, the deity is transformed back to the *bindu,* which in turn transforms back to the luminous blue space. This is then meditated upon as the source and nature of all experience.

The point is clear enough: you must be in control of the process. Ultimately, the god or goddess with whom you enjoy this unalloyed pleasure is a product of the power of your own mind.

The main reason for cultivating the other as a divine image is to promote the proper feeling in the heart. This feeling in the heart that is ideal for transcendental (or just plain great) lovemaking is one of quiet reverence, of high esteem, of deep respect with a touch of awe and childlike wonder. Due to the intensity of gratitude that is generated when the consort is viewed as a sacred figure, a strong quality of caring, compassion and kindness towards the consort is then a natural response.

There is really only one thing that trips us up in the sexual act—the fact that it is so difficult to generate feelings of compassion, reverence and kindness in the midst of the strong forces that move us in physical sex. When a god and goddess make love, the experience is certain to be uplifting.

GROUND AND STORE ENERGY

Lovemaking can generate huge amounts of energy. Perhaps you would like to collect and store this energy. Or you may open and expand so much that you want a way to empower yourself before facing the world again.

Personal grounding helps you to manage and keep the energy generated and reestablishes a sense of having both feet on the ground. In general, grounding centers you physically and psychologically.

You may experience a heady, spaced out feeling from energy-oriented lovemaking. If you are feeling uncomfortable or if you feel the need to be more down-to-earth, take a few minutes after making love to ease your transition with one of these grounding techniques.

Finally, to be fully grounded is to fully participate in the sensory present. Anything that will help you come to your senses, such as a shower and a rubdown after a prolonged lovemaking session, also helps to ground you (see *Hara, Taoist Circle Of Gold*).

Belly Power

One way to accomplish this is very easy. Place your attention on your navel. Move your right fist in a circular motion 36 times in one direction, then 24 in the other. Make the circles bigger gradually but not more than half a foot wide.

If you are a woman, move your fist counterclockwise first, then clockwise. If you are a man, move your fist clockwise first, then counterclockwise. In other words, if you are a woman you first spiral away from the navel, then spiral into the navel. Do the opposite if you are a man. Hold a watch at your navel to make this simpler for you.

In fact, this is only one of many techniques for gathering and storing energy in the navel region. The spiraling can be done completely in the imagination as if it were being done deep within the navel. Take the energy deep into the core of the body almost to the spine.

In all seriousness, we recommend a simpler version of this ancient Chinese exercise which we call the yummy tummy exercise. As you know, kids rub their hands in a circular motion around their tummy as they say "Yummy." Try it. If you can, watch a kid do it.

Another fun technique is performed on all fours (see *Cat Stretch*), only instead of stretching like a cat, you bark like a dog. Ellen likes to do this bouncing on the bed, kicking her legs behind her in the air. Of course, David teases her about this and has cautioned her that she will return as a canine in her next life. Nonetheless, it works and is lots of fun. The barking breath is deep in the belly, not the upper chest.

The lower belly region is the life force storage battery for the human body, at least according to Eastern thought. The Taoists believed that energy ascended up the back and descended down the front. To encourage upward energy flow without also encouraging downward energy flow was considered by them to be downright foolhardy.

Some people are concerned that they will accumulate more energy through prolonged lovemaking than they can handle. Taoist Chinese yoga teaches that the way to manage big energy loads is to store the charge in the lower belly.

Chopping Wood

A quick way to get more in touch with your body is chopping wood. In case you don't have any wood handy, the movement is just what you would imagine. Begin by standing and taking a deep breath. To start chopping wood, bend over vigorously, your arms performing the chopping motion as if you had an axe in your hands.

Breathe out strongly through the mouth as you bend over. Repeat several times. Make noise. This one is a real workout.

Deep Roots

A method taught in psychic development classes is to stand in a relaxed fashion and imagine that there is a thick and very strong cord of light extending from each of your feet down to the very center of the earth. Allow yourself to feel totally rooted as you do this. Some find visualizing that their body is a tree and the cords from their feet are roots works well.

Separately or in conjunction with seeing cords or roots extend from your feet, you can see a cord extending from the base of your spine at the tailbone down to the center of the earth. This may be easier to do sitting down. Some find that thinking the cord is like a monkey's prehensile tail works well.

I Am

Another simple method is to sit or lie with both hands on your belly. Breathing deeply from the belly, repeat "I-I" or "I am (your name)" with each breath. Do this in sets of three for a few minutes.

If you have entered a trance as a result of high-energy lovemaking—which can range from a slightly dreamy state to a full-blown hypnotic trance—a quick way to break the trance is to adjust your body position frequently. If there are behaviors that connect you to a dynamic state, such as waving your hands in the air while talking excitedly about a favorite topic, perform that behavior now. It will tend to induce the more dynamic, awake state.

Seal Your Field   This fast acting technique, developed by Betty Bethards, has the effect of sealing your personal energy field. Sitting in a comfortable position, place your hands on your thighs and make fists out of them. Visualize yourself immersed in an enormous globe made of brilliant white light. Do this for a minute or so until you feel noticeably more settled and collected.

Squat   The squat is another exercise that brings you down close to Mother Earth. Begin with your legs wide apart and your feet angled out slightly. As you squat down and slowly lower your buttocks, put your hands together in a prayer position and extend them in front of you. Then your hands will act as a counterweight to help you keep your balance.

When this is easy, bring the palms closer and closer to your chest and your feet parallel as much as you are able. This can be combined with breathing in and out of the genitals in the imagination. You can also try walking from the squatting position.

Touch The Earth   Another technique uses the earth itself, or a convenient floor, as your ground. We find touching the earth itself is optimal in grounding exercises. Bending from the waist, press the palms of the hands and the soles of the feet firmly into the ground. Bend your knees as much as you need in order to feel comfortable—this is not a yoga stretch.

Breathe deeply and rhythmically from the belly. If this breathing makes you dizzy, don't do it. Take your time.

This exercise is best done barefoot. Sunrise on dewy grass is said to be the optimal time and place.

INSPIRE YOURSELF   Below we describe a variety of special ways to breathe while making love. They are designed to heat up, cool down or sensitize your system (see *Co-Inspiration*).

Heating or yang breaths tend to increase arousal and may be used to bring on or intensify orgasm. Cooling or yin breaths tend to diffuse arousal and may be used to delay or expand orgasm. Sensitivity to the breath increases awareness of subtle energy and encourages energy recycling.

The skills described below are presented for solo use, though two people can certainly perform them together. If appropriate, check with your family physician before doing this or any other breath controlling technique in this book (i.e., heart trouble, high blood pressure).

Deep breathing is far more useful than most people realize. The average person is said to use only one-sixth of their lung capacity. Strive to breathe deeply and completely throughout your lovemaking.

Pelvic breathing coordinates the thrust, be it male or female, with the breath. When you thrust out from your body and to your partner, breathe out (exhale). When you pull in to your body and away from your partner, breathe in (inhale). This rhythm may feel uncomfortable at first, but it is definitely the way the pelvis and breath naturally move together. For more details, see *Pelvic Expression.*

Panting   To heat yourself up breathe with your mouth. Pant on purpose if you want to heat up rapidly. Breathe rapidly from your belly (not your throat) with your mouth open. You can extend your tongue a little. Panting helps bring orgasm on if you are close, but if you are not, it relaxes the belly and pelvis and delays orgasm.

Betty Dodson notes that the panting taught in childbirth class for coping with pain enables her to go to new levels of ecstasy and orgasm. The tendency is to freeze the breath and hold back. Instead, use the panting breath to leap to new levels of delight. One of the benefits is that supersensitivity of the clitoris immediately following orgasm disappears.

Breath Of Fire   By involving the diaphragm more, panting turns into another energizing breath, the Breath of Fire. Really pull the abdomen in and up. Breathe out forcefully.

If you do this breath through the nose, be aware that it has a cleansing effect and mucus may come out of the nostrils. It is also known for its ability to eliminate stale air from the lungs. Do the Breath of Fire a little before making love, so that this is not a concern. A box of tissues nearby is still a good idea even then.

Naturally, this breath can be done through the mouth. Then you may want to purse the lips a little. If the atmosphere is hot and humid, you will probably find breathing through the mouth more comfortable. Inhaling through the nose and exhaling through the mouth is another alternative.

The full cycle has three steps. Do the breath with forceful exhalation for 30 seconds, then take a deep inhalation and hold for 15 seconds. Focus on the solar plexus as you hold the breath. You will quickly build up energy there. Now take a couple of slow, relaxing complete breaths and repeat. It is recommended that you do this cycle for a maximum of three minutes only, about three or four times. However, you may find that just one cycle, in the context of erotic arousal, is enough to heat things up and expand energy.

As this is a forceful breath, you will really be pushing your envelope. Do not underrate this technique. It is an excellent way to get the energy out of the pelvic box up to the solar plexus. From there it easily spreads to the rest of the body, facilitating whole-body arousal and orgasm as well as the various energetic types of experiences that are possible.

Of course, you will want to have agreement with your partner that intensive breathing is allowed, or at least let them know what you will be doing. Doing the Breath of Fire together is fun, too. But co-breathing here is not a necessity. The Breath of Fire is something you do when you really want to and your desire to build up or move the energy is strong.

Men may find this useful for delaying ejaculation, achieving male multiple orgasm and intensifying climax. Women may be able to bring on or extend orgasm as well as bridge to multiorgasmic patterns with this breath. While we want to stress not overdoing the Breath of Fire, it is a very good yang breath that should quickly convince you of the power of the breath as a sexual stimulant and consciousness raising tool.

Chakra Charging
This Cherokee Chuluaqui Quodoushka teaching leads to an ecstatic, healing Tantric orgasm experience with or without genital stimulation (see *Energy Centers, Appendix*).

Lie on your back with your knees up and feet flat on the floor (see *Pelvic Expression*). Breathing through the mouth, draw energy deep into the first chakra at the clitoris (female) or perineum (male) until it feels charged. Tighten your PC muscle with each inhalation. Then inhale energy up to the second chakra, rocking the energy back and forth until they both feel charged up and full. Do the same between the second and third, then the third and fourth. Continue breathing the energy up through the throat, third eye and crown.

As the energy begins to move you, you may want to arch your back, moan, tremble, shake wildly. Go with it! You may experience movements typical of orgasm or do spontaneous yoga. Afterwards, relax and enjoy the pleasurable streaming through the body. A deep meditative state may result.

PC Muscle
Another way to increase arousal and bring on orgasm is to coordinate PC muscle clenching and deep breathing. Clench on the rhythmic exhalation or on breath retention. Pull up and in with the anal muscles for maximum effect. Add affirmations and/or visualizations if they work for you. Doing this to music can be fun as well as highly arousing.

Cooling Down To cool down, breathe slowly and rhythmically through the nose. Since the male tendency is to rapidly heat up and then explode, not unlike a volcano, men have searched for ways to stay cool under pressure. There are also women who are too "hot" and need to cool down and enjoy more peace and harmony when they make love. The ability to calmly experience and appreciate sexual arousal is a benefit of this technique.

Even more effective may be the cooling breath. Open your mouth slightly and part your teeth a little. Press the tip of your tongue to the back of your teeth or out between your teeth. If you can curl your tongue, then roll your tongue up to form a tunnel and protrude it slightly out your mouth. Inhale long and deeply through your mouth. Exhale lightly and serenely through your nose. Encourage the calm, cool feelings. You may want to close your eyes.

Also having a cooling effect is inhalation through the teeth. A hiss is created as you inhale. This breathing technique is called *sitkara* in the *Kama Sutra.* You may find the hissing sound that it creates quite sensual. You can experiment with the placement of your tongue, as this changes the effect slightly.

Air can be sucked or slurped or sipped in between pursed lips, which aids concentration. The sounds created in this way are considered quite erotic by some consorts. You will sometimes see actors inhaling through closed teeth or pursed lips in pornographic movies for dramatic effect. They are ways to have control over arousal, too. You may also want to experiment with breathing in and out of the nose and mouth at the same time.

Locking in the breath slows you down yet increases energy, preparing you for a deeper and fuller orgasm later. A simple version is to simply inhale and hold the breath while tightening the PC muscle and pulling up and in with the anus. The lock is released before the breath is released.

To increase relaxation of the pelvic and genital region, add the bearing down maneuver. Let the PC–anal contraction go and press down and out with your pelvic muscles. Then release the air. Relish the relaxed feeling that follows. However, either form of locking in the breath is not recommended for people with high blood pressure.

Do not do this when you are teetering on the edge unless you want to encourage orgasm. At that point, go limp with your whole body or relax in some other way without tensing first.

Potbelly breath is keeping the abdomen enlarged at both

inhalation and exhalation. It will enable both of you to contain more sex energy charge longer.

The lion breath is a fun variation. This is best performed when you are on top. When you exhale open your mouth wide and loll your tongue forward. Roll your eyes up into the top of your head and roll your head back. You may want to exhale quietly and gently, making a slight rasping sound. You may want to roar like a lion. If you prefer, just roar in your mind without making a sound outwardly. Stay with the exhalation for a moment and enjoy the expanded feeling.

The muscles of the body can be tensed or relaxed in time with the breath. Here is a technique that brings strength to the lower abdomen and genitals and increases vitality and endurance. Breathing through the nose, the muscles of the stomach are drawn in firmly during the exhalation, forcing a maximum amount of air out. After the exhalation is complete, allow the inhalation to happen on its own. The PC and anal muscles may also be tightened during the exhalation.

Another approach is to make the belly and pelvic region as soft and relaxed as possible, like cotton or jelly. Consciously release the anus as well.

The whole body can be relaxed or tensed in rhythm with your inhalation or exhalation. Imagine that the erotic energy is spreading through your entire body.

Finally, try just holding the inhalation or the exhalation on purpose without breathing in any special way. People tend to do this unconsciously. Doing it consciously during lovemaking will lead you to insights on how to use the breath to creatively color and shape the sensual joy you are experiencing.

Connected Breathing   This breath, made popular by Rebirthing, quickly leads to a heightened sensitivity. Ordinarily, people pause briefly after each inhalation and each exhalation. In connected breathing this pause is eliminated. Connected breathing can be performed via the nose or mouth. Breathe deeply from the belly. Stop if you experience discomfort.

Creative Breathing   Positive creative images can be coordinated with breathing. Imagine that you are breathing light if you want to feel inspired. Imagine a fire with its red flames leaping high around you if you want to heat up. Your inhalations and exhalations fan the flames. If you want to cool down, imagine making love in the snow.

Genital breathing uses the imagination to feel air or water flowing in and out of the genitals. The feeling of arousal can be encouraged to spread through the body as a whole by imagining that your exhalation is going out in all directions from your pelvic region.

Other variations of whole-body breathing include pore breathing and bone breathing. Imagine that you are breathing in and out simultaneously through all the pores of your body at the same time. In bone breathing you imagine that the air is entering your body through the soles of your feet and going out through the top of your head on the inhalation, then entering back through the top of your head and going out through the soles of your feet on the exhalation. Imagine that the breath flows up the bones in the legs, through the pelvis, up the spine and through the skull. Try to feel the breath moving through the very marrow of your bones.

A related technique is to place your attention at the soles of your feet. The precise point is in the center of each sole towards the toes just below the ball of the foot. Located here is a major energy focal point known as Bubbling Spring in Chinese acupuncture (Kidney One or *yong quan*). You may feel the gentle ebb and flow of your breath at the soles of your feet. You may want to enjoy the fantasy of a bubbling spring bathing the soles of your feet. This is the same point that is pressed as part of an aculoving foot massage. You can press it while making love, too.

Reverse Breathing Reverse breathing, sometimes called the cobra breath, is to be practiced only after you have worked with the complete breath for awhile. When breathing in, pull the stomach in. When breathing out, extend the belly out. You will notice that this is the opposite of regular abdominal breathing as practiced in the complete breath.

Start out by performing a few normal abdominal breaths through the nose. Then do the reverse breathing very deeply through the nose, forcefully moving the belly in and out as if you are using it as a pump (which you are). Do no more than twelve reverse breaths at a time. After the set, take at least thirty seconds to relax deeply and see how you feel. A pleasant floating feeling is a common response. However, dizziness is also a typical reaction, at least at first, so be sure to take it easy.

The benefit of reverse breathing is that it acts as a pump to move the cerebrospinal fluid and sexual energy up the spine to the pituitary and pineal glands and psychic centers in the brain. Besides the potential for enhancement of health and mental power, it is a powerful tool for sexual energy recycling and assists in achieving the Tantric whole-body climax without conventional orgasm.

You can coordinate PC muscle contraction with the inhalation, relaxing the PC muscle with the exhalation. It is enough to place your attention at the top or center of your head to start and simply encourage or will the energy to go up the spine. You can coordinate it with the *Elevate Energy* technique if you like.

You only need to do one to three sets in a lovemaking session to feel the effect. It is ideal if you do it together sitting upright in the YabYum posture during a *Full Stop*. However, it is important that you practice it beforehand on your own so that you become comfortable with it. This may take a few weeks.

After each set, relax into a meditative state as you allow the open feeling that occurs in your head and body to expand. Take some time to enjoy and appreciate the subtleties of this experience of expanded consciousness. You may want to utilize a grounding technique afterwards (see *Taoist Circle Of Gold, Ground And Store Energy*).

LOVE TAP   The valley between the breasts is frequently neglected in lovemaking. The entire valley is an erotic zone for men as well as women. At the upper end of this valley is the thymus gland, which is easily stimulated by forceful tapping, pressing, rubbing and so on (see *Love Spot, Aculoving*).

According to John Diamond, M.D., an expert on the role of the thymus gland in optimal health, thumping the chest with the fist instantly enhances your ability to handle stress, balances your left and right brain hemispheres and increases your available life energy. He reports that the Tongue Press has the same beneficial effects (see *Sexercises, Complete Circuits*).

Jacquelyn McCandless, M.D., a noted psychiatrist and sex therapist, emphasizes in her practice that opening the heart and loving yourself and others improves the health of the thymus and vice versa. A healthy thymus gland is crucial to your good health because the thymus is the manager of your bodymind's self-defense.

Ninety-five percent of the people tested by Dr. Diamond had underactive thymus glands. Arousing your thymus gland may be a strong preventative health step and may enhance your ability to love self and others. What better time to arouse the thymus than while making love?

In the *Kama Sutra*, an intercourse technique is described which stimulates the thymus in this way. After entering his consort, the man begins striking the valley between her breasts with the back of his hand, at first very slowly and gently, then more rapidly and more forcefully.

The *Kama Sutra* also suggests a potent technique for the woman to use. When she senses that the man is approaching ejaculation, she should slap his buttocks and his chest with her open palm. If she slaps with enough force, his ejaculation will be delayed (of course, do not injure him). She should repeat the technique until she achieves sexual orgasm. The *Ananga Ranga* advises that gently patting his chest with her closed fist will add to his pleasure.

Caressing or rubbing the *Love Spot* just plain feels good anyway. Caring feelings are transferred heart to heart with a tender touch. Music, spoken rhythmic poetry, singing and gazing at a painting of a beautiful natural scene are also thought to stimulate the thymus gland.

MAKE LOVE WITH YOUR MIND

Many people have sex from the viewpoint of body alone. But making love must be a joint creation of body and mind. Here we focus on some ways to enhance your mental involvement by using your thoughts and your imagination creatively.

Many experience an abundance of distracting thoughts while making love. Our favorite way of dealing with these freeloaders is to focus on staying in the sensory present (see *Making Love Is A Touching Experience*).

New Thought

One popular approach is to substitute positive thoughts for negative thoughts. If you are thinking "I feel tense," you substitute "I feel relaxed." A simple positive thought such as "I feel peaceful" or "Yes" can be substituted for undesired thoughts as they appear. Another approach is to insert a thought which has no meaning to you, such as "Mmmmm" or "Ooohhh." These counter thoughts can be coordinated with the breath. These are some strategies you can use in the privacy of your own mind (or out loud if you wish).

Affirmation

An affirmation is a short positive statement that is repeated over and over again. Negative or undesired thoughts are kept at bay. Unity of body and mind is encouraged.

Affirmations are quite popular with some people. You can make up your own or try a standard one like "God Is Love" or "We Are One" or "I Am You" or "You Are Me" or

"Love Is All Around Us" or "We Are Love." Affirmations can be coordinated with breathing and PC-anal muscle clenches. You can also use them with harmonious images of your choice. Affirmations are natural during lovemaking. Why not make a good thing better? Do positive affirmations privately or together, silently or aloud.

The best affirmation is one that is personally meaningful to you. Experiment with one of these: "Yes," "Oh God," "Fire," "Mygasm," "Come," "Yummy," "Mama," "Papa," or "One." We also recommend "You Love Me," which is the other and often neglected side of "I Love You," and "Thank You."

Affirmations can be explored in at least two different ways. One is to use the literal meaning. Another way is to play with the sound it creates. For example, "We Are Loving" is a powerful statement in the English language. The sound "Weeeh Ahhrr Luuhv-eeenng" has its own potency independent of the dictionary definition. If you use an affirmation from another language, contact an authority in your area who can instruct you in the subtleties of the correct pronunciation or attend group chanting sessions led by an expert (see *Sound Sex*).

Above all, do not engage in a struggle with any unwanted thoughts. If a thought insists on sticking around, then simply allow it. This may make you uncomfortable for awhile, but sooner or later it will leave due to your lack of interest.

As you approach the deeper level of lovemaking participation, you may find that your thoughts are like the skin on an orange: the skin must be peeled away in order to enjoy the delicious fruit beneath. Even the thoughts "I am a man" or "I am a woman" are discarded as consorts pierce deeper and deeper into the mystery at the heart of making love.

Though stray thoughts may distract or trouble you, the thoughts themselves are not the problem. It is good to understand that every thought we entertain is there because we claimed it and let it in. At the same time, we are free to dismiss any unwanted thoughts any time we wish, for our mind is our home.

Fantasies   Fantasy imaging is very effective for some people. How would you like to make love to a living, breathing god or goddess of love? How would you like to be that god or goddess? Well, you can—with your imagination (see *Dream Lover, God And Goddess*).

You can imagine blood, energy and arousal rushing to

your sex organs and enhance pleasure and performance. Make the image vivid, colorful, detailed and full of action for best results.

A very effective strategy is to use the breath with the fantasy, or visualization, you have created. Allow the image to expand and contract, appear and disappear as your breath flows in and out.

The possibilities available in the world of imagination are infinite. You can surround yourself with golden mist, transport to another planet, fly through the air, make love in the heart of the sun.

Fantasies can be done solo in the privacy of your own mind or together. If you decide to share a fantasy, you may want to choose one of you to act as guide or coach to pace the scenario. You may want to create it together, enhancing a familiar fantasy model or improvising new ones. Fantasies can be enjoyed silently or verbally, with or without music and other props.

Nowadays visualization is used to succeed at business, athletic competition and healing. According to some contemporary sex therapists, fantasy and visualization are the next frontier of sexual discovery.

Fantasies can be enhanced by carefully selected, evocative music, rhythmic co-breathing or a supportive environment. Take time each week to develop your imagination. Not only is it great fun, you will discover that there is no end to what you can accomplish.

Here are several easy fantasies that use simple images but generate a powerful effect.

Blue Lotus Flower   There is a blue lotus flower in the center of your chest. As you make love, it expands and radiates a beautiful blue light. It expands and contracts in rhythm with your breathing. As you reach a climax in your lovemaking (which may or may not include conventional sexual orgasm), this blue light expands to penetrate and enclose both you and your consort in blue bubble of peace, love and happiness.

You may prefer visualizing a brilliant blue jewel shining in your chest. During one lovemaking session, Ellen felt as if her heart was a rose which began to flower and open. Although this was spontaneous, feel free to visualize images like this.

Bubble   Imagine you are a bubble floating on the ocean. Wave after wave carries you higher and higher. At orgasm or another right moment, you burst into. . . .

Circulate Light   As you make love, see a circle of moving light that circulates energy and feelings between your bodies. See it pass out the top of your head into their head and out the bottom of their feet or genitals into your feet or genitals. Or you can see and feel light and energy being shared and exchanged in any way that your imagination wants to go.

Think of it as special effects for a movie, if that helps you to be more comfortable with the concept. Be creative. Have fun (see *Fusion Breath Sex*).

Effulgence   As you breathe in, draw radiant energy from an effulgent source above your head. Inhale this breath energy down the front of your body into your perineum (area between the genitals and anus). As you exhale, you release this breath back up your spine to the infinite, nameless source of effulgence above your head (see *Elevate Energy*).

Firecracker   You are a firecracker lit at the genitals. Your spine is the fuse. When it reaches your head, you explode. Or vice versa, you are lit at your head and when it reaches your genitals or feet, you explode.

Garden   You are making love in a tropical garden. You can hear the waterfall nearby and the distant ocean surf, too. Lush tropical vegetation, exotic birds and a perfect temperature add to the delight of this tropical island for two (see *Aural Sex*).

Golden Fog   A golden circle of misty light surrounds you. The light turns into a golden glowing fog which spreads all through and around your body. You melt into this fog until you are the fog itself.

Ruby Laser   Iridescent ruby red laser beams shine from your navel, *Love Spot,* throat and third eye, bonding the two of you in some unexplainable yet glorious way. Or the beams shine from your nipples.

Super Penis—
Super Vagina   His penis is a mountain or a thunderbolt or simply of enormous size. It is made of hard beautiful rock such as diamond or jade. Her vagina is the mouth of the volcano or a lagoon that opens to the boundless sea. It is made of bands of gold that grow in size and strength, so that they have tremendous gripping power (see *Pompoir*). Or she is taking him in and being penetrated deeper and deeper, impossibly deep. Use images that fascinate you. Do this privately if you wish. The more outlandish the idea, the more effective it is likely to be.

Temple

Your body is a temple. The *yoni* (vagina) is the door to the temple; the *lingam* (penis) is the one who worships in the temple. Together, you experience the bliss of sacred unity.

Ties That Bind

Generate a greater feeling of closeness and oneness by seeing ropes of light binding your two bodies together. You can see yourselves surrounded by a brilliant hue of violet or magenta (red-purple).

You can also expand and deepen your heart feelings by literally seeing your hearts open up. See a foggy golden light pour out of them, one into the other, yet surrounding each of you.

You can also imagine your bodies melting like pads of butter on a hot stove, first softening and melting into themselves, then, borders and boundaries dissolved, into each other. If you like to work with chakras, before or during lovemaking connect your *Energy Centers* with rays of light.

Visualization— Advanced Skills

While visualization is a skill that is developed with practice, neurolinguistics indicates that some people are more visual than others. Here are several advanced techniques that not only offer a degree of challenge but the possibility of a major breakthrough in consciousness as well.

Bodies of Light

Feel that your bodies are literally made of light. Go all the way with this visualization. Don't just fill your body with light. Turn your body completely into a pure light. Every part of your body glows and radiates and then actually becomes a blinding light. White or gold are best for basic work, though other colors such as red, blue or green, provided they are seen as very bright, pure and clear, can be very beneficial.

Your consort also becomes light. Once you are both light, it is extremely easy for you to attain a total merger that most people only dream about. This is the way it is done on subtler planes of consciousness.

It is helpful to sit calmly before making love and see not only your bodies turning into a blinding radiance, but your immediate environment as well. With your mind's eye, see the entire room and everything in it turning into bright light. When you feel your surroundings have turned into light, it is actually much easier then—you are going from the outside in—to turn your bodies into light. The ancient teachings are clear on this: the light is one, the light is love, the light is you.

When you make love, feel that with each breath the light intensifies, expands and brightens. You can make love in any style you wish, but it is best to go slowly, saturating each movement and sensation with the light, feeling its healing and blissful touch. An affirmation such as "I am light, love and bliss" may add, but if you are lost in the contemplation of light, you will not need it. Some people like to think of the light as coming from their heart or third eye.

Love Your Consort As Yourself   This is one of the most powerful techniques of the Tantric repertoire. Imagine that when you touch them it is actually them touching you. In other words, become them and be the receiver of your own touch. Experience kissing, the contact between your sex organs and bedroom eye language as well as caresses from this point of view.

This may sound complicated or silly, but this viewpoint is a very quick way to get into a deep state of psychic communion. It is usually best to keep your movements slow and deliberate, at least at first.

There are two ways to approach this. Quickly, while making love—your lovemaking can be very dynamic, very passionate—quickly, in an instant, switch and become your partner. Do this without thinking or rationalizing—if you think about it, either you will hesitate and not do it at all or do it only partly and miss the effect.

Do it in an instant, just make the jump and be them, feeling their sensations, including their penis or vagina. Be aware specifically of what it feels like for them to have your sex organ around or in their sex organ. It is a most intense, absolutely enthralling experience.

In the second approach, which is perhaps more difficult, you melt with them gradually and then, on some prearranged signal, you turn around within, and make love to yourself but from their vantage point.

The key here is to emphasize feeling without thinking. There is no "how" to doing it. Once you do it, though, you will realize a great truth—that you are them and they you—one of the most ancient keys to ecstasy.

Make A Good Impression   Imagine as you are making love that your fingers or emanations of energy from your fingers are going deep inside their body. Imagine that every contact penetrates deep into their flesh, perhaps even into their bone marrow, or even into their essence. If you wish to give a color to this projection, white, blue or rose are good.

Strive to feel that their touch and other tactile contacts penetrate very deeply into your body. Even if they are not doing the technique with you, you can imagine this for yourself. When practicing this alone, you can touch your own body in this way. Use the technique all over the body, not just on the genitals.

See What You Want In Bed

A good friend of ours is an excellent visualizer. She found that by focusing in her third eye before making love, by placing her attention on the mental television screen at the front of her brain, she could get her lover to do things he ordinarily does not do.

Although this raises questions of using the power of the mind to control others, it must be pointed out that all of these things were healthy and positive in nature. She did not want him to do anything cruel or humiliating.

On several occasions, she mentally rehearsed scenarios of things he would do that in the past he had refused to do for her. She wanted to have these pleasurable experiences and did not want to have to go to somebody else for them. She did this in a deep state of concentration just before seeing him while still over at her place.

When she saw him later that night at his house, they made love. Amazingly, he proceeded to do exactly what she had imagined movement by movement. And she never said a word to him!

PEACEFUL POSITIONS

Lovemaking can be made more fulfilling by taking time out to appreciate what it is that the two of you are doing. Stop moving and just hang out together. Take in all the sight, sound, smell, taste and touch sensations. Relax and allow your tender feelings to take root and blossom.

It is good to have several alternatives to the standard, male-dominant missionary position in your repertoire. Side-by-side and woman above positions suggest physical and psychological equality as well as providing comfort for long periods of time.

These positions are suitable for soft style, yin, Tantric lovemaking (see *Nights Of Tantra*). They can be transition poses between more active or tension producing poses. They can be enjoyed as a passive way to warm up to each other or as a way to share the afterglow that follows climax.

These peaceful positions are outward symbols of an inner peace and contentment. What you are looking for, be it in sex or success or self-knowledge, you already have. By outwardly assuming a peaceful position, you encourage an inward peaceful position or attitude. Motionlessness has the

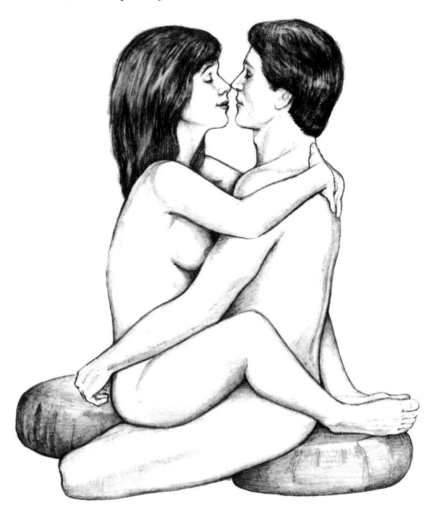

YABYUM *above*
We find that Zafus—Zen
meditation pillows—are
good for sex meditation.

psychological effect of slowing down the mind, reducing anxiety, thought activity and stress.

Each position is a sophisticated form of frozen body language, an hieroglyph of flesh. If you spend enough time with different positions, you will experience how each one has its own unique effect on the two of you and may even serve as a doorway to the mysteries of the deep mind (see *Full Stop, Stay Together, Tension Positions*).

Peaceful positions encourage a mood of mutual surrender. Surrender is perhaps a controversial, even scary word. But there is a joy to surrender that must not be missed. Surrender means the fighting is over. Peace prevails. You give in. You implode (rather than explode). You make room for a new fullness. You become the empty cup. Now you can be completely full-filled.

The key peaceful positions are Scissors, YabYum, Carriage and Seesaw (the "X" position). Scissors is illustrated in *Bio-Electric Sex*. Carriage and Seesaw are shown in *Soaking*.

To achieve Scissors, the man lies on his side and the woman raises her inner leg. For example, if he is on his left side, she raises her right leg.

YabYum is easy to reach from woman above positions provided she is facing him. Another way to achieve YabYum is to start out in missionary. Then, embracing each other, he pulls both up into a sitting position.

An effortless way to achieve Seesaw is to get into Yab-Yum and fall back away from each other.

To do the Carriage, she lies on her back and lifts both legs as he enters.

You will find illustrations of other peaceful positions in these sections: *Charge Up, Complete Circuits, Soaking, Stay Together, Creative Sex, Extrasensory Sex, Kabbazah Sex* and *Fusion Breath Sex.*

SOAKING

Lingam–yoni soaking is a deeply sensitizing practice taught by Tantra expert Sundar, which we elaborated. We prefer to use the Sanskrit for penis and vagina, which are, respectively, *lingam* and *yoni.* Using the Sanskrit names lends a certain elegance and mystery, which is certainly in place here.

Soaking starts as a visualization practice but quickly goes beyond that. The whole-body Tantric orgasm can be attained from this alone, far more easily than you may think. At any rate, you will quickly learn the difference between what Sundar calls inner sex and outer sex. It is important that you begin in a comfortable position that you can hold for awhile, such as Scissors, Carriage, Seesaw or YabYum.

The principle behind it is simple enough. The opening in the man that corresponds energetically to the yoni is the urethral opening at the top of the lingam. Just as the sensitive clitoris of the woman is at the top and forward, so is the highly responsive crown or glans of the lingam. Likewise, while the G spot of the woman rests down and inside, so does the prostate, its erotic equivalent, in the man.

Lingam–Yoni Exchange

There are three steps. In the first step, the lingam rests on the yoni so that the opening at the head of the lingam faces the clitoris. Then, instead of the usual sequence of events, where the man seeks to penetrate the woman with his energy, the couple performs the opposite. The man seeks to experience a yoni-like feeling in and through the opening at the top of his lingam, allowing his inner female (anima, in Jungian terms) to open and flower. He allows the feeling of space within the lingam to become greater and greater. He may feel this deep down in his body into the root of the penis, the prostate and beyond.

Similarly, the woman allows her clitoris to become and feel more and more like a lingam, erect, proud, powerful and pulsating, gushing forth masculine energy. She feels permission to have a hard, rock solid erection there that actually feels like it grows out of her body and stands tall—just like a fully aroused lingam. She can feel it literally emitting, as the lingam does as it ejaculates. Relax into this experience for awhile.

Polarity Switch   Now for step two. Gently, the lingam enters the yoni. Continue the contemplation, the man feeling that his lingam has become a yoni, the woman feeling that her yoni has become a lingam. Gradually, this will be what you actually experience.

He will begin to feel that he has a very deep, yet full yoni.

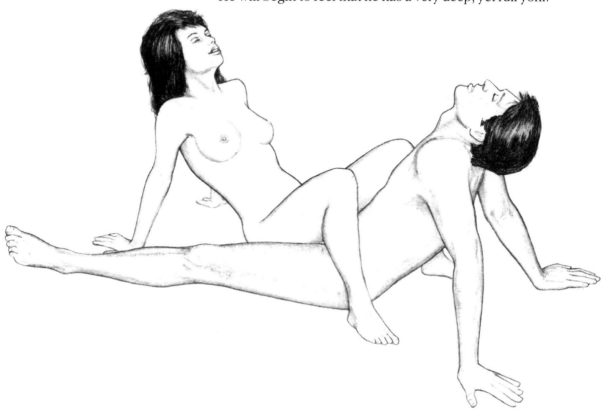

She will begin to feel that she has a very long, thick, powerful lingam.

As the process continues, a switching of polarity begins to take place. For the first time, perhaps, she can feel her male energy being accepted by a man. He, likewise, is experiencing being fed by a woman in a new way, for now he is so concentrated on feeling in a literal, physical way the receptivity of the yoni.

This technique works surprisingly well because the man is very comfortable focusing on his lingam. While it is conventional wisdom to say "Open from your heart," in fact this is not always the best way for the man. Therefore, we say try opening from the lingam. Use the natural opening at the crown to draw in energy rather than to just emit energy. Likewise, the woman will feel accepted and touched, appreciated and respected, at a new level.

Once in the yoni, the lingam has two places it can be. It can rest just inside, so that it is still at the mouth of the yoni. From there it can receive the emanations of the G spot. Or it can go in more deeply so that it is fully surrounded by the yoni.

Deep Soaking

Now for step three, the soaking proper. You can continue your union with the visualization developed in step two or switch to the imagery suggested below.

Many of us tend to think in a vague way that the lingam and the yoni are the two points of contact. The male, in particular, seeks to prove to himself the fact of the lingam in the yoni. He wants confirmation that he has not lost his lingam back to the woman who, according to Tantric teachings, unconsciously symbolizes his mother.

His tendency is to immediately begin thrusting as if to prove "Yes, I am in here alright. I can feel myself. I have not been swallowed up by the yoni." So it is rare that the couple rests with the lingam inside the yoni to experience what kind of contact there can be without the rubbing in and out. If the man wants this confirmation, he can simply ask his partner to squeeze her yoni around his lingam.

Once you are comfortable, imagine and feel that each organ is now completely sensitive all over. Strive to feel literally a thousand points of scintillating energy contact, eager to give and receive intensely pleasurable energy. It may feel as if each point is a balloon, a mouth, bulging and swelling, contracting and pulsing, each a miniature lingam–yoni exchange channel.

As this soaking process continues and deepens, patterns

SEESAW *overleaf*

CARRIAGE *opposite*

of energy develop within your bodies, much like the circular waves that emanate out from the central contact point between a thrown stone (lingam) and the receptive concavity (yoni) of a pond. A pulsation almost like a musical beat is experienced as the energy fields merge. Effortlessly, this intercoursing of life energies is consciously orchestrated in ecstatic flows within and between and through your bodies. Deep satisfaction is experienced because each has truly intercoursed with the other.

If you don't wish to try the first two steps, but want to go right into step three, that is fine. Some couples, once they hear the explanation, know exactly what to do. They are eager to go immediately into the soaking experience, feeling the merger of bodies as if the man's body is lingam only, the woman's entirely the yoni (or vice versa).

Practice Pointers   This process can be combined with *Kabazzah Sex,* which emphasizes the use of *Pompoir.* In fact, this is a very good training for that style, since a common complaint is that the stimulation is not great enough. For *Kabbazah Sex,* the woman's PC muscle must definitely be strong. However, the male contribution is to increase his sensitivity, as well as his own PC muscle strength, so that even a little stimulation is powerfully felt.

This technique helps considerably and men will find concentrating on opening the lingam a true win/win situa-

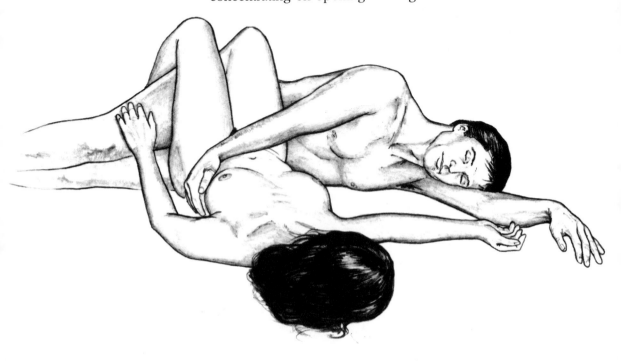

tion, as it enhances sexual pleasure and performance as well. Also, we have found that if women who want to open from their breasts instead of their yoni stay aware of both nipples at the same time, they will experience a deep and very natural opening.

There is another way to be drawn into inner sex. Imagine that the whole body of your partner has become a giant sex organ. The man visualizes his consort as a giant lingam. He clutches her close to him, striving to feel the sensations that such a contact might bring. Likewise, the woman imagines that her consort is now a giant yoni and surrenders to the feelings that brings.

The logic is simple. For outer sex, we approach the partner as opposite. Pay attention during lovemaking and you will see in deeply passionate sex you have become the lingam and the yoni; you have lost your heads and that is why it feels so good. So this technique is very deep, as it uses this identification to invoke non-duality.

SOUND SEX Sounds help to vibrate the body and spread energy, making sexual orgasm easier to achive. Getting into sound making with the whole body awakens and relocates the aroused energy so effectively that it can make male ejaculation effortlessly voluntary. Sounds enable alternative climax experiences, too (see *Make Love With Your Mind*).

Feel what you are doing and then allow that feeling to become a sound. Allow whatever comes out—a moan, a groan, a grunt, a growl, a sigh, a cry, a laugh. Use sound to send energy to your consort as well.

If you overlay a technique of making sounds onto your making love experience, you may miss the point. Some people are noisy in bed. Some are quiet. The quality of the sounds, rather than the quantity, makes them sounds of the whole body.

The impulse of whole-body sounds come from deep inside. The sounds seem to originate as much from your toes and your hair as from your vocal cords. The sounds may seem to appear independent of your will. The kinds of sounds you hear yourself make or kinds of emotions you feel may astonish you. Your experience of the act of making love may change to a startling degree.

The whole body is the human sex instrument. To make the beautiful music of love with that instrument, encourage sounds without forcing them. Perhaps making love, with its sounds, rhythms, full stops, slows, quickenings, crescendos, emotional tones and vibrations is, at some level, literally making music.

You may want to make the loudest, most primal sounds you can as a kind of therapy. It may feel artificial. But it can help you get over some of your inhibitions about making sounds during sex, and so it may be beneficial to you.

Make sounds that express your total feeling of being with your consort, sounds that come from your deeper feelings as well as your genitals. Use your voice to express your desire for oneness.

Ah "Ah" is a very special sound used since ancient times to encourage deep emotional, pleasurable whole body release. Sex therapists Kline-Graber and Graber suggest making the "Ah" sound deep in your throat. Just let it come out. "Ah" is an incredible sound that contains a whole symphony.

Ancient Hindu scriptures state that the sound "Ah" is the womb of the universal mother, which in turn gave birth to the famous "OM" or "AUM" ("Ahh-ooh-ohmm"). Stay with "Ah" for several lovemaking sessions and explore its many subtle variations. Feel it in different parts of your body, especially the chest and genitals. In particular, extend "Ah" as "Ahhh. . . . "

Animal Sounds Animal sounds are fun. Animals generally lack the self-consciousness that so often gets in our way. To feel like a tiger or tigress, sound like one.

Baby Sounds Among the most powerful of sounds are the first sounds we make: usually "Ma, Ma" for men, "Da, Da" for women. Try repeating these primal sounds silently or aloud as you make love. Once the shock wears off, this may become one of your favorite expressions. The phenomenon of moaning either of these during deep orgasm is not uncommon.

Body Stimulators A harder variant of "Ah" is "Uh!", which some prefer for its force. "Ooh" has a more pointed effect. You may find that it seems to emanate from the clitoris or the crown of the penis. "Eeh" seems to increase arousal.

These sounds may at first be most easily explored alone on all fours. Allowing the back to sag, relax the belly and spread the knees wide. As you make these sounds, you will feel an opening in your sex organs and buttocks. You may feel a pleasurable energy move from your belly to your spine and up your back.

Try the sequence "Uh! Ah! Ooh! Eeh!" at first and then play with them until you get the pleasurable wave in your body. Experimentation with this sequence, developed by Dr. A. Harris, shows that it effortlessly moves sound—and thus energy and pleasure—from the belly or sex center up to the head. The sequence works particularly well when you are making love doggie style or when sitting upright in YabYum.

Conservation Chant

A related way to use sound to spread energy through the body and achieve whole-body arousal is the Tantric mantra "Eee Ih Ohh!" Yes, this is the very same sequence of sounds that you hear on the children's song "Old MacDonald Had a Farm." (No, we can't explain the connection.)

The proper way to do this is to first tighten the anal muscles. Breathe in as you do this and imagine energy going up the spine to the center of the head. Use "Eee Ih Ohh!" as you breathe out, releasing the anal muscles at the same time. According to Tantric tradition, this easy mantra removes the energy from the semen or vaginal secretions, spreading it throughout the body and eliminating the threat of losing vital forces. Men who are concerned with losing energy through ejaculation will want to try this one.

Humming

The simple hum of two lips together and then making an expressive sound—a moan, a groan, a sigh—is also special. Let this kind of hum express many different feelings. It may surprise you by spreading over your entire bodymind, creating pleasant tingles in your toes and scalp. The hum can be combined with the Tongue Press, vibrating the brain and skull.

Laughter

Good-natured laughter before, after or even while making love really loosens things up. Of course, nervous laughter will only make matters worse. People do take sex a bit too seriously, don't you think?

Mantras

Some sounds seem to represent or evoke wholeness more than others. For example, you can do your personalized affirmations as if you are talking or you can do them as pure sound. "We Are One," for example, can become "Weeeh Aaahhrrerr Wuuuhhnnnnnggg." Note the extra sounds at the end of each syllable to make them vibrate more.

Eastern holy (wholly) sounds, or mantras, are now well-known. The mutually created harmonious vibrations of the mantra creates harmony in your union.

An excellent way to do mantras together is facing each

other, hands in a prayer position at the chest. This position vibrates the chest, opening the deeper feelings of the *Love Spot* and stimulating the thymus gland. Further resonance is achieved by adding a slight nasalness to your tone.

Mantras can be done before lovemaking begins, as part of for play or during a *Full Stop*. Chant 20 minutes or longer if convenient, but as few as five minutes is enough to open up feelings and harmonize your emotions.

In order to keep the sound going, creating a "surround sound" effect, alternate your breathing so that while one of you is inhaling the other is exhaling and making sound. On the other hand, sounding together and then silence together as you inhale is great, too.

Some of the best mantras are also the simplest. In this category are "Om Mani Padme Hum," "Om Ah Hum" and "Yum." The Tibetan mantra "Om Mani Padme Hum" is correctly pronounced in a variety of ways. These sounds are very old and variations have developed.

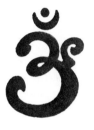

Here is one version you can get started on: "Ohhmmm Muhnee Pahdmay Ho-ummm." A breath is taken between "Muhnee" and "Pahdmay" and the sounds are, of course, prolonged. However, it can also be performed very rapidly with good effect.

We have found that doing this mantra before lovemaking has a very potent calming yet energizing influence, ideal for approaching sexual love as an ecstatic meditation. Naturally, as it means none other than "the jewel in the lotus" it is also an excellent sound for contemplation during sexual union. While the jewel referred to can signify the penis and the lotus the vagina, the mantra also indicates a blissful state of oneness awareness. It is said to create a resonance that touches all levels of consciousness.

If possible, attend a group chanting session where this mantra is being performed to expose yourself to the nuances of pronunciation and creative sound blending. Also, there are records and tapes.

The "Om Ah Hum" is a sequence of sounds that occurs in everyday life. For example, you run into someone after some years of being out of touch. You say "Oh" in surprise. As you tell the person what you are doing, he says "Ah" in agreement. Pleased with seeing you again, he utters a sound of contentment, "Hmmm." These sounds express feelings, needs and affirmations that are natural and universal as well as religious. Intellectual comprehension is not needed.

"Om Ah Hum" can also be sounded in the body in a specific way. Then, in order to really feel the sound driving into the pelvic region, it is good to replace "Hum" with "Hung."

While exhaling, say "Om" thinking of your forehead, "Ah" thinking of your throat or heart and "Hung" thinking of the your center of sexual energy. During the "Hung" clench your PC muscle tight. Repeat several times out loud, then do it for awhile silently to yourself. You can also do it together.

"Om Ah Hum" is a heart mantra as well. To bring the mind down into the heart, conclude by vibrating the "Hum" in the chest instead. This awakens feelings of great love and leads to the self-actualizing experience that "I am" the pure joy of beingness.

Another classic breath meditation mantra is "So-Hum" (or "Hum-So"). "So" (sometimes rendered as "Sah") is the natural sound of your inhalation, "Hum" that of your exhalation. Though simple in concept, "So-Hum" can quickly lead to altered states of consciousness, especially that of being beyond or out of the body. As it tends to induce a "spaced-out" condition, be sure to make full contact with your body afterwards (see *Ground And Store Energy*).

There are several levels of practice. To begin with, just think "So" with the inbreath and "Hum" with the outbreath. The next level is to feel the energy move from the navel up to the throat with "So," and back down with "Hum."

This is followed by focusing on the flow up and down between the root center and the third eye as you explore their intimate connection. Finally, your attention flows from the root center up the spinal cord through the crown center on "So" and back down deep into the root center on "Hum."

If "So" and "Hum" start switching back and forth, do not be concerned. This is a typical experience. Also, your mind may relax and spontaneously drop the mantra, drifting into a peaceful, thought-free state. This, too, is a good sign that the mantra is working.

"So-Hum" is perhaps the most natural mantra of all, for it is the instinctive sound of your own breathing. Since the breath is continuous and automatic, some people find this technique wonderfully effective. "So-Hum" can be practiced before or during Tantric lovemaking. It is said to be most effective when the body is completely still.

Another favorite is "Yum." This is a mantra for opening the deep feeling center at the heart, the *Love Spot*. What is interesting about it is that when you get going fast with "Yum" it turns into "Yummy," the familiar sound of contentment. "Yum" is probably an example of a well-known spontaneous sound that was turned into a technique.

SURRENDER *opposite*
Sometimes, the most special moments happen right after you make love.

Power Sounds Power sounds are grunts, growls, howls and hollers, and emotion-laden percussive words like fuck. Their key feature is gut level response. Two sounds that are noted for their ability to release power from the solar plexus area (the storehouse of vital energy) are "Gah!" and "Kiyai!" Power sounds build arousal and can be used to trigger or intensify orgasm.

Release Sounds Making love can act like therapy, healing the inner child. Buried emotional material may surface. Strong feelings of need, of loneliness and neglect, of fear, may rise up. Allow them to surface and give them a voice. You may discover that this improves your ability to handle stress or to drop undesirable habits as well as making you a more fulfilled lover.

STAIRWAY TO HEAVEN Conventionally, the more active role is assumed by the male partner, the passive role by the female partner. Not only can this be reversed, it can be exchanged. The effect of going back and forth from active to passive can result in what we like to call the Stairway To Heaven (see *Creative Sexual Orgasm*).

The key to this technique is that the passive partner is stimulated to near orgasm by the active partner, then the roles are reversed. Male ejaculation orgasm brings an end to the ascending cycle but female orgasm does not. Stimulation is achieved via your preferred means.

The final climax of the session allows for simultaneous male and female orgasms. Of course, this is only one of several possibilities.

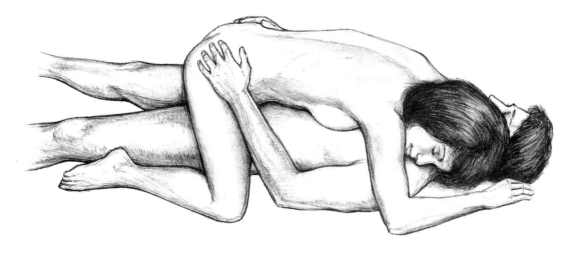

You can also incorporate this give and take into your lovemaking without a particular format or goal in mind. The man may find the experience of being the passive receptive partner a welcome relief. The advantage here is that not only does the female get a chance to be dominant and aggressive, but the male is less threatened by the role reversal by knowing that his turn is next.

STAY TOGETHER   After you have made love, stay together. This is a precious time. Even if one or both of you should fall asleep, you are strengthening the bonds of your intimacy.

Making love is like everything else in life. It takes time to get into it and time to get out of it.

The entree of a gourmet meal is heralded by a great variety of lesser dishes. Following the entree is dessert, coffee and perhaps a liqueur. To arrive just in time for the entree, then bolt it down and leave immediately is simply not proper. But this is precisely what people do at fast food restaurants.

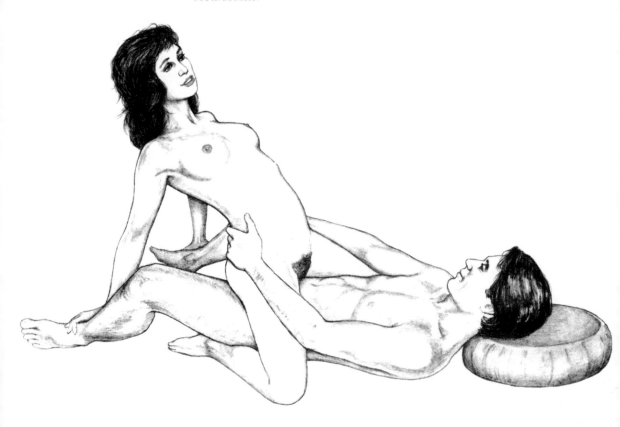

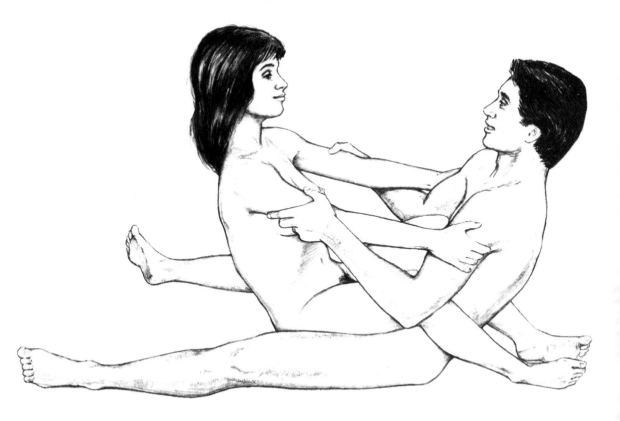

This time that you spend together after making love, still genitally joined, is the dessert, coffee and liqueur. You may argue that the orgasm is the dessert. That may be, but the sweetest part of lovemaking is the sweetness of the hearts that have melted.

We find that the peaceful position Surrender, with her on top and him on his back, is ideal for this tapering off time. His legs may be extended or bent at the knees. She lies on his stomach and chest, her knees bent (see page 245).

Next time you make love, try this cycle. Start with a man above position, switch to a side-by-side position or YabYum or Seesaw, and finish with a woman above position. Feel free to practice your position sequences beforehand. This preparation can become quite light and playful.

Allow at least 10 or 15 minutes, if not 20 or 30. If ejaculation has occurred, keeping genitals connected may be more difficult, especially in a woman above position. If you have had an unusually moving or profound experience, this cooldown time is needed so that your system has time to digest what just happened.

Unless the woman is heavier, a woman above or side-by-

COBRA
opposite

AROUSING SEESAW
above

side position will probably offer the most comfort (see *Bio-Electric Sex*).

Staying together is the ideal time to expand and prolong your genital orgasm. After the initial intense phase, direct the waves of enlivening pleasure, perhaps experienced as a glowing warmth or electrical tingles, throughout your body. These waves will respond to your will, multiplying your pleasure and enhancing the benefits of sexual orgasm.

Of course, if AIDS is a concern and you are using a condom, it is best to separate soon, for when the lingam detumesces it may slide out of the condom. However, you can still hold each other afterwards, focusing on the pleasure waves that continue to course through your bodyminds after orgasm.

TENSION POSITIONS

Tension positions offer a thrill that neither serene *Peaceful Positions* nor dynamic thrusting positions can offer. You may want to hold the position or you may want to move with tantalizing slowness.

Tension positions are designed to be stimulating. After resting in a peaceful position, they can be used to build up arousal while maintaining feelings of closeness and calmness. Another benefit of varying your poses is that energy and attention are drawn away from the sex organs, prolonging intercourse.

Here are some examples.

○ *Cobra:* the female arches back as far as she can (woman above facing man)
○ *Lover's Rack:* man or woman above with all your arms and legs stretched out to the maximum
○ *Penetrator:* male superior with the man pressing powerfully into the woman by pushing against a wall behind him with his feet
○ *Rear Entry:* with both consorts on knees (stimulates G spot for some women)

Some of the *Peaceful Positions* have arousing variations. The Seesaw, for example, offers a delightful active version in which lovers lock hands and wrists and slowly frictionate each other to genital orgasm by seesawing back and forth. It can also be held as a stationary tension position (see illustration on page 247).

The Seesaw is the YabYum unfurled and the transition is

STIMULATING THE G SPOT
below
Make love "doggie style"
or woman on top to
arouse this magic spot.

smooth. In YabYum you can create a feeling of intensity by maintaining eye contact for five or more minutes (see *Pair Bonding And Tuning*).

If you are fairly limber, you will enjoy going into and holding stretches like the Cobra (see illustration on page 246). This may stimulate her clitoris. The male can do the Cobra stretch also. She can push on his chest to increase the stretch. The feeling that goes with doing the Cobra is that you are stretching yourself open wide. The Cobra can be combined with *Elevate Energy*.

Many other yoga-type stretches can be incorporated into lovemaking, combining the sheer physical delight of elegant movement with the erotic fire of your merger. In fact, many of the postures that make up yoga routines can be transferred whole to the bedroom. An example of an advanced position would be woman above and facing away from him as she performs the splits on his prone body. This is only briefly held, of course.

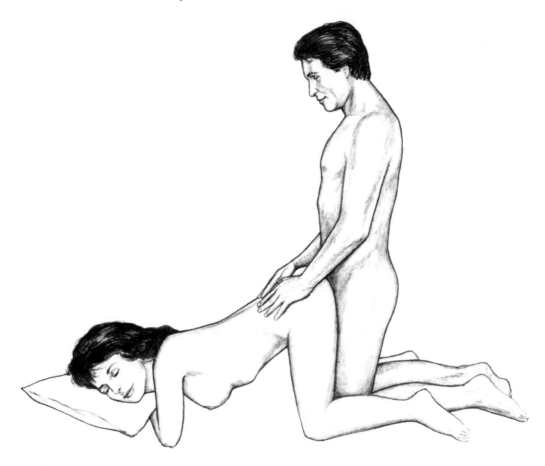

Quite apart from the exotic positions that symbolize yoga to many people is the attitude of yoga, of union. Just as holding, exploring and breathing through tension positions has its place in the yoga class, so it has its rightful role in the bedroom. Just as the physical approach to yoga is called *hatha* yoga, *ha* meaning "sun" and *tha* "moon," so does sexual yoga seek union of masculine and feminine forces. Tension is part of the primordial whole.

Tension positions emphasize forceful physical contact. There are many ways to make this work for you. In your mind, trace the outlines of your bodies together as one unit, quite literally as if the two of you are a permanent yet mobile sculputure in stone. Feel the enormous weight of your finely sculptured forms.

The highest practice is, perhaps, to be completely in tune with the moment, following no preconceived technique. Whatever your approach, the challenge will be to cooperate consciously with the life force, as it has its own intelligence and way of doing things.

When you are able to go with that intense, vibratory ecstasy—tension is concentrated vibration—the results are reliable and remarkable. Ultimately, focusing on bodily tension can result in a deeper awareness of energy, as the way in is either shake convulsively into energetic nothingness or become absolutely heavy and go with gravity to the Source.

Climax

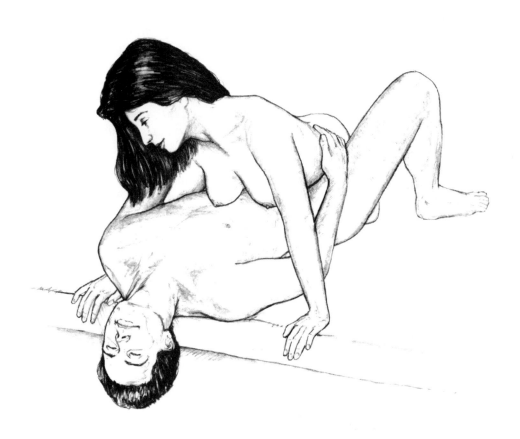

WHERE DO YOU GO?

When you come, where do you go? It is now scientifically established that orgasm is an altered state of consciousness. In other words, orgasm really is a natural high. Some people have reported that at the Peak Of the Peak of an orgasm (POP) that their thoughts stopped completely or that their ego sense of self disappeared.

When you are having an orgasm, especially such an intense orgasm, who are you? What are you? Where are you?

During a moment of no thought, what sex are you? Do you exist?

The moment is, of course, very brief.

But being brief makes it no less real.

We could say that anybody who is having such an intense orgasm, so intense that they really lose themselves in the experience and reach the POP, is a momentary mystic.

Even the crudest sexual relations offer such a possibility for mystical experience, of this mystical moment.

Naturally, most people cover it over as quickly as possible. A moment of no mind can be quite unnerving, especially when you weren't looking for it and haven't been preparing for it.

On the other hand, some people, people who seek this mystical freedom beyond the mind, do cultivate this potential of sexual intercourse in general and of sexual orgasm in particular. Of course, just because people have sex doesn't make them mystics.

Sex is one of the few activities in life which more or less automatically draws us into uninhibited yet fully focused participation. So, the next time you orgasm, ask yourself where you went.

CREATIVE SEX

when you want to make a baby:
procreative sex
when you want to make love:
creative sex

the function of procreative sex is to create babies

the function of creative sex is to create
whatever you want
with the energy that becomes available to you
such as
more harmony and wholeness
better health and better life
or just more fulfilling lovemaking

use the tools in this book to be
a creative couple
not just a couple
choosing
or avoiding
procreation

physical creation
through sexual union
can take many forms
of which a baby
is only one

sexualove healing
of bodies and hearts
can happen too
especially
when you invite the Power of Life
by whatever name you call it
or with wordless feeling
into your union

remember
results can be yours

without doing or believing anything
that runs contrary to
your present understanding

at the time of orgasm
or just before

see in your mind's eye
whatever it is
that your heart desires

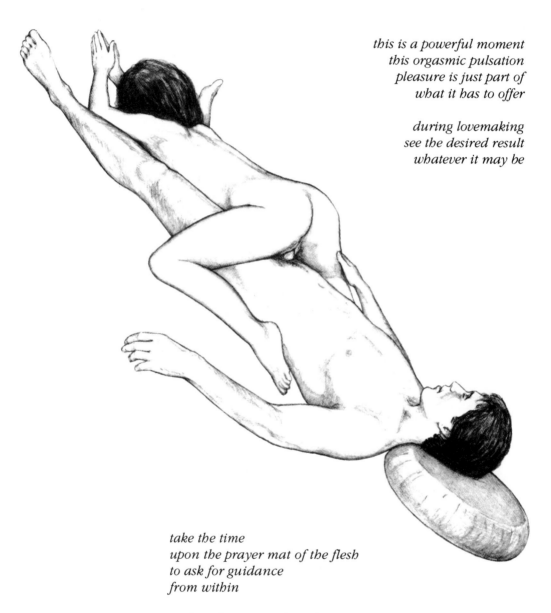

this is a powerful moment
this orgasmic pulsation
pleasure is just part of
what it has to offer

during lovemaking
see the desired result
whatever it may be

take the time
upon the prayer mat of the flesh
to ask for guidance
from within

making love is "making love"
from this basic fact
everything else follows

PEACE OF ASS   *"What I wouldn't give for a piece of ass tonight!"*

The words are right; the usual meaning is wrong.

What good will a piece of a woman's body do for that man?

When she wants to give him a "piece of her mind," he doesn't want that.

He wants her mind whole—a piece of someone's mind can be dangerous.

No, he wants peace of ass.

His orgasm will most likely be short-lived.

Intensely pleasurable yet unenduring, such is the usual orgasm.

How can it be his goal?

The greatest gift of woman to man is her peace.

Peace, contentment, relaxation, release, warmth, well-being, serenity.

Ejaculation orgasm he can have more or less at will.

The sweet serenity of her boudoir, the calm contentment of her ecstatic peaks, the indescribable peace of her ultimate Jade Palace, her sacred open O, her transcendental mouth, her incredible resting place, her temple of flesh that overwhelms the mind of man.

Here he can bathe in the waters of wholeness. The waves of her passion are the caress of an ocean's peaceful depths. The whole of lovemaking can be this ecstatic peace that is depth, absorption, surrender, descent into nature's endless valley of gravity, just like what is meant when we say fall in love.

Still, after man's orgasm, always, comes this peace he seeks.

This is the moment to be awake. Stay with her. Be with her now.

Here is what you were seeking.

The sweet, cool peace, the soothing lotion of love.

Look in her eyes. It is there. Even if she has learned to hide it, it is still there. It is there.

Peace of ass.

PRAYER MAT OF THE FLESH
opposite
If the body is a temple, then
making love is a prayer.

VOLUNTARY CREATIVE CLIMAX

The word climax has its origin in the Greek *klimax,* meaning "ladder." Climax implies that an ascension has taken place, that you have climbed the ladder of sexual energy to a higher level, towards heaven. The climax to a sexual act can be something other than a conventional sexual orgasm (see *Sexual Energy Ecstasy* and *Tantric Orgasm*).

Including the kind of sexual orgasm that is familiar to you, your perfect climax may range from experiencing wave after wave of ecstastic oneness to falling into a deep and wonderfully restful sleep. Also, there are ways to vary your subjective experience of the conventional orgasm itself.

Climax, whether it is of the kind studied by Masters and Johnson or not, can be a fantastically original and expressive act. Like painting or playing music, creative climaxing is an art. As with any other art form, skill and feeling are both essential. With very little effort, you will have immensely satisfying new experiences. Just a slight change in your concept of sexual climax, based on the approach of this book, may trigger these new experiences.

If you want bigger and better sexual orgasms, the skills in this section will help you do just that as well. Voluntary orgasm skills will make mutual genital orgasm during intercourse more likely.

You have a unique sexual potential which is maximized in a unique way. Become intimate with your erotic organs and with your individualized patterns of sexual response. Pursue peak physical, emotional, mental and spiritual well-being. Strive to fulfill your highest potential as a human being. In this way, you fulfill your highest orgasmic capacity as well.

Be all that you can be and you will understand the place of sexual orgasms in your life. You will be at choice about the sexual orgasm. You will be free to take it or leave it. You will be free to explore and enjoy voluntary creative climaxes, whether it is in the form of sexual orgasm or not. Ultra-intimate ecstasy will be yours.

ANGER AND ORGASM

Is there a relationship between anger and orgasm? It may be that people who find it easy to feel and display anger also tend to be more orgasmic. Difficulty with achieving sexual orgasm may be related to a suppression of the feeling or expression of anger. Perhaps developing a better relationship with anger enhances sexual orgasm for people who already orgasm with ease.

Rage and orgasm are very similar physiologically. When a person goes into an expressive rage, the blood rushes to the organs of expression, such as the face, hands and feet. The voice increases in volume. They may make moaning and groaning sounds. Their face may contort, as the faces of many do when they orgasm.

Some people who are skilled at getting angry acknowledge that it can feel as good as a genital orgasm. Getting angry and expressing it very dramatically may be a socially acceptable way of having an orgasm-type experience in public, a sort of "angergasm."

Maybe hitting a pillow before *Selfloving* or staging a mock argument before making love will enhance your orgasm. Keep it light. At some point, you will probably laugh at yourselves. Expressing anger in this way will liberate energy without hurting anyone.

When stored anger is released, orgasm may become fuller as well as easier. The release of anger liberates energy from the adrenal glands and the solar plexus. The next stop for this invigorating flood of life force is the *Love Spot* and the thymus gland in the chest. From there, a tingling warmth, energization and a feeling of well-being may flow to the rest of the body, the neck, head, hands and feet especially. When orgasm is allowed to expand out and up and down from the erotic organs, more of its healing power is released.

Anger is a beautiful emotion that can accomplish a great deal under the right circumstances. By making anger more consciously a part of your love life, you will be able to use hidden energy for your chosen purposes, including genital orgasm.

CREATIVE ORGASM

Genital orgasm is an opportunity to be creative and inventive. It is a state of both mind and body. You can extend and enhance the conventional orgasm by changing the quality of your participation in it.

A sexual orgasm can add to your growth as a person. It can be a peak experience that will be remembered as one of the most dramatic, rewarding and beautiful moments of your entire life.

You can use your imagination to enhance orgasm apart from being sexually stimulated. Practice remembering the orgasm sensation while relaxing in a sitting or lying down position. Spread the feeling throughout your bodymind with your imagination. Psychological research has shown that

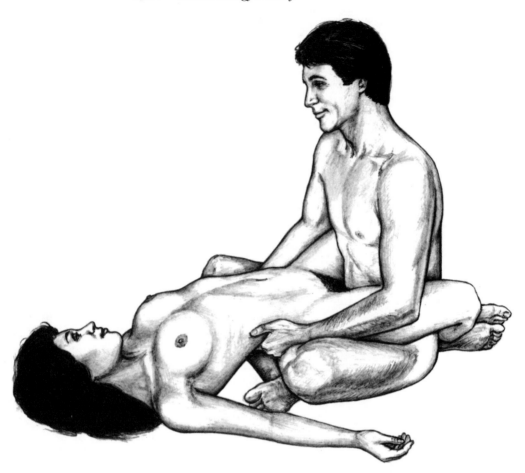

vividly imagining an experience affects the nervous system nearly as much as the actual event.

Here are some powerful techniques that are aimed at changing your state of mind as you enter sexual orgasm. Just as you have eating habits and talking habits, you have genital orgasm habits. With these techniques you will be able to develop new orgasm habits and increase your options for ecstasy.

Affirmation Mentally repeat "We Are One," "I Am You" or similar thought as you enter and ride the orgasm wave. You can agree on and practice ahead of time a oneness thought and image to share at mutual orgasm.

Afterglow As the intensity of your peak fades, encourage the waves of life-giving pleasure to spread through your entire bodymind, filling your chest, your belly, your arms, your legs, your head. Feel the tingling or other pleasant feelings spread to the very top of your head and the tips of your ears, fingers, toes and tailbone. These waves of energy can be imagined in the form of rolling waves of white light or a shimmering golden mist that fills and surrounds you.

Afterglow is one of the best parts of making love. Lie still together for up to 20 minutes before you separate. Some of the most beautiful sensations happen after genital orgasm. Consorts who quickly move into activity tend to miss out on this unexpected bonus.

Bach Flower Remedies

The flower essence remedies developed by the late English physician Edward Bach are experiencing widespread acceptance. The potential sexual benefit of these remedies is great. Holly is said to eliminate suspicion, negativity and helps to open your heart and keep it open. Aspen may be taken for anxiety. Walnut is said to assist supersensitive individuals. These remedies, especially Holly, may be of value in achieving orgasm for the first time, more consistently or more fully.

Crying Release

This is not really a technique, but it is a wonderful thing. Men as well as women may cry as part of having an orgasm. Emotions are being released as the pulse waves of the orgasm loosen up internal blocks. Tears may fall afterwards, too, sometimes many hours later. This is a special sign that the deep feeling core, or heart, is opening, that you have tapped the hidden power.

Dream Come True

Choose a visual image or symbol of something you would like to have in your life, such as a car, a vacation, more love, a higher state of consciousness. Imagine this image rushing out the top of your head on a wave of orgasmic bliss and winging away like a carrier pigeon to do your bidding. Use this technique to bring into your life whatever you like, but not at someone else's expense.

Emotional Climax

If you yield with sufficient sincerity and emotional intensity to your consort, you may experience what we call an "emotional climax." The intensity of your feeling is so great that it eclipses interest in or need for conventional orgasm on that occasion. Even if genital orgasm occurs, it may only be barely noticed as it melts into the larger drama of emotional surrender with the consort.

Expand It

Expand the size of the pleasurable sensations of orgasm with your mind. Make them much bigger. Use your imagination to puff them up like big balloons. You will feel that these

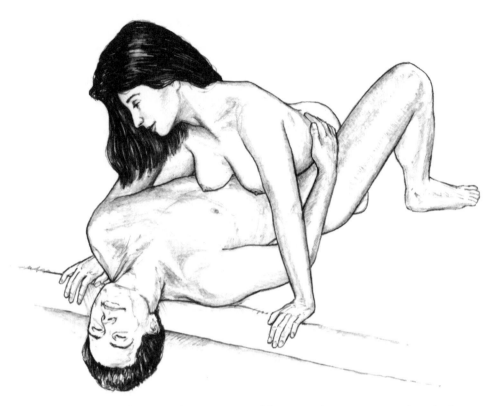

pleasurable sensations fill up much more space than before. The feelings of expansion and spaciousness may seem to extend far beyond your physical body. A related technique is to imagine that the explosion of your orgasm extends far beyond your bodymind to fill up the whole room, perhaps even the whole house, the whole world, the universe.

Eyegasm   Maintain eye contact during sexual orgasm. Orgasm does not have to be mutual. This technique may provide some of your most intimate and thrilling moments.

Flying High   Genital orgasm is often compared to a rocket in flight. Encourage the feeling of flying or going through space that may occur. See if you can go beyond the usual limits of your bodymind space. You may have the experience, for example, of being an eagle circling through the air high above the earth.

Give Your Orgasm   The pleasure of genital orgasm expands when it is given away. Rather than focusing on the pleasurable sensations in your genitals, give the bliss and energy you are feeling to your consort. Completely remove your attention from your

UPSIDE DOWN *opposite*
Go inside and let go.

own pleasure and concentrate on transferring your enjoyment to them. You can do this for each other, which can create a truly amazing climax of blissful unity.

It may help if, as you approach orgasm, you place one palm over their *Love Spot* and one on their head. Identify with them as completely as possible. Become them. Give everything that you are feeling to them as if they literally are you and their bodymind is your bodymind. In religious language, you are blessing them.

Go Fast Yes, go on a fast! Fasting tends to create emotional and physical serenity—and sensitivity. We find that making love while fasting is usually an exceptional experience. Make love in the evening or the following morning after one day without food.

On a one day fast, avoid liquid foods like fruit and vegetable juices as well. Just drink water or herbal tea. Longer fasts intensify the effects. We usually avoid conventional orgasm during a fast, but that does not mean you have to. Please consult your physician or holistic health practitioner before fasting (see *Diet For Sexual Well-Being*).

Hang Your Head Be pleasured to orgasm by your consort as you hang your head over the edge of the bed. This is not just a matter of the blood rushing to your head. This position really facilitates letting go. We especially like it when we want to internalize and go deep within during climax.

Ignorance Is Bliss The next time you are about to have genital orgasm, blank from your mind all thoughts of expectation. Forget everything you learned about what orgasm is or is supposed to be. Approach the orgasm as if you've never had one, as if it is entirely new to you and you have no idea what to expect. If you can, empty your mind of all thought.

Jellogasm If your usual way of enjoying an orgasmic rush is to tense and tighten your bodymind, try the opposite next time. Go completely limp. Become like jello. The orgasm is simply happening. You are not trying to control it in any way. You are just jello. If your usual habit is to go limp, then try tensing your whole body instead. Yet another variation is to make your bodymind completely stiff. Be as rigid as a metal bar.

Let It Go You may find that one ticket to memorable orgasm is to avoid concentrating on the sensations localized in your genitals. Keep your attention on another part of your body, such

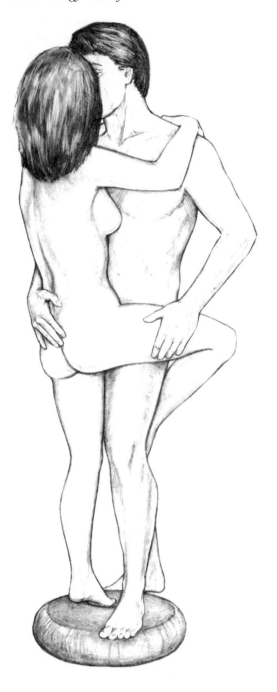

as your *Love Spot,* or the top of your head. This may take
some will power, a lot more, in fact, than you might expect.
In our experience, concentrating exclusively on the genital
sensations during orgasm prevents the spread of energy to
the rest of the body, reducing pleasure and benefits.

Passive   One consort is completely passive and is brought to genital orgasm by the other. The passive consort is given total permission to internalize and use whatever means he or she likes to deepen the experience and eliminate distractions, such as listening to music through headphones, a blindfold, ear plugs, entering a deeply relaxed state or meditation.

Seal The Crown   As your partner approaches orgasm, place the palm of your hand firmly on the top of their head. Cover the indentation towards the back. They should roll their eyes up vigorously and jam their tongue firmly into the roof of the mouth, strongly willing the energy up. They can think of becoming one with an ocean of loving yet impersonal energy. Sealing the crown leads to intense, deep release orgasms with a long afterglow period (up to half an hour) where blissful waves overtake and melt the body. Do this while selfloving, too, for equally stunning results (see *Complete Circuits*).

Sit Up   Sit up in YabYum. This is one of the keys to successful sex meditation, as the energy of the climax is then naturally encouraged to ascend. In general, variations in position create variations in the orgasm experience, although these differences may be subtle.

Stand Up   Stand up in Statues. Or be pleasured to orgasm while standing (in the shower, perhaps). It's fun in the water and you may find you feel closer to nature.

Surrender   Just to think in terms of total surrender makes a difference. Your attitude determines your experience. You experience what you believe in.

Surrender and unzip your body completely to the experience of orgasm. Be willing to let the energy blast open your navel and whistle through your skull. Use the genital orgasm to increase your capacity to feel, understand and enjoy energy. You get what you give.

White Light   Imagine that your body is an open tube and your orgasm is a blinding white light that roars like a river or tidal wave or volcanic eruption or laser beam through your body. Feel the energy rush through the core of your body, entering through the feet in a torrent and pouring out your head, ripping the top of your head right off.

STATUES *opposite*
Standing or sitting up encourages the energy to rise, intensifying bliss.

Or visualize a cosmic sun energy sphere a few feet above your head which you merge into. Try electric blue, solar gold and ruby red light, too (see *Elevate Energy*).

GRAND ORGASM   Even if you like to have sexual orgasm every time, build up the juice before you let it loose. Make the universal tension-relief principle work for you. One of the best ways to guarantee a grand sexual orgasm is to build up plenty of tension, or energy charge, beforehand.

The intercourse strategies of the *Imsak* and *Kabbazah* styles are great for building up that erotic tension. Even if you plan on having a conventional orgasm, try not to think about it. Fool yourself into feeling you have no back door. Then, when sexual orgasm does arrive, it will be fantastic.

You have a pleasure threshold much like you have a pain threshold. The more pleasure you can sustain, the more energy ecstasy you will be able to enjoy. Make a commitment to go past your usual tolerance level.

Sexual orgasm can be planned or be a surprise. Our experience has been that avoiding orgasm on some sessions will make it all the sweeter other times. Reserve the non-orgasm sessions for when you are low energy, working hard or just not in the mood.

Taking a break from having genital orgasms is not self-denying at all. You are just exploring other dimensions of your lovemaking world. When you go back, you can pretty much count on it being a grand orgasm.

One way to get more out of a quicky is to stop and wrench apart from each other as steam is building up for the actual genital union. This can be done before or after he has entered her. Since there is so much drive under these circumstances to get to orgasm, brief dramatic separation has the effect of driving you both crazy. If you stop too long, you could start analyzing, which may flatten your jungle fever beyond repair.

METASEXUAL   Strange de Jim, fascinating being and masseur extraordinary,
ORGASM   is the innovative creator of Metasexual lovemaking. He advises taking a professional level massage course and giving 100 free massages. Then, he claims, you will begin to understand the sensitivity, energy and state of mind that lead to extraordinary lovemaking.

In particular, he recommends two techniques. Remember, though these assignments may seem absurdly out of reach (or just simply absurd), the benefit is less in achieving the goal and more in what you discover on your way there. Treat these rather advanced games like Zen koans, if you like.

Both games are based on both partners becoming extremely still. They are structured so that one partner is active and focused, the other completely relaxed and receptive.

The first game is to turn your partner on so much that they climax from you touching their feet only. Adopt the premise that no part of your partner's body is more personal or sexual than any other. Indeed, out of each and every pore of their skin the same person is looking at you. The best way to explain it, perhaps, is that you listen closely to every nuance of their response as you touch them.

True sex, claims Strange de Jim, is awakening that quiet, exquisite being, not with the body on the outside but inwardly, from the inner to the outer. If you try, it is even more difficult. The climax must arise on its own from out of the silence.

To begin the second game, you, as the active partner, breathe deeply three times. You then put your tongue at their root chakra, that is, on the perineum between the anus and the genitals. This is identical to the Prostate Point of the man. Here is a center of primordial force, emanating powerful vibrations.

With eyes closed, enter the stillness. Encourage the place of connection to grow bigger in your awareness. Let it grow until it becomes your total world.

Look for, sense, taste in your partner that special mood or feeling state that is orgasm. Suck it into your own body using your tongue. Then send it to different places in their body.

Create orgasms in a thumb, an elbow, an eye, a toe, a knee, the brain, the eye, the heart. The most powerful will be at their third eye, the point between the eyebrows. But this will open a door to another reality, so it is to be approached with gravity.

Create orgasms that crackle in a series. Blow their whole body away in one great explosion. Music like Tchaikovsky's *1812 Overture* or Ravel's *Bolero* may be appropriate.

Outrageous? Perhaps. Thought provoking? Definitely. Is it worth trying? Of course.

PEAK EXPERIENCE The concept is sound: we can reprogram our minds during the orgasm because it is a gap, a rift into another dimension, and thus a period of supersensitivity. What if your lover were to affirm in your ear "You are beautiful. You are special. You are a genius."? You would definitely benefit.

Affirmations can be programmed in any subject, not just romance related ones. Health, prosperity, love, confidence, even losing weight. You can silently affirm to yourself at the orgasm breakthrough as well as having your partner talk to you. This may seem awkward at first, but this will soon pass. After all, you are loving yourself in doing this. What better time than climax?

If you are into the affirmation approach to improving self, you will soon discover that peak experience programming leads to rapid imprinting of the positive attitudes you want in your life. Our research suggests that what you say or think at this epochal moment—avoiding the thoughtless, encouraging the caring—will have a more lasting impact than at almost any other time. It is no accident that some people call out "Oh, God!" during an intense climax!

TOTAL ORGASM

Total Orgasm is the title of a classic guide to body awakening by therapist Jack Rosenberg (see *Pelvic Expression*). We want to alert you to a pivotal concept of his: replace your mental picture of your orgasm with real, uncensored, sensory experience of it.

This concept may seem superfluous. Not so. Many of us approach orgasm as an effortful task that we achieve by pushing hard on ourselves. While this seems to enable orgasm, the drawback is that this very act of pushing tends to interfere with the intensity of the orgasm as well as its intrinsic nourishing qualities.

Once it is understood that orgasm is a natural reflex, then we can approach having an orgasm in a different way that allows maximum energization. We can directly know what this orgastic reflex process is like for us individually.

To do this, we need to reawaken sensitivity in the body, especially in the pelvic region. Then the image that we had of the orgasm process, an image usually based largely on speculation, vague theories and the ideas of other people, is replaced by vivid, personal, felt experience.

Now the orgasm is not restricted to just the genitals. We are swept away by a tidal wave. The earth moves beneath our feet. In place of the presumed loss, we have energy; instead of *le petit morte,* the little death, we participate in a greater life.

Furthermore, it is our tidal wave, our earthquake; we need not compare notes with others to know if it was good enough or if we did it right. There is an inner certainty, a

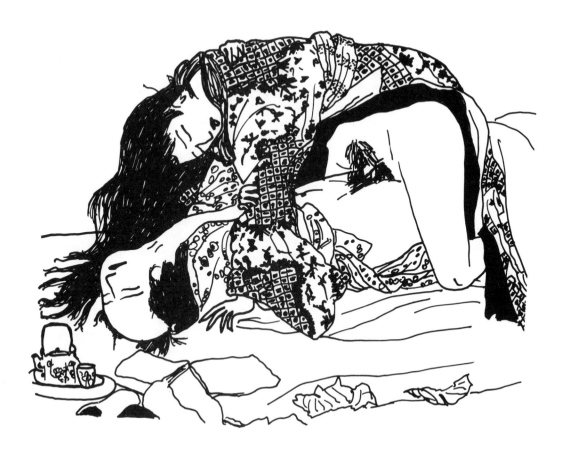

knowingness, a sense of connectedness with our own healing process and deeper self.

One of the best ways to work with total orgasm is to relax totally while your partner pleasures your penis or clitoris. You are completely centered. Your only concern is to fully experience building up to, having and enjoying orgasm, including the delicious states that follow it.

Research indicates that in this way or via *Selfloving* the most intense orgasm possible is achieved. Free to focus within, internal barriers to ecstasy are overcome. Even with AIDS, this kind of deeply erotic loving can be practiced with the appropriate safeguards, such as latex gloves and a water-based lubricant such as Astroglide® or K-Y jelly.

There are schools of Tantra which teach, in effect, that "an orgasm a day keeps the doctor away." As an act of full surrender, of sacrifice, orgasm opens us to the loving energy that surrounds us. While some philosophers have compared this brief, ecstatic giving up of the body to physical death, we like to think of it as a crash course in the fine art of letting go.

TOTAL ORGASM *above*
After a Japanese painted
album by Uemura Shoen.

VOLUNTARY
ORGASM
FOR MEN

The male genital orgasm usually combines ejaculation, pulsations of the prostate gland and contractions of the PC muscle with intensely pleasurable but short-lived sensations. Pleasurable alternative male orgasm experiences do occur and are discussed elsewhere in this book, but so far scientific investigators have concentrated their research on the conventional male genital orgasm.

Ultimately, the orgasm is a gesture of surrender with profound political and spiritual implications. However, men need to explore the deeper levels of their feeling being for this to be actualized. While this journey entails a rediscovery of the inner feminine, it is, nonetheless, a way of renewing an ancient and powerful masculinity that nurtures as it expresses. Paths that encourage this way include Tantra Yoga, Taoism, Shamanism, the men's movement and some contemporary psychospiritual methods. See *Voluntary Orgasm For Women, OTV, Tao Of Sex, Imsak.*

Voluntary
Ejaculation

Voluntary ejaculation is a useful term introduced by Michael Castleman. It replaces the older and less descriptive term ejaculation control. The word control implies a state of tension to many men, when in fact the key to making ejaculation voluntary, to having control, is relaxation. This is true whether you seek to delay or achieve ejaculation.

The purpose of voluntary ejaculation training is to make ejaculation a choice, a voluntary act. This does not mean you no longer can be surprised by the ejaculation orgasm. You can choose that, too. Masculine self-esteem usually gets a boost as ejaculation becomes more voluntary.

An important first step in making ejaculation voluntary is to realize that you do not need to ejaculate every time you have intercourse. If you believe that you must ejaculate every single time, then for you ejaculation is involuntary. To paraphrase Shakespeare's Hamlet, you can enjoy freedom of choice "To ejaculate or not to ejaculate?" Among those that criticize the "every time" belief are Michael Castleman, who was the founding Director of the Men's Reproductive Health Clinic in San Francisco, and prominent sex therapist Bernie Zilbergeld.

A young man attended one of our workshops who delays ejaculation by creating a map of the United States in his mind and mentally visiting each state. Men who try to use mental concentration techniques usually become spectators instead of participants and miss out on a lot of fun and satisfaction. Many times the technique fails anyway.

You can let go and still last as long as you want.

Getting to that place where ejaculation is voluntary is not just a mental activity. It is a bodymind process. Below we look at some of the skills that will help you to maximize your penis power, whatever your individual need.

The Training
You must be ready to work out regularly, daily if possible, for at least a month or two. You may choose Kegel exercises, the male Deer exercise, the Root Lock with the Thunderbolt Gesture. Some kind of regular training program for tuning into and developing the muscles used during sexual intercourse is a must. These muscles are the pubococcygeus (PC) muscle and the muscles of the anus. If you have a sedentary job or drive a great deal, why not do your sexercises then?

The little-known key to making ejaculation totally voluntary is to tune into and develop control over the smooth muscles of the prostatic urethra (the tube that begins at the bladder, passes through the prostate and exits at the tip of the penis). The spasmodic, involuntary contractions of these little-known smooth muscles play a major role in ejaculation. They can be more easily felt if you apply internal pressure by contracting the PC muscle and holding your breath in the lower abdomen (see illustration in *Pleasuring The Lingam*).

The PC-anal and urethral muscles *must* increase in tension and contract for ejaculation to take place. If you learn how to consciously control these muscles, then ejaculation will truly become voluntary. Of course, control includes the ability to achieve and maintain erection as well.

However, achieving this degree of mastery takes a lot of work. Even though you may not be interested in becoming a sexual adept, we wanted you to know this valuable secret.

This technique is the modern equivalent of the advanced *Vajroli Mudra* of ancient Tantric yoga. In that risky practice, which included blowing air into the penis as a training discipline, part of the goal was to learn how to draw ejaculated semen back into the penis.

Though hazardous, the strategy did accomplish a vital function: the internal pressure produced by the air acted as biofeedback to help the yogi identify the smooth muscles of the prostatic urethra. A crude parallel is to sit with a rolled up towel under your perineum. This increases the pressure on the PC muscle and up through to the prostatic urethra above it, enhancing biofeedback of sensations.

Once you are in tune with these muscles and can keep them completely relaxed, this approach is virtually infallible. As pure relaxation is more difficult to apply when on top, try the Push Out if these more complex strategies fail you.

Make an effort to maximize your skills. You probably place lovemaking near the top of your list of favorite activities. How much time did you spend last year learning how to become a better lover? Compare that with how much time you spend improving your job skills or learning how to play a sport better. A little homework and do-it-yourself training will go a long way.

There is another trap, though, and that is to emphasize skill too much. Men already tend to believe that all they need is the right technique at the right time. Just push the right buttons and sexual fulfillment will follow automatically.

You may be a great performer then, a fact some partners will certainly appreciate, but your experience will probably stay on the surface. The depths of pleasure will escape you.

Skill is not at all the only thing that matters. What and how much you are able to feel matters at least as much. The ability to feel—and to express those feelings with a degree of sensitivity—is what being human is all about. There are, in fact, men who are able to feel so deeply and share so much of those deep feelings that women are drawn to them like thirsty desert travelers to an oasis.

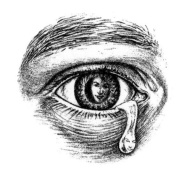

George Leonard illustrates this point beautifully in his book *The End of Sex*. Charles, an old black jazz pianist in the North Beach area of San Francisco, was renowned for his success with women. When asked about his secret, Leonard was astounded to hear Charles reply that he cried. His tears flowed, Charles said, because of their beauty, because it felt so wonderful. Charles said he couldn't help it. He covered their bodies with his tears, and they loved it. No man had ever cried for them before.

If you are already emotionally vulnerable with women, you have probably found that they respect and desire you greatly for it. Emotional vulnerability increases your personal and sexual magnetism. The word vulnerability has a scary sound to it, but in practice it simply means to relax and soften the mind, the emotions, the body. Soft style lovemaking makes vulnerability easier.

On the job, competition is fierce. Vulnerability like that is undesirable. When it is time to make love, it is time to make a shift from invulnerability to vulnerability.

In medieval times, a knight had to take his armor off to make love to his lady. This didn't make him a target. To take your armor off just means that you are willing to be affected by your consort, ready to make love.

Maximum penis power is based on a lot more than emotional vulnerability, though. It is a synergy of many seemingly unrelated factors, including your awareness of your bodymind, general health, diet, drugs, allergies, exercise, hormone levels, energy level, self-suggestion, life stress level and consort chemistry.

Exquisite Ejaculation

Take some time out to experiment with arousal, erection and ejaculation. Probably the most convenient way to become more aware of what is happening within you is *Selfloving*.

Using a lubricant, selflove for at least 20 minutes. Approach orgasm at least three times. You may ejaculate at the conclusion or you may allow your erection to subside.

Do this on several different days. If you do not thoroughly spread the excitement (which, on the whole, seems more difficult for men), then we suggest an orgasm at least every other session. Do it dry, without lubrication, also.

What do you notice happening in your body as you approach orgasm? What is your breathing like? Are you holding your breath? Are you panting? What muscles are you tensing? Are you contracting your pelvic and genital region? These are ways of speeding up ejaculation orgasm.

Men often learn how to achieve orgasm under stressful circumstances. Did you furtively borrow one of your dad's pornographic magazines and masturbate in the bathroom, making no noise in order to avoid being discovered? This is only one pattern out of thousands, but the result is the same. Adolescents learn to achieve ejaculation as quickly as possible, to build up tension rapidly, reach the peak and quickly go over the edge into the relief and pleasure of orgasm.

The high school sex scene probably wasn't much of an improvement. Once again, time seemed short. Having sex in the car meant make it fast. You might get caught. Sex was in short supply and when you got some, you wolfed it down, whether your love object was a real person or a two-dimensional fantasy in a sexual fantasy magazine.

The most valuable step you can take is to develop a detailed knowledge of how you achieve ejaculation orgasm. This means taking it slowly. Be aware of the tendency to rush, the compulsion to get there. Enjoy the preliminaries. Explore the delight of just very mild arousal, the pleasurable feelings that occur long before ejaculation feels inevitable. Though we cannot promise it, this training may double or triple your pleasure at the ejaculation orgasm.

Do this by yourself and/or with your consort's help. Pay special attention to how your breath, your muscles and your thoughts work together to build up arousal and bring on your climax.

Prostate Pointers   Sexual stimulation causes the prostate to swell up with its own juices. At this point, the prostate must be relieved. It can pump itself, or you or your consort can do the pumping manually. When the prostate has reached this stage and begins pumping or emitting on its own, you are approaching ejaculation. Soon the urgency in the prostate for relief will reach a peak, helping to trigger ejaculation orgasm.

Provided you begin doing the pumping for the prostate well before this peak is reached, and pump frequently and firmly, your ejaculation can be delayed indefinitely. If a man's PC and anal muscles are exceptionally strong, he may be able to accomplish the same result by flexing his sexual muscle. In this way, the need for external intervention is eliminated.

The male prostate is a muscular gland the size and shape of a chestnut. It is located at the root of the penis inside the body. It contributes to the pleasure felt during arousal and ejaculation orgasm. The neck of the bladder passes through there.

One side of it can be felt manually through the wall of the anus facing the penis. A physician will do this when performing a prostate examination. Pressure can also be exerted on the prostate through the perineum between the anus and the scrotum. This is the location of the Prostate Point (see illustration in *Pleasuring The Lingam*).

The prostatic fluid secreted by the prostate is the main ingredient found in semen. The prostate performs a mixing function, combining secretions from the epididymis in the testicles and the seminal vesicles with its own. Secretions from Cowper's glands, which lie just in front of the prostate along the urethra, are then added. Together, these four ingredients make up what we call semen.

Ejaculation is a two-stage process. During the first stage, emission, the prostate gland and the seminal vesicles begin contracting and empty their ingredients into the urethra. The second stage is expulsion, the muscular pulsations that move the sperm out of the body, usually accompanied by intensely pleasurable sensations.

Emission and expulsion can be experienced separately without difficulty by selfloving close to the point of no return and then relaxing. The contractions of the prostate and seminal vesicles will be clearly felt. A clear fluid may appear at the end of your penis, part of the emitted substances.

Although the Prostate Point technique has been around for a very long time, it has not been medically tested. It is an experimental technique. You may want to consult with your physician before altering your sexual patterns to incorporate this technique (see *Pleasure, Health And The Anus*).

The technique itself is easy. You or your partner push firmly with one or two fingers up and into the perineum. The correct point is central between the anus and the scrotum just behind the root of the penis. Acupuncture locates a major point (CV One) there. According to Chinese sexology, if the man does it for himself he should use the index and middle fingers of his left hand. Some couples will find this technique easier to apply if the man withdraws briefly.

The push can be a long and firm pressure, accompanied by exhalation. Encourage yourself to feel a sense of relief as you do this. Or the push can be a rhythmic pulsing action. You will probably find it more pleasurable when she applies the pressure and does it for you.

As an added bonus, the manual pressure causes the penis to swell and emboldens the erection, a fact which she will find delightfully noticeable. For this reason alone, her application of the technique in the middle of the heat of lovemaking fits right in. This further reduces the male need for self-conscious controlling in order to delay ejaculation.

What happens to the unejaculated contents of the prostate? According to one Oriental physician, the male body readily recycles the preserved seminal ingredients via lymphatic ducts, which in turn delivers these hormonal treasures to the blood for the service of the whole body.

Rhythmically pushing on the Prostate Point imitates the rhythmic pulsation of the prostate when it is approaching or participating in climax. The method can also be applied directly to the prostate by inserting a lubricated, rubber gloved finger into the anus and pressing towards the penis. In addition to reducing prostate tension and thereby delaying ejaculation, these novel techniques are quite pleasurable provided you are suffcently aroused. The appearance of small amounts of prostatic fluid at the tip of the penis is quite normal and is not a cause for alarm.

For many men, it is pleasurable to have the prostate stimulated via the Prostate Point or directly through the rectal wall. This stimulation tends to delay ejaculation orgasm when the man is not yet close. The stage of excitation and arousal that he enjoys well before he reaches the point of no return is prolonged.

Prostate stimulation can bring on an orgasm if a man is highly aroused. However, it can also extend the orgasm if his partner rhythmically alternates between manual stimulation of the penis and the prostate.

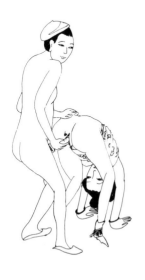

THE DONKEYS OF
LATE SPRING *above*
Ming Dynasty.

If you have not ejaculated in the course of a vigorous lovemaking session or have no intention of doing so, it is common sense that you or your consort employ one of these techniques to reduce the swelling of your prostate gland. Repeated acts of intercourse in which you push yourself to the verge of ejaculation without actually ejaculating, however, may result in a congested prostate, enlarged prostate and/or prostatitis. If, on the other hand, your lovemaking is very leisurely and you are not approaching the point of no return, frequent ejaculation may not be necessary.

The Prostate Point technique is different from *coitus saxonus,* which is advocated by some Eastern sex experts. *Coitus saxonus* is accomplished by pressing on this same point just before ejaculation. The ejaculate is blocked and forced into the bladder.

Although we believe, based on our research, that loss of energy is largely prevented by *coitus saxonus,* we do not agree that the technique is without danger. We believe that it should be used in a clutch by the man who is committed to conserving and recycling his life force (see *Tao Of Sex*) or as a fun experiment to try a few times. It can change the way a man's orgasm feels in some interesting ways.

A "look ma, no hands" version of *coitus saxonus* is what we call semen stopping. This can be performed during intercourse, more easily if you are on your back. Immediately before ejaculation, clench your PC and rectal muscles and hold your breath. You will experience all of the sensations of orgasm with very little if any ejaculation.

This technique is much more dramatic when performed during selfloving because nothing comes out even though you felt the orgasmic sensations. Like *coitus saxonus,* this is an interesting item to play with; however, you can overstress the prostate and other parts of your urinary and genital system doing this. If nothing else, though, semen stopping is a vivid demonstration of the power of the sexual muscles in the man.

Neither *coitus saxonus* nor semen stopping should be used as a means of birth control. Both can be used in a pinch for the conservation-oriented man, but their place is in the early stages of training. They should not be used repeatedly under any circumstances.

The techniques that follow should increase your ability to enjoy intercourse and satisfy your consort. They are not just techniques for achieving and maintaining erection and for making ejaculation more voluntary. They invite your full mental and emotional participation as well.

Breathe Through Your Nose

The man's tendency is to rapidly heat up and explode, not unlike a volcano. The single most effective way to stay cool under pressure is to breathe slowly and deeply and rhythmically through the nose. To make this work you must breathe very deeply and completely and be consistent.

A few deep breaths here and there while making love may help, too, but don't count on that being enough. Some men find this technique is made even more effective by concentrating on extending the exhalation time.

Clove Oil

Apply a very tiny drop of clove oil to the head of the penis is before intercourse and spread it around with your fingers. Avoid the urethral opening. Do not do this just before entering her as you may get clove oil on her genitals. This may not be to her liking, so you should ask first.

You may enjoy the tingling sensation. The mild anesthetic effect may help delay ejaculation. Some men apply Nupercainal® Anesthetic Ointment or similar non-prescription products to achieve this effect. This technique is not a substitute for developing ejaculation control, but it can be a fun variation on occasion.

Condom Sense

Aside from their birth control and safer sex applications, condoms offer the advantage of reducing the stimulation to the penis, delaying ejaculation. Some ultra-thin Japanese imports offer protection with only a slight loss of penile sensitivity. Don't use a petroleum base cream at the same time. Astroglide® or K-Y lubricating jelly are excellent.

Avoid condoms in a packet that is not perfectly sealed. Buy condoms that have the nipple-shaped receptacle at the end. Put the condom on before you go in. It is possible for her to accidentally pull the condom off the penis when she is on top (see *Safer Sex*).

Emotional Detachment

Emotional involvement is certainly stressed in this book, but emotional detachment has its uses, too. The excitement and pleasure that is felt in sexual activity is largely emotional for both sexes. Play with this fact. Be cool, a little detached, a bit flip in your attitude and see what happens. Don't be cold or selfish, just be, well, cool. These seem to be attributes that make some men very sexy. Most of the macho superstars of the movie screen display these qualities in their characters.

Here is one piece of advice that works best in very small doses. Some of the old Chinese schools told the male *Tao Of Sex* aspirant to think of the woman as unattractive, even ugly, to avoid overheating and ejaculating involuntarily.

Enter Soft

This is possibly an obvious one to most readers and it is one of the best. With a little practice and adequate lubrication, be it nature's own or not, entry while completely or partially soft is perfectly feasible. The advantage is you are starting from scratch. The treat for some women is to feel his manhood grow inside. Vegetable oil or Astroglide® on either or both sex organs may ease penetration.

Soft entry may be easier if she lies on her side and he enters her vagina from the rear. The ancient Chinese formula for ejaculation control was "Enter soft, leave hard." Typically, men enter hard. By entering soft instead, time spent achieving erection is time spent stimulating her as well.

Fellatio For Dessert

We would all like to be sexual supermen and first be fellated for half an hour and still be able to give the woman who has just so expertly honored our instrument the best time of her life. Let's be realistic. It all depends on what you want, both together and separately. If what both of you want is for you to last as long as possible inside her, so that you can orgasm together or succeed at *Karezza,* fellatio as dessert or fellatio solo may be necessary. You rarely see fellatio illustrated in the ancient Chinese erotic art for this very reason—it is so arousing for a man.

Fierce Face

Making fierce expressions is one of our personal favorites simply because it is such a crazy thing to do while making love. We inherited it from the old Chinese experts. Make a face that embodies the "Rahrrr" feeling that you may have bottled up inside you during lovemaking.

Yes, go ahead and roar. This roar is not only a tension release but it is also your cry of victory and exultation at taking your woman. You may feel timid the first few times, but most women will love this.

Here is a fierce face. Open your mouth wide, stretch out your tongue like a lion, and bug out and roll up or cross your eyes as you tense your facial muscles. If you've seen the horrific faces of Oriental temple guardian statues then you know what this expression looks like.

The logic behind this action is that the face is one of the areas of the bodymind most under the control of our self-conscious social ego (as in the phrase "to lose face"). It may need loosening up for you to get in touch with the irrational primal powers released in lovemaking. A facial massage before making love has much the same effect. You can make a game out of doing these grimaces alone or together as a way of working out negative emotions before intimacy, too.

Focus Physically Focus on your physical movements with all of your attention. Be aware of your physical position at all times. Focus on your physical sensations fully, especially your sense of touch (see *Making Love Is A Touching Experience*).

Frequent Intercourse Frequent intercourse with or without frequent ejaculation orgasm is helpful. What would be frequent for you is not necessarily frequent for another man, though. The key is to establish a steady rhythm in your sexual relations. To a point, having a routine is beneficial, just as going to work at the same time makes life smoother—but only to a point, of course.

Heavy Belly A heady uprushing sensation can often be felt just before ejaculation takes place. This is just one bit of evidence that ejaculation requires a shift in the direction your personal energy is moving. In an ordinary ejaculation, that direction is first up and then out.

Imagine that your bodymind is a well and you have thrown a small but very heavy stone or iron ball into it. This ball sinks deeper and deeper and deeper into the well of your bodymind. As this ball sinks lower, your attention goes with it. It continues sinking and sinking and sinking. Finally, it hits bottom with a resounding and very solid thud. It is there to stay.

The location of your physical center of gravity is about two inches below the navel. Called *Hara* in the martial arts, this is also the location of the pelvic body mass center point. You may have seen the dolls that are heavy in the base and so can not be knocked over that are popular in Japan. As long as you stay collected at your body's center of gravity, your energy will not move from its place.

A striking similarity between ejaculation and fully expressed anger is that both seem to require this upward energy movement followed by an explosive dispersal of the energy. This can be observed if your physical center of gravity is maintained under these circumstances.

Here is a special breath to help you stay in your center of gravity. When you exhale, pull your lower belly in firmly. The muscles of your stomach will force almost all of your air out, and your inhalation will happen automatically.

Hoo Hop A bit like wild dancing but more structured, here is a fascinating technique developed by Osho Rajneesh. Jump up and down with your hands above your head, breathing deeply as you shout "Hoo!" from your root center.

Make the "Hoo!" sound each time you land. Do this for 10 minutes and go for your second wind, as you may be tempted to stop after a couple of minutes. More than just a crazy thing to do, it balances your energy, maximizing performance and pleasure. Try hopping together, too.

In Deep And Circle In and out again and again is not necessarily the winning thrusting strategy. Put your hands underneath her buttocks. A pillow there may work as well. It helps if you have something to push against with your feet, such as the wall. The clitoris may be more stimulated. You can even grasp her shoulders and pull if this is comfortable for her. Circle and dance with your pelvis. You can also enter without thrusting, pressing your pelvis firmly against her as she does *Pompoir*.

Intensive Exercise One of the best ways to prolong erection and easily control ejaculation during intercourse may be to regularly engage in an exercise program. Cardiovascular exercise is not the only kind of exercise that offers this benefit. Hatha yoga, T'ai Chi, Chi Gung and other soft exercise styles have a similar effect.

Exercise contributes to voluntary ejaculation by releasing mental and sexual tensions, balancing and harmonizing physical energies and burning off toxic accumulations in the system. Pelvic tension, in particular, is burned off or recirculated as energy.

Focused exercise just before making love has also been reported to increase potency and performance. The key does not seem to be any particular kind of exercise. Choose movements that bring you real enjoyment. Concentrate mind in body as you move. Be sure to obtain your physician's consent before embarking on any exercise program.

Perineum Point Here is a concentration technique that successfully delays ejaculation orgasm. It may lead to some unusual and most delightful alternative orgasm experiences. Midway between the anus and scrotum visualize a small red dot. Concentrate on this dot. The Prostate Point is also here.

The root center in men is located just above this point. The equivalent point in women is located at the cervix.

Alternatively, concentrate at the end of your tailbone. Feel the gentle pulsation there as you breathe in and out.

Pull Out That's right, just pull out. Pulling out while the penis is still hard is an effective easy way to reduce ejaculatory urgency and prolong intercourse. Not only that, it can add to the erotic tension, a factor *Imsak* translates into a fine art.

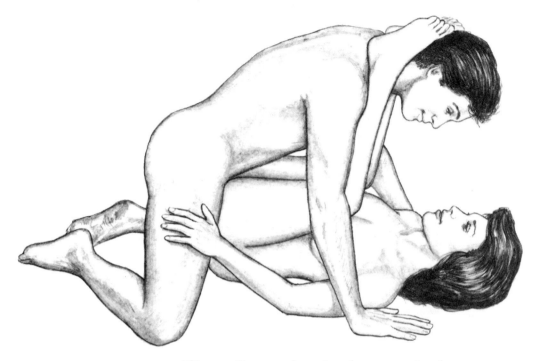

If just pulling out doesn't reduce your ejaculatory urgency enough, apply the Masters and Johnson squeeze technique. She puts her thumb behind the head of your penis and squeezes firmly. In other words, her thumb is at the top of the penis on the side facing your body and her fingers are on the side facing the other way. This can be done with one or two hands.

She needs to do this firmly. Your verbal feedback is helpful if for no other reason than she may think she is hurting you.

This method of pulling out is used if you want to re-enter her. There is an acupressure point on the pubic region immediately above the penis that helps delay ejaculation (see *Aculoving*).

Push Out   During a natural pause when thrusting in or out, or at a *Full Stop,* push down and out as if to have a bowel movement. As the muscles cannot be relaxed and tensed at the same time, this prevents ejaculation. Without straining, exhale or retain the breath to increase the effect.

Well worth mastering, this simple technique brings quick results. It is especially handy when you are on top. Other relaxation techniques can be difficult to apply then due to the muscular effort required by the position. Practice the Push Out as part of your regular PC muscle workout.

HE PUSHES OUT *above*
A young man told us the Push Out technique had made him one of the best lovers in the world.

Relaxed For Loving   It can take hours to prepare a good meal at home so why not take half an hour to prepare for making love? Part of the problem is that taking time to relax just isn't that well understood by our society. Massage, muscle relaxation techniques and meditation are just a few of your options. Hot baths and jacuzzis relax but tend to devitalize, so don't overdo. Follow with a cold shower. In fact, a cold shower or bath by itself just before making love stimulates erotic drive.

The next time you have a chance to vacation a week or two, try a tropical vacation where you do absolutely nothing except lie on your beach chair day after day—and make love night after night (see *Educe Each Other, Spreading*).

Swallow Saliva   This may seem like nonsense but the principle is sound. A man burning up from being in the sun all day will really be helped by a glass of water. Likewise, saliva will help cool a man down in the heat of lovemaking. Swirl the tongue around the mouth to get more saliva. Pressing the tongue against the soft palate will increase saliva flow.

According to tradition, you swallow the saliva in three gulps. It may seem more genteel to reach for your glass of sparkling water with a twist of lemon, but this is not always good form during the pleasurable conflict. Also, recycling saliva is believed to have healing properties. Sharing saliva when you kiss is also said to be good for both of you.

Testicle Tug   For some reason, this feels much more pleasurable when your partner does the tugging. She will want to get a firm grasp and then tug harder than she thinks she should. This helps delay ejaculation because the testicles must elevate close to the body for most men to ejaculate, though this tends to be less true in older men.

Thrusting Sequence   Thrusting sequences put a method in your madness. This stylistic choice has been receiving rave reviews from women for many centuries now, so on that basis alone it is worth trying. What we call Chinese Nines translates in practice to nine shallow–one deep. Three, five and seven shallow is also good. Variations in depth, angle of penetration as well as speed of thrust or withdrawal are also worth exploring.

Mentally divide vaginal depth into three or more levels, such as shallow, middle and deep. The ancient Chinese experts set up eight divisions. The deepest was called, appropriately enough, North Pole. Angle of penetration can be varied on both entry and withdrawal and can be straightforward, diagonal, zigzag and so on (see *Imsak*).

Turtle Stretch   The Turtle is an ancient Chinese health exercise so named because it imitates the craning movement of the turtle as he sticks his head out from his shell. To perform the Turtle, pull out so that you are just barely inside the vagina. Arch your back, stretch your neck, roll your head back and lower the shoulders. Close your eyes and mouth, mentally go within, press the tip of the tongue against the soft palate (the Tongue Press), flare your nostrils and take several complete breaths. Perform the Turtle when you are highly aroused to delay ejaculation. It is said to send energy up to the thymus, thyroid and brain.

A simpler Taoist technique is to suddenly lift your head, pop your eyes wide open and look to the right, left, up and down. At the same time, contract your lower belly. This should help delay ejaculation.

The Taoist sex experts also advised the man to roll his eyes counterclockwise in circles and to click or grind his teeth 24 or 36 times during intercourse to avoid ejaculation. In *The Classic of Immortals* grinding teeth, long exhalations and pressing firmly on the Prostate Point with the index and middle fingers of the left hand are combined for the purpose of returning semen energy to the brain.

These techniques were believed to move the vital force up into the brain and around the bodymind rather than leaving it stuck in the genitals. If nothing else, the novelty of these techniques will distract and entertain you.

Vaginal Veneration   Cunnilingus is an oft-neglected art. Based on current research, women need to be aroused for an average of 20 minutes before they can achieve orgasm, at least during intercourse. Fully arousing her well before you have your ejaculation orgasm may turn out to be more satisfying for you as well.

This may take more time than you would like, but your unselfishness will probably be very amply repaid. Skill with the penis during intercourse is important, but you must be sensitive to her unique needs to satisfy her. Ask her what she would like you to do. Even if she is the assertive type, she may need convincing to believe you want to do this for her.

A simple reliable technique is to very gently and lightly move your tongue or moistened middle finger (use oil or saliva) side to side on the clitoris. The Taoist sex experts rated cunnilingus very highly as they believed that lapping up the woman's "tide of yin" (genital orgasm) added masculine force and healthy years to the lucky male's life (see *Pleasuring The Yoni*).

VOLUNTARY ORGASM FOR WOMEN

Achieving orgasm is a major concern of many women today and rightly so. Some women can achieve orgasm on their own but have difficulty orgasming during intercourse. Below we make some practical suggestions for achieving conventional orgasm more voluntarily which may be new to you. Methods for achieving alternative orgasmic experiences are discussed elsewhere in this book.

The issue of voluntary orgasm cannot be separated from the personal, economic, political and spiritual realities of woman's place in the world today. As individuals, it is important for women to become more assertive and expressive, to develop their own identities apart from the expectations and demands of men and of each other.

As a group, women can support and guide each other, creating an expanding circle of feminine force that benefits not only women, but men and society as a whole. As men and women express more ecstasy and intimacy privately and publicly, the world will become happier, freer and more peaceful (see *Pompoir, Sexercises, Selfloving, Kabbazah*).

Easy Orgasm

There are several excellent guides that focus on achieving orgasm, including *Woman's Orgasm* by Kline-Graber and Graber or *For Yourself* by Lonnie Barbach. Qualified sex therapists are located in your area. The American Association of Sex Educators, Counselors and Therapists publishes a *National Register of Certified Sex Therapists* if you would like assistance (see *Appendix*). Studies show that short-term sex therapy offers a success rate of about 80 percent.

"Know thyself" is the cornerstone of voluntary orgasm. Vaginal self-examination especially can be an important step towards increasing orgasmic capacity. The feminist movement has created a valuable network of services and resources. When you claim your climax, you assert your power.

How Do You Orgasm?

You are probably familiar with the Masters and Johnson four-stage model of human sexual response (excitement, plateau, orgasm and resolution). Valuable though this model is, it leaves out the fact that orgasm is a two-step dance for the nervous system. The part of your nervous system most involved in building up to and delivering orgasm has two divisions, only one of which is usually dominant at any time.

The parasympathetic half of your (involuntary) nervous system is mainly responsible for the excitement and plateau phases. The crucial transition from plateau to orgasm, however, is handled by the sympathetic half. Look at the light switch on your wall. To turn on the light, you must flip that switch. To turn on orgasm, you must flip the switch that moves you from the parasympathetic to the sympathetic.

The sympathetic nervous system handles your fight or flight responses. Anger, stress, survival, aggression and so on are under its management. Though a form of stress and tension like anxiety may interfere with the achievement of orgasm, stress in the form of force or intensity that is under your control is very desirable. Muscular, emotional and mental force applied at just the right time is the hand that flips the light switch and turns on the light of orgasm.

Force at the right moment will trigger the transition from plateau to orgasm. Applied too soon, focusing force will tend to reduce arousal. An example of focusing force is tensing the whole body, especially the muscles around the vagina, and moaning out loud.

Another way to look at the situation is in terms of how soft or hard and how cool or warm you are. The bodymind energy of a woman who is experiencing difficulty achieving orgasm may be too soft and too cool. She may need to toughen up physically, emotionally, mentally and display more energy overall.

A hardening activity such as martial arts, hard (yang) style hatha yoga classes (such as Iyengar style), working out with weights or assertiveness training, preferably taught by a woman, may help release your inner forcefulness and heat. Aerobics classes are good, too. Kegel clenches can be done with the butt tucks.

The additional forcefulness, inner heat and ability to focus mind and will can contribute to sexual arousal and take you over the edge into orgasm. It will make orgasm more voluntary if you already orgasm frequently. Of course, a few women are too hard and too hot and need to soften and cool down. This may be the result of too much smoking and red meat.

Hatha yoga is especially good for maintaining hormonal balance, and may be of special value for the harder, hotter woman who likes intense cardiovascular exercise. Too much of a good thing is still too much. Find the balance between hard and soft, warm and cool that is ideal for you.

Blood plays a major role in making orgasm possible, and your blood flows where your attention goes. Improvement in your ability to focus thought and emotion in your sex organs makes orgasm more voluntary for you. Since the oxygen carried by the blood is also vital for pre-orgasmic buildup and orgasmic release, deep complete breathing in one of its many varieties may be helpful. You can visualize the robust, cherry red, healing blood full of oxygen and erotic feeling rushing to and engorging your sexual organs in the buildup phase.

The PC (pubococcygeus) muscle is the star of the genital orgasm achievement team. Your voluntary contractions help build up arousal to the necessary peak, and will further strengthen them. They bring blood, feeling and energy to the vagina, clitoris and G spot. During genital orgasm, the PC muscle contracts once every .8 seconds. If you want to make your orgasm more voluntary, PC muscle exercises are a must (see *Sexercises*).

Training the PC muscle will eventually give you control over the smooth muscles of the vagina. This is the key to *Pompoir*. Development often leads to stronger physical sensations, intensified arousal and longer, stronger orgasms.

Set up the right conditions and you will orgasm. By paying attention to the sequence of events that leads to orgasm in your bodymind, you learn how to repeat the experience again and again and again.

Orgasm results when excitation builds up sufficiently in the genital and pelvic areas. Orgasm is based on the tension-relief principle: in order to feel relief, you must first experience tension. This is not tension in the sense of stress, of course, but rather the muscular tension of a clenching fist. Allow your clenching genital fist to expand into explosive orgasm.

Some women who are able to achieve orgasm while selfloving have difficulty doing so during intercourse. There are many reasons for this. Sexual scientists are not certain that every woman is able to achieve orgasm during intercourse even under ideal conditions. In several recent surveys, for example, less than half of the women reported having orgasms during intercourse. It is possible that some women who frequently selflove with vibrators have raised their tolerance for erotic stimulation too high for orgasm during intercourse to occur (see *Selfloving)*.

The notion that orgasm must occur with every act of intercourse may be part of the problem. This expectation sets up unrealistic goals that only succeed in creating more undesirable stress. The pursuit of such a goal can take on an obsessive quality, which may take you even further from real total sexual fulfillment.

One of the best ways to be assured of having an orgasm during intercourse is to forget about the whole idea and just get into it as sensuously and feelingly as you can. By being totally in the here and now you may eventually find yourself

CLAIM YOUR CLIMAX
opposite
Rajarani Temple, 12th cent.
It is a spiritual and political act of great power for a woman to assert that she deserves ecstasy.

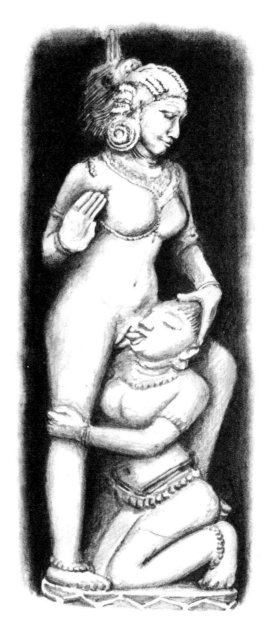

having an orgasm. You are now feeling so good that you couldn't care less if you had one or not. Though the skillful application of force may help you achieve genital orgasm when and how you like it, relaxed bodymind awareness is ultimately the key to voluntary sexual orgasm.

The biggest obstacle our pre-orgasmic clients seem to have is lack of motivation. Claim your climax! Prioritize your pleasure! The ability to achieve orgasm seems to develop naturally as you experience more finely and deeply your personal arousal states, especially those that take you into orgasm. Strive to focus completely on the sensations that you are feeling in your body. Be open to their fiery beauty.

Practice the *Sexercises* described in the beginning of this book. Everything you do to tune and tone your bodymind contributes to your success. Voluntary orgasm is a self-assertive act. Work with your bodymind at least a few times a week, if possible. Relax it, strengthen it, develop it, get to know it better.

What at first may seem like burdensome discipline will become your path to freedom. Behind the issue of voluntary orgasm for women is the issue of fulfilling self-expression for women. You can network now with other women more freely and more extensively than any recent time in herstory.

There really are many beautiful lovemaking climax experiences that are possible which are not genital orgasms. But the first step for you may be to achieve a personal peak of genital orgasm expressiveness that you feel really good about. Then you can ask yourself "What's next? Is there more? Do I have other options for sexual ecstasy?"

As you continue to experiment with your orgasm options, you may begin to enjoy delightful energies during lovemaking and apart from lovemaking that are not connected to the genital trigger at all. By fully exploring the potentials of your genital generator, though, you can get in touch with these blissful, healing energies of the bodymind. You discover wonderful reasons to love and esteem and trust yourself. You become you.

Here are some holistic suggestions that may help you set up the right conditions more easily. You may find this information helpful regardless of the ease with which you currently reach orgasm. Genital orgasm is a combination of physical, mind and heart participation.

Practicing with these techniques will also show you how to delay genital orgasm. You may want to delay it in order to assure mutual orgasm, to build up more charge to get a bigger bang or to store the accumulated energy if your health, energy level or mental attitude are under par. The ability to orchestrate orgasm includes learning how to start, stop, delay, alter, extend and multiply orgasms, all skills which you will acquire as you continue to experiment with the techniques in this book and explore the endless variety of genital orgasms and of climaxes of other kinds. You may want to look at other sections including *Voluntary Orgasm For Men, Diet For Sexual Well-Being, Sexercises, Selfloving.*

Arousal Before Union   The more aroused you are before coitus, the better chance you will have of orgasming when he is inside you. Be verbally specific about what you like. For example, suggest that he massage your vaginal lips and clitoris very gently dry or with cocoa butter. Let him know exactly what feels good, and thank him for it. Also, you don't have to be shy even about stimulating yourself. Some men love to watch and can learn a lot this way.

Suggest that he tease you with his penis at your vaginal entrance for awhile before before entering, long enough to get you asking for more. Also, be willing to do something to relax him first.

You can also use fantasy to get you in the mood. For some women, this is unconscious. They are so turned on with anticipation that they are already warmed up by the time he enters her. Whether they realize it or not, they probably use self-talk, mental pictures and fine attunement to body feelings to generate a state of high arousal.

This kind of arousal can be achieved on purpose by creating the words and pictures and encouraging the body sensations that go with making love and feelings of intense arousal. Since they did not wait for the man to turn them on, many women who become adept at this are able to have orgasm during intercourse frequently. One study indicates that it takes about 20 minutes for these women to achieve the ready state, the same amount of stimulation time that the average woman is said to need before or during intercourse if orgasm is to take place.

Belly Dancing   Belly dancing training develops awareness and strength in many of the muscles vital to full sexual satisfaction. It is a beautiful whole-body exercise approach. If belly dancing is offered in your area, leap at the chance. *Nauli,* a yoga exercise, offers a similar benefit (see *Sexercises*).

Breathing Energetically   Continuous deep energizing breaths during lovemaking can be an enormous help for increasing arousal and bringing on genital orgasm. Hyperventilation will not occur if breath is rhythmic and easy. Open the belly and chest and take in plenty of air, but stay comfortable. Straining and over efforting only delays good results (see *Complete Breath, Inspire Yourself, Co-Inspiration*).

Cervix Point   During intercourse imagine a red dot at the entrance of your cervix or just concentrate your attention in your cervix, which is the location of your root center. This can greatly

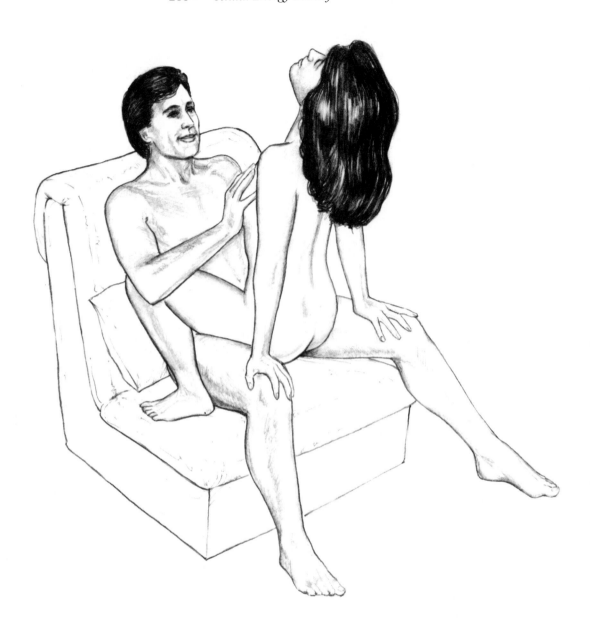

increase the intensity, duration and pleasure of your orgasms. You may also have more alternative climax experiences as a result of intense concentration here.

Crescent Pillow In missionary position, a crescent-shaped pillow under your buttocks affords maximum penetration and stimulates your clitoris. He can place his hands under your buttocks instead, though this tends to limit movement.

Energy Level   Genital orgasm is a release of energy. Your bodymind won't want to release energy if it doesn't have enough to begin with. A surplus of energy ranks with PC muscle training as one of the major secrets of sexual fulfillment. Women are, unfortunately, conditioned from an early age to behave in a subdued fashion. Claim your energy via exercise, nutrition, relaxation, meditation, women's support groups and so on.

Es Sibfahheh   Get on top and face him. This is the position known as *es sibfahheh*, "swimming." The position gets its name from the ease with which the clitoral bud is manually stimulated by you or him and intense arousal is achieved, especially in conjunction with *Pompoir*. This position enables you to control your arousal level with your own movements, too. It may also stimulate your G spot (see *Imsak, Tension Positions*). A pillow under his hips usually adds to the pleasure.

If either of you are uncomfortable with the change, try a little psychology. Tell him "I really want to feel you, to absorb your penis and drink it in. It just feels so good to have you inside me. Go slow and let me savor this excitement of having you inside of me." Most men really enjoy this kind of talk.

Focus on your feelings of containing your man, of completely surrounding him. Don't be concerned about performance. Opening to these feelings takes you to the heights of erotic power and joy.

Another advantage of being on top is the experience of absorbing the penis rather than being "stabbed" by it. Now it is you who *choose* to take him into you. You may feel like you are accepting the whole of him, absorbing the person as well as the penis to which he is attached.

Approached with sensitivity, this position reversal transforms sexual union. Known by the special name *viparita maithuna* (inverted intercourse) and declared by the *Kama Sutra* to be a sacred posture that should be performed rarely in conventional intercourse, it is in itself enough to open the door to the joys of Tantra for some couples. A powerful path for female empowerment, this simple gesture benefits your partner, your relationship and, ultimately, the world.

Free to move back-and-forth and side to side and up and down, to circle with your hips, to squeeze and release with your powerful vaginal muscles, you really will feel like a goddess. Plus there is the added treat of a longer lasting *Shiva* (illustrated on pages 215, 237, 246, 260, 267, 343).

Wild and free, shaking with ecstasy, you are the goddess of love, *Shakti*. The universe is yours to enjoy and explore

SHE LIKES BEING ON TOP
opposite

and—if the mood hits you—to destroy as well! Still, your consort need not fear. You will swiftly rebuild it, bigger and more beautiful than before, for your greatest joy is to create.

You will need his cooperation to explore *es sibfabbeb.* Some relationships cannot handle this demand, for it challenges his commitment. But if this is so, why not let it go?

You are the sacred *devadasi,* the temple prostitute who initiates him into mystical joy. Once again, as in ancient times, your bedroom is the temple. To transform lovemaking in this way helps to heal our planet! Of this, have no doubt.

Speak frankly with him. Show him. Be direct. What you ask is good for both of you. You are not being greedy. You are following the ancient way of the wise women, the way of Mother Nature. You are being a healer and a guide (see *Do It Rite, Kabbazah Sex, Pleasuring The Yoni*).

Female Pleasure 101

You may have to educate your man in the art of *Pleasuring The Yoni*. After all, where is he going to learn? It is certainly not taught in school. Be patient with him and encourage him to ask questions.

Understand that he probably feels inadequate in this area. This almost certainly accounts for any reluctance he may seem to show. As a picture is worth a thousand words, a selfloving demonstration in which you show and tell will probably help immeasureably.

Naturally, after you have had some success with clitoral stimulation to orgasm, you can take on the G spot. The female orgasm can be extended by rhythmically alternating manual stimulation of the clitoris and G spot.

Give your man the benefit of the doubt—he really does want to give you pleasure.

Histamine

The research teams of Pearson and Shaw and Walker and Walker report that the vitamin supplement niacin can assist in achieving and enhancing orgasm. For some women, healthy diet is a decisive factor in sexual fulfillment and prevention of premenstrual stress (see *Diet For Sexual Well-Being*).

Iron

The presence of richly oxygenated blood is essential for orgasm to take place. Adequate iron is needed for blood to carry oxygen. Yet nine out of ten women were found to have iron deficient diets in the first Health and Nutrition Examination Survey mandated by the United States Congress in the early 1970s. Take a minimum of 10 or 15 mg supplemental iron a day to replace the iron you lose during menstruation. Women can exceed 50 mg a day but men should not.

Martial Arts   Aside from increasing power and heat, self-confidence and self-defense skill, martial arts training teaches you how to focus the bodymind for a brief, intense moment, the same skill that is used to go over the edge from pleasurable arousal to resounding orgasm.

Pompoir   This is the key to maximum orgasmic potential. Our society undervalues it and suffers the result but you don't have to. Coordinate PC clenches with inhalation or exhalation, affirmation, visualization and so on (see *Pompoir, Imsak*).

Prostate Point   His Prostate Point is located in the middle of his perineum just in front of his anus. Although he can press the Prostate Point himself, the pleasure for him is increased if you do it for him. The advantage of this easy, unobstrusive technique is you can delay his orgasm considerably without making an issue of it. You can even present it to him simply as something that feels good to men and leave it at that.

Applying pressure there during his orgasm may extend and intensify his experience. This ancient technique has been practiced in China and Middle Eastern countries for centuries. Oriental prostitutes use this technique to guarantee repeat customers (see *Voluntary Orgasm For Men*).

Soft Styles   The soft or Tantric styles and *Pair Bonding And Tuning* skills described in this book may attune the two of you more deeply and sensitively than the more familiar hard style of lovemaking. Many women find that this attunement with their consort is a prerequisite to having an orgasm with him, especially through genital intercourse.

It is easy to get trapped into excessive efforting and block the natural high that is intrinsic to sexual communion. Just settle back in body and mind and the richness that you seek will be yours. You can have the best of both worlds and enjoy ecstasy with intimacy (see *Nights Of Tantra* section).

Wild Woman   A popular theme in today's books, songs and movies is the wild woman. There is an old saying: the ideal woman is an angel in the kitchen and a devil in bed. The great Mae West, a legendary, self-assured and liberated woman, was best noted perhaps for her glorious statement "When I'm good, I'm very good, and when I'm bad, I'm better!"

Be a wonderful, caring, nurturing woman outside of the bedroom, of course. But in the bedroom? In the bedroom, go crazy, go bananas, go nuts, go mad, go for the ultimate, supreme, mind-free ecstasy. Tibetan teachings state that the highest level of orgasm reached by woman is identical to the fully enlightened state. They do not say this about the man.

Lovemaking taps the most primeval—and powerful—forces available to the human race. Lovemaking is an atomic explosion. Allow your wild woman to emerge. Synchronize your erotic awakening via sexercises, meditation on sex energy, *Selfloving* and plenty of lovemaking.

Be willing to take the lead in a sensuous, non-verbal way and be assertive (see *Educe Each Other*). Aggressiveness, by the way, is different. Aggression involves interfering with the other person's space, integrity and freedom of choice and expression. Assertion simply means that you have expressed exactly what it is that you want from that person and that situation. Share this consciousness with your sisters.

However, at stake here is much more than being a little more self-assertive. We are talking about the fate of our beautiful blue planet. At one time, women were worshipped as direct emanations of the Goddess. Sexual union with a woman was considered holy, a profoundly spiritual act. At that time, too, we lived in harmony with our planet, for respect for women and nature flow from the same spring.

It is time to return to this way of balance. Woman must assert her goddesshood, and there is no more direct way than by making love. Abandoning yourself to ecstasy, initiate him into the soft, nurturing way of Tantric love. Let him discover, through your example, the invincible power of living life as a joyful, radiant lover. *Kali Asana,* the position sacred to the Tantric goddess Kali, also called *es sibfahheh,* greatly facilitates this transmission (see page 343).

The *Devi Mahatmyam,* "Glory of the Divine Mother," describes an ancient time when the world was so overrun by demonic forces that the gods would soon be defeated. Combining their forces, they called upon the primordial force of the Divine Mother to protect them and conquer the great demons. Divine Mother appeared and swiftly dispatched the terrible *asuras* who held the gods and worlds captive.

A time of great danger is once again upon us. We must call upon the Goddess to save us from our modern demons, from our self-created path of social and ecological destruction. We call upon you, sweet emanation of the Great Goddess, to draw down your powers and assert your majestic, overwhelming beauty. More than ever, we need you.

Make love. Claim your climax. Abandon yourself to the ecstatic ways of the Earth Mother. Teach the sacred secrets of erotic love. The world needs you now, sweet goddess of peace and love, to be a Wild Woman.

Nights
Of
Tantra

**MAKING LOVE
IS A MODEL
FOR LIVING**

Making love involves both pleasure and pain. A certain amount of pain often accompanies making love, such as bites and nail scratches. Somehow, these usually painful events are experienced as enjoyable.

During sexual intercourse, what was pleasure a moment ago can suddenly become pain, as well as what is ordinarily painful become pleasurable.

The meaning of pain can be transformed. This is shown during sex.

The futility of pleasure is that it will end, just as orgasms do. The reality of pleasure is that it will be transformed.

Pleasure becomes Pain. Pain becomes Pleasure. And then there are neutral states, also.

What has made the pain experienced while making love pleasurable? It is the intensity of the involvement. We are most fully involved at the time, more than almost any other time in our daily lives.

Can it be that a truly maximum participation in this sensory moment has the power to transform pain and extend enjoyment? Can it be that there is a condition of being that is beyond the cycle of pleasure and pain, yet not above or below them, but right there in them?

Making love is a model for living. Live as if you were making love every minute. Make love to this moment, to the car as you drive it, to the book as you read it, to the food as you eat it, to the bed as you sleep in it, to the clothes as you wear them.

Make love with the world and it will make love with you.

NIGHTS OF TANTRA   Tantra, a controversial Sanskrit word with a wealth of definitions, has emerged as the best single term for consciousness-raising sexual activity. For some Hindus and Buddhists, it is a serious religious path. However, Tantra type practices are known around the world. The Chinese, Native American, Polynesian, Egyptian, Scandinavian and African cultures all have their own versions of Tantric sex.

Tantra, of course, is not just about sex. In fact, one review of traditional Tantric scriptures found that only about five percent of the literature associated with Tantric theory and practice actually concerns sex. Nonetheless, Tantra has distinguished itself for all time as the only major religious force that openly emphasizes and works with sexual energy as a powerful vehicle for self-realization.

Tantra is also distinguished by its emphasis on the Goddess, on the Divine Mother. Tantric scriptures are neither vague nor shy in expressing their feelings for the Goddess: "Wherever one sees the feet of woman, one should give worship in one's soul even as to one's guru." "All the women in the world are the parts, the form of the Goddess. Each and every woman literally *is* the Goddess incarnate." "Be ever among women in thought."

These Nights Of Tantra represent the cream of Tantric lovemaking styles from a wide variety of cultures. Approach them in the form and mood that is most natural for you. Tantra is the way of action and experience. Theorizing will prove valueless.

Enjoy these Nights Of Tantra with total commitment. Shiva, the Father of Tantra, advises "Your body will understand long before your mind puts words to it."

Trust your innate intelligence. Seek the inward balance point of pain and pleasure, love and death, ecstasy and serenity, emptiness and infinity.

Sexual energy is the natural high. If you follow it back to its source, you will discover *the* Source.

Trust yourself. Be yourself. Feel free to do whatever you want, to experiment according to your spirit, only do not knowingly or intentionally harm another or interfere with their growth. Love—self-love and loving the other as yourself—is the law of Tantra.

Why Styles?   If the Tantric, soft styles of lovemaking are new to you, be prepared for one of the most exciting and satisfying adventures of your life. Even so, you may find this to be true only after you have broken through the inertia of old habits. There may be a period in the beginning when it all seems like complete nonsense and an utter waste of time. This is to be expected, for our culture does not prepare us to be lovers.

The process is not unlike what author Mary Shivanandan reported happens to couples when they go on a "natural sex" birth control program. This program required up to two weeks of abstinence from sexual intercourse every month. Though they had agreed to the concept in theory, in practice couples often went through stages of confused separation, then anger and finally self-deception before reaching the fulfillment stage.

Don Kramer, a Natural Family Planning Center director, outlined these stages after observing hundreds of couples. He found that men especially have difficulty making the adjustment. Still, the rewards were great for the couple who went all the way.

Many of these couples experienced the fulfillment stage as a profound deepening of their erotic life. The voluntary abstinence period became a blessing as the couple passed beyond the usual dependence on simple physical release into a realm of loving communion. A simple touch, which before may have only meant an invitation to intercourse, now expressed a universe of tender feelings. A kiss became a magical life-giving act.

Mutual respect and commitment grew in the light of this elevated enjoyment. What before seemed like much to give up was now eclipsed by an intimacy so rich some couples felt embarrassed when they recalled their old habits.

Following a natural cycle of indulgence and abstinence, they tapped a mysterious power which enabled them to feel—and this is almost a miracle—those feelings of wonder, glory, excitement and awe that they shared in the very beginning of their relationship. By accident or design, they discovered a universal secret for restoring the virginity of their union. Sexual relations became fresh, exciting, magnetic again.

The way of Sexual Energy Ecstasy makes use of voluntary abstinence and enjoyment, too, but this is just one of the many strategies you learn in the Nights Of Tantra. Sexual Energy Ecstasy is a way to redefine and refine the way we make love so that the reality of sex in our lives becomes a growing source of joy and clarity.

The principles that bring success to the refinement of the sexual drive are universal, as the experience of the "natural sex" practicioners illustrates. Dozens of examples could be given, but what good would that do? What is left is for you to do it.

Based on our own experiences in making the transition, we decided to take this approach of giving instructions for a wide variety of styles. The reasoning is simple. Hard style habits are often so strong that only direct intervention will bring about changes.

It will not be enough to suggest some exercises. Would you do preparatory exercises at home? Possibly not. Or if we say "Breathe deeply, go slowly, feel, really feel your consort," you may think to yourself "So what? Big deal."

We really want you to do it.

Why do we want so much for you to do it? Because it's wonderful, simply wonderful. But you've got to get past the rough terrain at the beginning somehow.

Of course, you can use the techniques and principles of the different styles immediately. For example, you can apply the key to the *Imsak* style—the man pulls out and re-enters several times to build up erotic fervor—right away.

Conservation of the genital orgasm is more likely with soft, yin styles. You may find that Tantric, yin style sexual union without orgasm energizes, uplifts and inspires you. It may bring you and your consort closer together. However, it is very important that you take certain actions if you are having arousal without orgasm. Do *Spreading,* practice deep relaxation, direct the life energy with your attention, share energy with each other. The practice of meditation, prayer or some other method that brings you peace and insight is also good.

If you are without a consort and want to practice these styles, you may want to try *Selfloving* without genital orgasm on occasion. We have found that this can greatly increase personal and sexual magnetism, quickly drawing a suitable consort to you. When you selflove, place attention on the *Love Spot* and draw energy to that area, then the third eye, through the crown and back down to *Hara* for storage. Do *Spreading* of the energy with your hands. Relax and breath deeply during and after each session.

The other side of sexual freedom, of the sexual adventure, is exploring the subjective dimension of lovemaking with each other. You may find that one touch can literally be an explosion of mind-bending textures, a ripeness of sensation that is as overwhelming as an orgasm.

There really are no limits other than the ones we have in our minds.

Recipes For Ecstasy

Reading the styles is a little like reading a cookbook. Each style is a recipe for ecstasy. You don't have to read one recipe after another. Feel free to skip around, as you would in a cookbook. When you find a recipe that you like, then it's time to cook.

We recommend that you follow a recipe for ecstasy to the letter the first few times you try it, since there may be much in it that is new to you. Then play with it, create variations, improvise as you make love. Design new recipes, new styles, that are tailored to your appetite. Here is a quick overview of our recipes for ecstasy.

Sleeping Together   You can make love without making genital contact. This time-honored tradition is said by some to lead to sublime experiences of intimacy, ecstasy and energization. Since the Sleeping Together style does not require genital or even oral contact, it is, perhaps, the ultimate form of safer sex. For celibate persons, it offers energetic intimacy.

Extrasensory Sex   If you unite genitally and then do absolutely nothing for half an hour, the result can be a memorable lovemaking experience of a different kind or at least deep relaxation and energization.

Bio-Electric Sex   You can combine *Extrasensory Sex* and moderately active intercourse in equal amounts and enhance both, especially if you stay in a position that accents consort equality.

War And Peace   One of the secrets for delighting the senses is to alternate between extremes, such as very active and very passive lovemaking, concluding with relaxation and release (unless genital orgasm is preferred).

Magnetic Sex   By massaging each other in specific ways you can reach into each other's biomagnetic energy and relax and energize so much that making love becomes a new experience.

Karezza   The man moves only enough to keep his erection. As heartfelt and energy-giving caresses are shared, a quality of intimacy and aliveness so delightful is enjoyed that many devotees of this style describe it as a spiritual experience.

On The Verge   The moment of being on the verge of orgasm can be made to last much longer with practice, resulting in intense, exotic pleasure.

Tao Of Sex   Assuming the role of a pilot, the man guides the woman through nine stages of arousal until she reaches the fulfillment of total letting go. He delays his climax in favor of multiple almost-ejaculation orgasms.

Ragamaya Tantra A completely original and very imaginative approach to Tantric sex from a contemporary Tantra Master.

Imsak With or without the erotic incentive of vaginal muscle contractions, a strategy for erotic intensification is put into action in which the man withdraws, an affectionate break is enjoyed, he re-enters, another break follows and so on in a rising spiral of erotic fire that ends only by your choice.

Slow Motion By going more slowly than ever before from the very beginning of your love session, you enter a new depth of pleasure and union.

Fusion Breath Sex *Co-Inspiration* is taken to the ultimate degree in these advanced techniques. Complete fusion is the result.

Tantric Ritual Sex Step-by-step the traditional ritual induces a subtle state of mind that is ideal for Tantric sex meditation. Kundalini is safely awakened and the consorts merge into cosmic consciousness.

Kabbazah Sex Development of the circumvaginal muscles enables an extraordinary lovemaking experience in which sexual arousal is created and controlled by the woman alone. Maximum relaxation is artfully combined with maximum arousal, to make Tantric orgasm more likely.

Third Eye Sex Switching attention to the third eye is the top secret of enlightenment through sex and coming "Om."

SLEEPING TOGETHER Is it unmanly or unwomanly to hold each other and just fall asleep together? Do you have to "have sex"?

What is really happening when you "just" sleep with someone?

Although, obviously, not as overwhelming as genital union, a form of "sexual intercourse" is taking place. Mahatma Gandhi, for example, is reported to have slept with several young women—while remaining celibate—to boost his energy level during long protest fasts.

According to the story, Gandhi slept with a young virgin in front of him and one behind him. Whether this story is true or not, the message is clear: bodies asleep in a bed together are sharing, or "intercoursing," life energy.

It is recorded that in eighteenth century Paris, elderly men paid good money to a Madame Janus in the hopes of experiencing rejuvenation by sleeping in exactly this manner with two young women. Is "sleeping together," in other words, a form of very subtle sexual union?

There is a long-standing, quietly suppressed tradition in the West of "just sleeping together." More than 1500 years ago in Europe, some Christian monks were in the habit of sleeping with young Christian women. Although nude caressing, embracing and sleeping together was often all that took place, some of the monks probably also practiced a form of *coitus reservatus* (sexual intercourse without ejaculation). Evidently, this kind of relationship satisfied their need to elevate sex to the level of a sacred act.

This practice of monks enjoying *agapetae* or *virgines subintroductae,* as the young women were called, was eventually stamped out as the organized Church grew in power. Around the twelfth century, a similar practice popped up in Europe.

Young knights offered "courtly love" to women who were not only married but wedded to a nobleman or other male power figure. This was known as a *donnoi* relationship.

Again history is vague as to the details, but in addition to sleeping together in the nude, nude caresses, nude embraces and ravishing the naked noblewoman's body for hours with their eyes, the young knights may have also practiced *coitus reservatus* on occasion or even frequently.

Were these monks and knights torturing themselves and their lovers?

According to their own reports, these relationships fired their imaginations and lifted their psyches to planes of feeling much higher than ordinary sexual relations usually did. In fact, the knight's "courtly love" relationship is probably the predecessor of our contemporary romantic love ideal.

The lyrics of many pop music songs are about some of these very same emotions. What is lacking is the practical knowledge of how to go about maintaining such a high pitch of emotional intensity. A thousand years ago, this may have been common knowledge, transmitted by troubadors (who also practiced a form of *donnoi)* across the Continent.

It would appear that by not getting what you want you can get something even better.

Experiment with features of the *donnoi* arrangement that

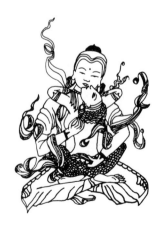

TIBETAN YABYUM
above
Sacred sexuality is a
global tradition.

appeal to you. You may discover it is more fun—and more natural—than you thought. Romantic passion is, after all, a form of creative tension.

As for "sleeping around," the next time you want just to sleep with somebody, why not?

You may discover that the urge we tend to automatically label as the need to "have sex" is in fact a rich bundle of basic needs. Included in this bundle are needs to be touched, held, caressed, cared for, breathed upon, smiled at, and perhaps even to smell each other.

If it would endanger your primary relationship to have sex with someone else, definitely give this idea your consideration. You may discover that a lot of what you are looking for in your exotic encounter is not physical intercourse but intimacy.

Sleeping Together is a wonderful way for two good friends to share a new level of consciousness and closeness without endangering the warm bond of affection they share. People who are celibate can enjoy the richly nourishing joys of energetic intimacy without violating their vows.

Holding each other, cuddling, can be a profound sharing. Some happy harmonious couples share a feeling of oneness or confluence (flowing together) by simply holding and feeling each other for 10 minutes or so. In fact, they may find this is more fulfilling than genital intercourse usually is. Talk about safe sex—we can't imagine it any safer than this!

Some people find that breathing in unison while holding each other brings them closer. Others find this too artificial. You will notice, though, that when the two of you are already in tune you tend to breathe together without trying.

One ancient sexual practice takes this a step further and recommends an hour-long embrace during which man and woman tune into the river of energy moving back and forth between them. This natural flow is already happening. The challenge is mainly in becoming aware of it. Back to back or belly to back contact, instead of the usual embrace, will also do the trick.

By allowing the breath to slow down, by actively imaging this force between and around you, by feeling or sensing internally for this flow, tuning in is achieved. Physical stillness is needed.

Usually, mind and body are prepared for several days in advance by contemplating the beauty and mystery of life. The special event is looked forward to with delight and respect, even awe.

The end result can be a peaceful, luminous ecstasy that

even poetry does not describe. The experience may linger for days, weeks or even months, permanently enhancing the quality of life for both consorts.

This really is an experience that ordinary people have had. The crucial ingredients are patience and a desire to really be with the person.

Whatever you experience, you will soon discover that there's much more to sleeping together and cuddling than keeping each other warm.

EXTRASENSORY SEX

Sexual intercourse is complete when you join genitals. The word coitus is simply the Latin for "meeting." To copulate, according to its roots, means to create a bond or link.

The word intercourse has come to us from the Latin *intercurrere,* "to run between." What is it that could be running between lovers? Life energy, love feelings, bioelectric impulses, hormones and glandular secretions, to name a few good things.

Another word for running back and forth is exchange. Some kind of valuable exchange between lovers is an automatic outcome of genital sexual union. No movement is necessary for "sexual intercourse" or "lovemaking" to be complete.

However, if you believe that the act of uniting genitals without movement is incomplete by itself, then, naturally it will be.

We first heard about "stuffing," a therapeutic technique taught in sexual surrogate training, from a medical doctor who took one of our workshops. The sexual surrogate and the person he or she is working with stuff the man in the woman. Then they watch TV or share some other low stress situation together.

The resemblance between this technique and Extrasensory Sex is on the surface only. Even so, some of the benefits of Extrasensory Sex may take place anyway. This probably accounts for some of stuffing's effectiveness. Though the form hasn't been followed to the letter, stuffing does encourage the most important ingredient of all, relaxation.

The bare bones of the Extrasensory Sex method is that a man and a woman unite genitally in a position that is extremely comfortably for both of them and lie completely still for about 40 minutes (see *Peaceful Positions* for YabYum on chair illustration). In order to get your energies moving, though, we recommend that you *Charge Up* first.

Curiously enough, once the couple are securely united genitally, the penis doesn't slip out. The vagina contracts around the penis, assuring continuous genital union. Also, it isn't necessary for the penis to be buried deep within the vagina. If just the tip of the penis is within the vagina, even if only mere contact between the organs is maintained for 30 to 40 minutes, that will be enough to produce results.

What are we looking for in an experience like this?

You can forget about conventional genital orgasm.

How many times have you come home from work too tired to make love yet wishing you had a way to unite and harmonize with your consort? Extrasensory Sex says unite genitally and fall asleep. The magic of sex is still at work even when you're not.

Extrasensory Sex can be wonderful. Some couples report that they share a beautiful natural high in this way. Lovers may discover that it deepens their feelings of intimacy in a way that hard style lovemaking does not.

Extrasensory Sex is thought to offer a number of practical benefits as well. For example, some people have reported that sexual dysfunctions disappeared, that stormy relationships found peace, and even that health problems vanished after taking up Extrasensory Sex on a regular basis (once a week). It's an exceptional style for a woman in the last trimester of pregnancy.

Extrasensory Sex consists of three simple steps:

○   Unite genitals (*Charge Up* optional)
○   Find comfortable positions, lie back, relax and enjoy
○   Remain motionless for 30 to 40 minutes (or longer)

Practice Pointers   You may want to prepare by taking a cold shower together (yes, cold). Semi-soft and even soft entry are feasible provided lubrication is adequate. To ease insertion, use saliva, vegetable oil or Astroglide®. Other kinds of lubrication may be too greasy or slippery and the penis may slip out.

If full insertion is not feasible or desired, simply place the penis just inside the lips of the vagina. The moist membranes of the two organs will then be in contact. This is all the genital union that is needed.

Do Extrasensory Sex after active lovemaking if you like. If male ejaculation has just occurred, though, the penis may slip out.

It is essential that neither one of you fidget or move. As the senses fatigue and the body image defocuses, you may, for example, experience the sensation that the two of you are one body. But this probably won't happen unless you stay motionless as well as relaxed.

Unconscious movements, such as hand twitches, can distract your consort much more than you. Simply rest your hands on your stomach or on the bed next to you.

Following a suggestion of a Bengali teacher, recorded in Omar Garrison's *Tantra: The Yoga of Sex,* you may want to imagine currents of life energy flowing between you during the long stillness phase. See this flow mostly but not only at the genitals. Also, the teacher recommends an effortless, almost indifferent, reverie state.

However, you may find that any kind of mental activity, visualization included, makes you less able to let go and enjoy the experience. Feelings very new to you may appear. Tuning into and encouraging these new feelings will be more than enough activity. The key is, after all, to relax, let go and allow your natural state of fulfillment to reveal itself.

Extrasensory Sex is a deceptively simple technique. It can be a very powerful experience even though it does not depend on the more familiar genital arousal and orgasm for its results. You may discover that you become very "high" or "spaced out" using this method. If this state is uncomfortable for you, try some of the grounding skills offered in this book (see *Ground And Store Energy*).

Feel free to use Extrasensory Sex, with or without the *Charge Up,* as a prelude to or aftermath of more active lovemaking.

BIO–ELECTRIC SEX

The late Rudolf von Urban, M.D., prominent psychiatrist and Tantric pioneer, devised his own approach to making maximum use of the subtle sexual energies. He made a number of claims for his technique based upon the physical, emotional and mental benefits he observed in his patients who used his "bio-electric" method of intercourse. We will call his method Bio-Electric Sex.

For example, von Urban reported that health problems as diverse as high blood pressure, skin disease and sleeplessness were totally cured in some patients after just a couple of weeks of Bio-Electric Sex. He also reported that the technique was found to be extraordinarily relaxing.

Von Urban writes that some experienced renewal of their marriages. Those who were in love became even more so. Some long-term relationships that had been full of discontent suddenly enjoyed peace.

Some lovers shared a special ecstasy during the Bio-Electric Sex sessions. Von Urban realized that something very valuable and wonderful was taking place. Beyond any immediate personal pleasures a man and woman might experience with this technique, startling benefits were being experienced by some participants that they had not enjoyed with conventional hot, hard style intercourse-to-orgasm.

At some point, von Urban developed a theory to explain these effects. Von Urban had worked out his theory and was prescribing this technique to patients as early as the 1920s in the United States.

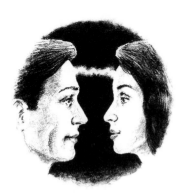

In brief, von Urban's theory was that the cells of the male bodymind and the female bodymind are of opposite electrical polarity. Via prolonged contact of the skin, particularly between the moist areas of the body, i.e., the genitals, the bio-electric quality of the skin changed.

This change in the skin attracted the unique bio-energy in the cells of the male and female forms to the surface, where they could be exchanged, resulting in benefits and perhaps ecstatic experiences.

Today science has confirmed the electromagnetic character of the human bodymind as a whole and of the human skin in particular. Von Urban's notion of male and female electrical cell polarities will remain a mystical non-explanation until it is studied scientifically. However, his intuition that the best scientific explanation of this process would be in terms of human bioelectromagnetism is remarkably contemporary.

Von Urban also explored the issue of contraception from his bio-electric point of view. He believed that barrier contraceptives made of rubber (an electrical insulator) such as diaphragms, cervical caps and condoms, block the energy exchange at the genital juncture. Technically, Von Urban was probably right. But emotional and psychological resistances create much more significant barriers. Your openness and high energy level easily overcome this technical obstacle.

Von Urban gave precise, easy to follow instructions:

Take a shower or bath.

Completely naked, cuddle, kiss and otherwise turn each other on.

Adopt the Scissors position with the man on his left side.

With or without an erection, his penis is placed just inside the outer lips of her vagina.

Lie in this way for at least 30 minutes. Focus intensely on any genital feelings. Keep attention on the exchange of male and female polarized energies taking place at the genitals.

SCISSORS *below*
This peaceful position
is ideal for any style of
soft or Tantric sex.

After the 30 minutes is up, have regular intercourse with genital thrusting but stay in the Scissors position. This should also last for 30 minutes. Male ejaculation is to be avoided. (Note: von Urban said nothing about ejaculation after the second half hour was over.)

Should male ejaculation occur, the couple stays genitally fused for 30 more minutes from that point. This is to insure that the bio-electric interchange between the lovers is complete.

The beauty of von Urban's approach is it proves that knowledge of or belief in Eastern mystical concepts is not a requirement for success with Tantric sex. His emphasis on the practical value of Tantric lovemaking techniques is quite appropriate. The most important thing, as we have tried to say many times in many ways, is to just simply do it. Take the leap of faith and try a technique such as Bio-Electric Sex.

Granted, it is a formula, and that will turn some people off. What we are dealing with here is the art of synchronizing energy. There must be some method to your development, at least in the beginning. Ideally, you will unite in a style such as this—energy, not performance, oriented—at least once or twice a month, perhaps on the new and full moons.

If you analyze or question it, you may never do it. Just take our word for it and try it for three months. That's only six sessions. Based on our experience and the feedback from our students, you should see definite practical benefits, such as greater relationship harmony.

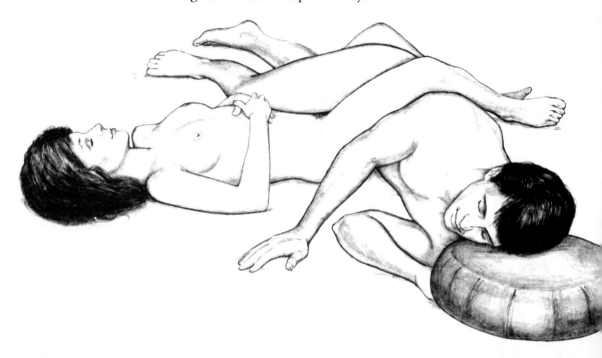

With no more effort or thought on the matter than this, you will see positive changes. Even issues that seem totally unrelated to sex and intimacy, such as finances or health, may improve, as doing Tantra intensifies and balances your energy fields. This is very powerful stuff, and the role your conscious mind plays can be quite minimal.

Tantric sexual loving works in mysterious ways. The deep, inner satisfaction the woman seeks through love is achieved internally by these methods in a way that conventional lovemaking styles, no matter how affectionately performed, rarely match. Paradoxically, some couples find that, regardless of the man's skills as a lover, his most satisfying performance for her takes place when they are genitally united and he does absolutely nothing!

Doing Tantra together is the best way to insure a deep, lasting, faithful relationship. Often, the woman must initiate the Tantric unions, at least at first (she *is* the Goddess, after all). Once he sees the results, though, he will look forward eagerly to the next time. If he is resistant at first, point out that doing Tantra is relaxing and reduces stress.

A writer acquaintance of ours and his wife have followed von Urban's instructions to the letter for many years. Over breakfast one morning, he described their experience with the method as "the Orgasm beyond the orgasm, the High beyond the high."

WAR AND PEACE   The gist of this approach is to alternate stimulation and relaxation in repeated cycles that last a total of about an hour (or two or three) and conclude in a final relaxation which ends in blissful consciousness and/or sleep.

You will be asked to relinquish the familiar and reliable certainty of sexual excitement leading to orgasm for the unfamiliar and unpredictable joys of ultra-intimate polarized communion and other possible benefits.

Remember, though, you always have the option of orgasm. The enormous energy you build up by shifting back and forth between arousal and relaxation virtually guarantees a great orgasm as the grand finale.

This unique approach to building up energy may also provide the necessary ingredients for a woman who has been pre-orgasmic during intercourse to achieve orgasm then. A woman can hold on to her level of arousal during the tranquilizing stages, increasing her momentum with each stimulating stage.

War And Peace gets its name from the repeated cycles of conflict (arousal) and resolution (relaxation). The final and deepest relaxation may take you beyond all dramas of conflict and resolution within and between each other into a wonderful oneness. Certainly, many believe that a power is built up by making love in this way, a power that this final relaxation releases for the healing of body and mind.

Each sub-cycle of War And Peace is like one complete cycle of *Extrasensory Sex*. The arousing phase in War And Peace corresponds to the *Charge Up* phase in *Extrasensory Sex*.

Peaks And Valleys   The purpose of the first arousal phase is to achieve genital union fairly rapidly so that the second phase, relaxation (meditation), can begin.

Just as the first arousal phase of the first cycle is brief (5 to 15 minutes), so is the first relaxation (5 to 15 minutes). It is preferable to keep these two phases on the short side in order to get things rolling. In particular, don't extend the arousal phase or you may never complete your first cycle. It's often a fast track that takes you to orgasm.

After you've completed the first cycle, the time that you spend topping (arousing) and bottoming (relaxing) depends to a large extent on whether you have 45 minutes or two or three hours. Arousal and relaxation phases of not less than five minutes and not more than 20 minutes should be ideal for most couples. However, the final relaxation phase should last at least 30 minutes (as in *Extrasensory Sex*) to allow time for the deepest feeling of communion to take place.

You can discuss these details before you actually make love, since this kind of lovemaking requires real teamwork. We find meditation techniques are quite useful during the relaxation phases (see *Deep Relaxation*).

War   You may want to decide in advance if you want to conclude with orgasm or final relaxation. If you want to conclude with orgasm, you can do so at the peak of your second arousal phase and never complete a second cycle.

You can complete two cycles and follow the third arousal phase with orgasm and not finish a third cycle.

Even though lovemaking during this phase can be quite vigorous, take your time. Go much slower than you do when you have orgasm in mind. Give much attention to the whole of your consort's bodymind.

Be like a king and queen vacationing on a luscious isolated island making love in an elegant open-air boudoir surrounded by swaying palms and painted skies. Your every need is taken care of. All you have is time, time and more time to enjoy each other. Life is a dream of sensuous peace.

Absorb all the sights and smells and sounds, the tastes and caresses and bites and moans. Especially explore the world of touch together. Tantalize each other. Celebrate your senses. Make love in a truly leisurely way, as if there were nothing else in your life but this moment.

You will find that when you are fully in the present with your lover, you have all the time in the world.

Unless you intend to take an arousal phase to sexual orgasm, avoid pushing yourself to your limit. In particular, it's not a good idea for a man to push to *OTV* again and again without concluding in ejaculation. His prostate is a delicate organ which may become inflamed or enlarged as a result of such practices.

After going through several cycles together, a couple usually generates a substantial surplus of energy. The orgasm at this point, particularly if it is consciously directed, will probably not be experienced as an energy drain even by the more sensitive. However, if one or both of you are making love in order to summon and store up vitality, you must avoid sexual orgasm in order to fulfill such a purpose (see *Ground And Store Energy*). Nevertheless, we recommend ejaculation after most vigorous lovemaking sessions to avoid any undue stress on the prostate.

Peace
The duration of the peace-filled phase(s) is completely up to you. In our experience, though, a minimum of five minutes and a maximum of 20 minutes works best in practice. This will allow for several complete cycles even if you have only an hour or less. As beautiful as the journey along the way will be, all is still a preparation for the final relaxation, which will be 30 minutes long or longer.

Follow the guidelines given in the discussion of *Extrasensory Sex*. Penile insertion will offer no difficulty as arousal will be complete.

Bliss
By using the War And Peace format you build up your mutual energy to an invisible and pregnant maximum, which you then fully and sensitively relish during the final relaxation.

The final relaxation, then, is a climax of a different order.

It's best to keep your expectations and ideas about what you may or may not experience to a minimum. Avoid using the experiences of others as your model. The way for you is unique. To follow it, listen to yourself.

Preparations And Positions

People think nothing of spending months and thousands of dollars in preparation for a legal wedding.

Making love in this fashion is a wedding of a different kind. It is a wedding of energies and dreams, of aspirations and evolutions.

A little preparation, at least, is recommended.

Improvise your preparation as the chemistry and the occasion dictate (see *Boudoir Basics, Do It Rite, Erotic Massage*). If you opt for a long encounter of two or three hours, you will find that a repertoire of many positions is optimal. You can practice these ahead of time, just as if you are dancing together.

Tension Positions shows some great arousing positions that need not involve movement. *Peaceful Positions* shows postures that are ideal for the relaxation phase.

Investing in an illustrated manual of positions designed for movement is worthwhile if you find that you are running out of ideas. We like to use variations of hatha yoga poses. Some are rather unadaptable and quite difficult, but we have lots of fun trying!

There is a delight to exploring position variations as a form of non-verbal communication in stillness and tension as well as through movement. We experience a precious satisfaction in exploring and contemplating various two-body postures that do not encourage, much less require, vigorous thrusting. The challenge in many of these tension and peaceful positions is maintaining them conscientiously. Arousal is created through a whole body effort that includes the genital avenue but does not emphasize it.

You have the option of assigning one person the role of leader for the duration of that lovemaking session. This simplifies the transitions, which can be choppy and break the mood.

Another option is practicing your positions and transitions ahead of time. Some people make a dance-like sequence out of several positions that flow easily from one to the next. If this sounds like a lot of work, remember that once you've stored these sequences and transitions they will add to all of your lovemaking. This kind of practice is also a good warm-up for what's ahead.

Your movements are the dance of life. We tend to personalize positions: on top, on the bottom, male-dominant, female-dominant. Consider the Yin-Yang symbol illustrated on page 18. Among other points, it seems to be saying that the interaction of male and female was invented by impersonal, cosmic forces, which we now imitate as we celebrate.

MAGNETIC SEX   Psychologist John Heider, Ph.D., has developed an innovative approach to Tantric loving, which we call Magnetic Sex.

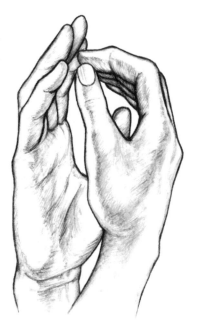

Heider stresses that there are major differences between, in his words, "electric" and "magnetic" sexual intercourse.

In electric intercourse, lovers concentrate on sexual push buttons: the most sensitive part of the penis (the head) and the clitoris. The arousal caused by stimulating these two push buttons increases until the genital orgasm, in the form of a rapid and pleasurable electrical discharge, brings relief.

The exciting electrical style of lovemaking is the most common approach to sexual intercourse in the West. The journey from genital arousal to genital climax can be a short ride and, judging from modern surveys, usually is. Electric push-button sex definitely brings quick impressive results, i.e., the "big bang" of conventional orgasm.

Magnetic intercourse, in contrast, is subtle and energy-oriented. There is no question that it takes more time. Sexual feeling and excitement must permeate the whole bodymind, though the sexual organs still play a major role.

Heider claims that the most magnetic regions of the bodymind are the base of the penis, the perineum (the area that stretches between the anus and the genitals) and the vagina. He believes that when these areas are massaged in a sensitive way, the resulting aliveness can spread throughout the entire bodymind. The lovers will then be truly and deeply touched by each other.

Heider recommends the regular practice of meditation and movement disciplines and/or body work over a period of time to enhance your enjoyment of Magnetic Sex.

Provided the couple is sufficiently in the flow, what can they expect? Heider asserts that the lovers will have the sensation sooner or later of falling backwards or dropping through the air. The feeling of having separate identities then begins to dissolve.

This process of falling or dropping continues until the couple really feel as if they are completely one. Instead of the familiar electric orgasm, they experience sensations that resemble orgasm but roll through them again and again like waves on the ocean.

Heider claims the experience is not only wonderful in itself but also healing and nurturing. He stresses that when the couple finally chooses to end their union, they should do so with extreme slowness. They have built up a powerful energy field together. If suddenly torn, this field could create an unpleasant backlash effect.

In Touch With Space

Here are Heider's simple yet elegant directions. We made a few changes based on our own practice of Magnetic Sex.

Sit and just be with each other for awhile. You may meditate together if you wish. As you sit, make an effort to become aware of and to feel the life energy that fills the space where the two of you are sitting. Try to get a clear sense of what your personal presence or personal space is like. How far from your bodymind does it extend? What color is it or is it transparent? Once you have this sense of your personal space, be it real or imagined, choose to extend it to include your consort and the space surrounding the two of you.

This is only one way to go about it. Another tactic is to simply stretch the tactile sensitivity of your skin slowly out away from your bodymind, as if it were expanding like a big balloon. There are many techniques. What is most important is that the technique you use suits you personally and makes use of your unique talents and inclinations.

Using stroking movements, softly and tenderly caress and massage each other's bodies. We recommend using the flat of the hand, with both the palms and fingers. Feel or imagine life energy filling your hands and perhaps flowing through your hands as you do this.

How do you know how much to do? One good way is to stroke and caress until you feel that more would simply be too much.

Using your hands in the same way execute the same stroking movements only now gently caress and massage the space near your bodies at a distance of two inches. In other words, four open hands slowly sweep over two bodies at a height of two inches above the skin.

You will feel the life energy around you build up and become thick and compacted as a result. The space between and all around your bodyminds will be experienced as being filled with this life energy. The high density of life energy in the air will feel tangible and solid. You will feel with certainty that it is as real as your own flesh.

Union Now you genitally unite. You move only a little or lie motionless. Movements should be only enough to sustain his erection and her natural vaginal lubrication. By staying still in mind and body, breathing and relaxing fully again and again, the genital energy will not build up as tension but instead spread throughout your bodies.

At some point the feeling of falling backwards or dropping through the air occurs. The usual sense of having separate identities begins to dissolve. Eventually your sense of oneness becomes total. The two of you (at the life energy level) have literally become one. Thrilling oceanic wave-like feelings that are like orgasm yet different course through your bodies over and over and over again. This is a classic orgasm of total relaxation, the Tantric orgasm.

Eventually, you disunite, very tenderly, with sensitivity and caution. Avoid suddenly disrupting the powerful energy field you just created.

It can be quite a shock if one of you decides to get up abruptly and leave the scene, even psychologically. Even physically moving apart a little too quickly at this point can feel distressing. Your energy fields are still literally one at this stage. Oneness is oneness, and it makes sense that your separation following such intimacy should not be a casual affair.

KAREZZA Karezza or Carezza, pronounced "kuh-*retz*-zuh," is an Italian word which means "caress." It first appeared in English usage in 1883 in a privately printed book, *Tokology,* written by a pioneering female physician named Alice Bunker Stockham. Her views later appeared in slightly revised form in *Karezza: Ethics Of Marriage.*

So widespread was the excitement this little self-published book generated that it was translated into Russian by the great novelist Leo Tolstoi, and German and Swedish also. Letters of gratitude poured into her office in Chicago.

Many of the letters were variations on a single, exciting theme: now, at long last, husband and wife can celebrate the sexual act as a form of sacred communion.

This lovemaking technique was by no means Stockham's original discovery. But the name she gave it has stuck ever since and appropriately so. The concept and practice of the sexual caress is nowhere more highly developed than in Karezza.

Stockham was not the first American to stumble across

this approach. In fact, she almost certainly owed the essentials of the method to a socioreligious revolutionary by the name of John Humphrey Noyes. Himself the author of a popular pamphlet entitled *Male Continence,* Noyes claimed the technique came right out of the *Holy Bible.*

The Putney, Vermont minister was not the sort of man to just publish a pamphlet or two. In 1846, Noyes founded the famed utopian social experiment that found a place in history, the Oneida Community. This group made the well-known silverware of the same name. The 250 members of the original Community practiced a form of open group marriage Noyes christened "Complex Marriage."

The practice of male continence as described and championed by Noyes supplied the glue which held the radical sexual experiment together. Though Noyes may have first developed the practice as a new birth control measure, he quickly discovered that something new and wonderful was happening for him and his wife. Though the method did offer some birth control advantages for these pre-contraception pioneers, Karezza thrived when it proved to be a technique that promoted exceptional harmony and fulfillment between man and woman.

Holding On To Your Love

The basic prerequisite for Karezza, discovered by Noyes and promoted by Stockham, is the ancient Roman practice of *coitus reservatus.* The value of male continence or retention in lovemaking had been rediscovered.

As none other than Xaviera Hollander points out, continence doesn't mean denial but refers to the ability to contain something. For thousands of years, men and women, but especially men, have believed that containing the forces of Eros within the bodymind tabernacle is a wise and healthy thing to do.

Karezza advocates have developed the art of the loving sexual caress to an impressive degree. Male non-ejaculation simply sets the stage for up to an hour or more of exalted and highly refined interplay between man and woman.

In Karezza, there is no dancing on the brink as in *OTV.* In contrast to the pyrotechnics of that style, a gentle celebration of the very act of sexual communion itself prior to and distinct from the sexual orgasm is enjoyed.

The point is not containment for its own sake. In the words of Karezza master J. William Lloyd, "Try to feel your utter unity with him or her. This is the real ideal and end of Karezza. You will finally enter into such unity that in your fullest embrace you can hardly tell yourselves apart."

J. William Lloyd. *The Karezza Method or Magnetation.* Hollywood: Phoenix House, 1973, page 60.

Science Of
Ecstasy

Though the psychophysiology of human arousal and orgasm has been studied, this remains an area of major mystery to modern science. Briefly, the current understanding is that in the beginning stages of sexual arousal the parasympathetic nervous system is dominant, while in the culminating stages of sexual arousal, i.e., during pre-orgasm and orgasm, the sympathetic nervous system is dominant.

The parasympathetic nervous system is more associated with relaxed and "I feel good" states of bodymind. The sympathetic nervous system is more associated with survival and the "fight-or-flight" reaction.

This description is obviously an oversimplification. The interactions between these two halves of the autonomic (involuntary) nervous system during sexual arousal are far more complex than this. However, these convenient descriptions are accurate enough to make our point: the Karezza practice has a sound biological basis.

As odd as it seems, in order to complete the sexual act through conventional orgasm, consorts must switch over from the pleasant parasympathetic sensations to the stressful sympathetic sensations.

As we interpret the scientific basis for the claims of Noyes and Stockham, what they are saying can be rephrased in this way: "Stay with the parasympathetic arousal in the beginning. Explore and enjoy and celebrate that." Noyes called it the "social" stage of intercourse.

If you don't shift over to sympathetic nervous system dominance, if you don't shift over to the "fight-or-flight" response in which your hearts race and your lungs pant, then it isn't particularly stressful to either of you to delay or avoid genital orgasm.

To Caress You
Is To Bless You

The word caress comes to us from the Latin *carus,* meaning "dear, precious." *Magnetic Sex* uses the sexual caress as a way to condense and dynamize the life energy in the immediate vicinity of the two lovers during the arousal before genital union.

In contrast, Karezza uses the energized hand to send energy, feeling and arousal to the consort during sexual union. Man and woman are conceived of as two halves of a profound battery of life.

The hands, which are in some fundamental way extensions of the heart, of the deep feeling capacity in the core of our bodies, act as mobile contacts for the mutual electricity. The arms extend like wires, the hands offer living, moving, flexible connections.

Many advocates of Karezza conceive of it as a spiritual act and seem to enjoy couching their descriptions of this unique method in religious language.

In their way of Karezza, to caress you is to bless you.

Stockham's Karezza

Being a physician, Stockham was of the opinion that to practice Karezza promoted health and wholeness. In particular, she recommended it in cases of sterility. She definitely believed that a wide variety of beneficial biochemicals, secretions and vital forces were exchanged during a Karezza session.

Stockham was quite specific about how to prepare for a Karezza lovemaking session. A few days or even a week before the Karezza union, the lovers are especially kind in their daily dealings with each other.

During this preparation period, they read to each other uplifting writings and contemplate their meanings. Ralph Waldo Emerson, the noted philosopher, and Elizabeth Barrett Browning, acclaimed author of love poetry, were two authors she recommended.

They meditate on surrendering their individual will to the cosmic will. They seek to lose their individual consciousness in the cosmic consciousness.

She was also quite specific on how to do Karezza.

She recommends an hour of quiet sexual union. Movement is slight. Arousal stays pleasurable and undemanding. The mood is serene and contemplative. Relaxation is total. Genital tension beyond pure and simple arousal is given little opportunity to develop. As a result, the need for orgasm is not experienced and the relief that it offers is not felt to be necessary. When genital friction is light, the need for orgasm is diminished.

She also recommends religious affirmations. A contemporary example is "God Is Love." Or, "We are spiritual beings and this intimacy of our bodies symbolizes the union of our souls." She recommends doing this before and during the Karezza lovemaking session. This is also the time to practice a religious devotion, to pray, if this is your way. She makes it quite clear that both affirmations and devotions are completely optional.

Stockham summarized her approach with these poetic words: "At the appointed time, without fatigue of body or unrest of mind, accompany general bodily contact with expressions of endearment and affection, followed by the complete but quiet union of sexual organs. During a lengthy period of perfect control, the whole being is merged into the

KAREZZA *opposite*
Khajuraho, Parsvanatha Temple, 11th century, India. Success at Karezza requires innocence, not technique.

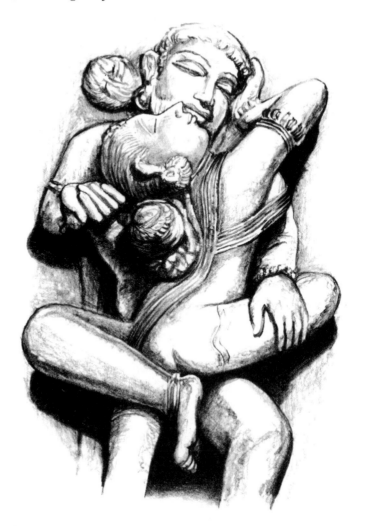

other, and an exquisite exaltation experienced. In the course of an hour the physical tension subsides, the spiritual exaltation increases, and not uncommonly, visions of a transcendent life are seen and a stirring consciousness of new powers experienced."

Of course your state of mind at the time—how bright, how clear, how concentrated, how calm, how contented, how centered you are—is very important. In fact, your state of mind in your life as a whole, past and present, has an effect.

Compassionate Climax

In Noyes' Karezza, the man does not have genital orgasm but the woman may or may not.

In Stockham's Karezza, neither the man nor the woman have genital orgasm.

Karezza master J. William Lloyd wrote that if you opt for the conventional sexual orgasm you end up dumping most of the "wine" you have contained in your body bottle. It rushes through you so fast you can't take advantage of it.

The chief benefits obtained through intercourse without sexual orgasm are an increase in personal energy and well-being, an intensification of the interpersonal bond and an alignment with the higher forces of personal evolution. All agreed the male ejaculation orgasm was an undesirable dispersal of this accumulated benign energy. In Stockham's view, the female sexual orgasm was also undesirable for the same reason.

Noyes points out in his writings that though men tend to think of ejaculation as being what having sex is really all about, the event of seminal release is the aftermath of the sexual act, actually following after it. When a man begins his ejaculation, he has already reached and gone past his point of no return.

What is it that he is unable to return to?

He cannot, after passing that point, return immediately to the act of making love. He is now committed to a roller coaster ride as quick as it is intense, self-involving and mind-boggling. Making love has become making orgasm, yet the two can be as different as day and night.

If you stay at the beginning, it doesn't have to end.

Our Karezza   In the style of Karezza that we do, the man moves just enough to maintain his erection, just every now and then. The rest of the technique is to relax and let go of everyday thinking mind (see *It's The Thought That Counters*). From deep within ourselves we reach out for and into each other, melting in the ever increasing feeling and sensitivity. The woman uses *Pompoir,* too, as needed.

We are not of the school that teaches the orgasm per se must be conserved. Instead, we believe in encouraging unconditional openness. We trust and follow the deeper intuition of the moment.

If conventional orgasm feels appropriate, then it is enjoyed. If it does not, if satisfaction is sweet and complete without it, then we choose to not have conventional orgasm. In either case, no sense of deprivation occurs. Nothing is missed.

Ultimately, energy is unlimited. It is our receptivity to that energy that, at least for the moment, limits us. Provided enough energy is accumulated while making love, climax is simply joyful overflow—and there are many kinds of climax.

Lovemaking—
Peacemaking

Too often, the instruments of sex are used as instruments of war, however subtly. The goal of Karezza is to transform the penile sword and vaginal sheath into instruments for the cultivation of food and nourishment.

The sword becomes the plowshare. The vagina becomes the field of plenty.

The Karezza relationship, in which the energy of life is accumulated, escalated and recycled, offers the possibility of an insoluble mutual magnetic bond, lasting beyond even the body, or so it is believed.

Ultimately, the issue is not whether to avoid the conventional orgasm or not.

Hopefully, ultra-intimacy and Tantric orgasm will not become the kind of elusive frustrating goals that bring more sadness than success. Since they are the experiences of real people, these ideas may be useful as gentle guidelines. If these concepts get in your way or cause you distress, just drop them.

The mutual and unquestioned commitment of heart-felt vital energy between man and woman is the condition unconsciously sought by most consorts. It offers sufficient fire with or without the intentional avoidance of the orgasmic act. You want to love and be loved, to feel ecstasy, to be free. Acknowledge this and you will find it.

What To Expect

What you will experience is impossible to predict. Veteran practicioners of Karezza describe it as thrilling, inspiring, blissful, ecstatic, regenerating, exalted, spiritual, transcendental, and . . . indescribable.

To find out for yourself, you must do it.

If you don't get results the first time, then do it again.

Every time you make love in this way, or simply try to make love in this way, you will grow a little bit as a human being.

You are integrating sex and love, man and woman, hard and soft, wisdom and power in yourself a little bit each time. Karezza lovemaking is an intentional act of conscious self-evolution.

In fact, any kind of lovemaking, even the hardest, fiercest kind of lovemaking, can have this effect. The key is in the attitude.

Yet, at least at the beginning, it seems easier to reap these benefits from yin, soft style lovemaking. It's like learning to meditate, which is much easier when you begin by sitting quietly. With practice, you are able to retain your center as you move and fully participate in the events of life.

Viva Karezza   Without a doubt, Karezza is one of the most enduring and internationally popular soft or yin sexual love styles of all time. The great Chinese physician Master Sun described Karezza type lovemaking back in the seventh century. In his version, the lovers adorned their navels with a big imaginary red egg but the basic style was pure Karezza.

Those who find the arousal with a Karezza method inadequate may have neglected one of the essential skills of Sexual Energy Ecstasy: *Pompoir.* The art of *Pompoir* boldly applied heats the oven and firms the ol' jelly roll well indeed.

Karezza offers a practical do-it-yourself way to reconcile the age old conflict between love and lust: stay in the first, parasympathetic stage of arousal and emphasize deep heart-felt feelings. The quality of the sexual union may change vastly. Regardless of their background, people are moved to describe the experience as sacred, holy, spiritual, uplifting, transcendent and so on.

Always feel free to improvise and change. The methods of Stockham and Noyes may strike you as a bit formal. Personalize them and they will feel natural to you.

Put simply, the Karezza advocates believe that love is the principal food of life, and that one of the principal ways of feeding love to each other is unselfish lovemaking. Here is the Karezza secret: in order to be deeply touched by Karezza, be the person who gives that touch to another.

OTV—
ON THE VERGE   Making love on the verge (OTV) can be your ticket into a twilight world of mind boggling erotic magic. What you are on the verge of is, of course, orgasm. Paradoxically, the significance—though certainly not the pleasure—of orgasm as a climactic event tends to fade a bit when the entire act of making love becomes saturated with orgasmic intensity.

Let us share with you just one experience of erotic madness provoked in this way. Imagine, if you will, literally riding on top of a volcano as it explodes and explodes and explodes. Imagine skiing or surfing on the rolling fury of a mountainous molten red lava flow. Imagine that all around you, even with your eyes wide open, all you can see is red, red, red. Imagine your bodymind is consumed with a head spinning erotic fire that burns all of your flesh at once. Imagine pleasure so intense that you beg for it to end.

For us that day in Topanga, California, it was not imagination. It was real. (And, yes, it was a high from sex—not drugs.)

Riding a volcano is, of course, just one metaphor for the erotic ecstasy which can be enjoyed when the timeless world that lies between arousal and orgasm is entered. Those who dare to try this technique may discover that the word "erotic" takes on an entirely new meaning for them.

Whenever transiting from one kind of reality to another, as from night to day or from day to night, there is a period of time when it is not the old reality and not yet the new reality. You are in between.

Take a moment now to recall the indescribable appeal of dawn to sunrise and of sunset to dusk in a natural setting. These twilight times of earth have long been felt to offer special value. It is as if what lies normally hidden becomes more visible.

The mysterious transitional time from peak arousal to orgasmic release is such another special time. Experimenting with this interval shows that it can be extended indefinitely.

Reaching OTV   Begin an OTV session from a place of real relaxation. A depth of relaxation will make it much easier to notice the finer gradations of arousal as they show up. This noticing may feel quite rewarding in itself.

Remain relaxed, particularly in the pelvic region, the genitals and the buttocks. Also relax your hands and feet. When you approach peak arousal, don't squeeze your PC or anal muscles.

Spread the sensation of arousal throughout your entire bodymind as much as possible. A casual, almost indifferent, dream-like attitude works for many people.

You may want to breathe deeply and concentrate on your feeling center at your heart (see *Love Spot*). You may feel waves of energy surge up or you can visualize this happening if you wish. Again, relax.

Another technique is to visualize the energy from the genitals spreading thoughout your whole bodymind. Use your breath to send the energy flow to other parts of your bodymind. Of course, you can always orgasm.

After a few weeks or months of this you learn to love feeling close to orgasm without orgasming a lot. Just listen to your own energy needs. Don't be surprised if your attitude about having orgasms changes a little.

Rhythmic, stroking movements with your hands help a great deal to spread the erotic fire down the legs, up the trunk and to the extremities (see *Spreading*). The extremities include the tips of the ears, the top of the head, the soles of the feet, the palms and the tips of the toes and fingers.

Your breath and your heart-felt emotions can be directed with the intention of enabling a whole body response in both you and your consort. To use your breath and feelings in this way, invest them with a quality of expansion, a feeling of spaciousness and brightness, as you give them to your consort.

Also remember to fully take in what your consort is offering you.

Colors Of Arousal

In a sexuality seminar given in Los Angeles, psychologist Paul Bindrim made an analogy between the green, yellow and red traffic lights and the situation of someone gradually approaching the point of orgasmic no return. We liked the analogy but found it useful to fine tune our awareness of genital excitedness into five subdivisions, each with its own color and significance.

Green is the first level. Green means all systems are "Go." Yellow would ordinarily be next, signifying "caution," but it is helpful to identify a new level in between green and yellow, the "lime" level.

In the lime level, it is already time to put your sexual energy management strategies into action. In practice, this means you will successfully undermine the compulsion to rush and bring your lovemaking to an end. You will nip it in the bud, so to speak.

Beneath this compulsiveness lies a vast oceanic space of peace and energy. If you make the transition now, early enough, you may move into a new level of mastery you never dreamed possible. Men, especially, who often are concerned with "lasting longer," will be pleased with this new ability level.

You celebrate the thrill of skill in a moment of great challenge. Like a master surfer or race car driver, your thrill comes from playing the edge. Part of that thrill is a product of the real possibility of a wipe out or a crash. However, with OTV the consequence of going over the edge is having an orgasm!

The yellow level of arousal is the true caution level. At this arousal checkpoint, you decide the outcome of that particular union. If you're doing OTV, now is the time to ever so gently ease into the orange level.

The orange level is the realm of OTV. Since red is the level of orgasmic certainty, to be in the orange level is to be on the verge or at the threshold. When a man enters the red level, he is at the point of no return, or ejaculatory inevitability.

Love Magic At Orange Level

When you are in orange level, the slightest sudden movement can set either or both of you off. You do move, but you move with tremendous tenderness, with supersensitivity, so that you remain pre-orgasmic. You will find that every sensation is magnified. Because of the enormous expansion of your passion, even a tiny movement, though it doesn't set off an orgasm, results in earthquakes of sensation, in floods of feeling.

Success at OTV requires top notch teamwork. All the sensational fanfare aside, the joy of cooperating so intimately with another is substantial reward in itself.

When your lovemaking is flowing in this way, you won't feel any sense of strain at all. You will be like entranced firewalkers, dancing in the flames and feeling only warmth and love.

Of course, you can always exercise your orgasm option. It is fun, though, to choose when and how you will have your orgasm(s), to make it an act in which you exercise complete freedom of choice.

If you are constantly having to use force to hold your bodymind back from orgasmic release, then you have already passed through the orange level and are just fighting off the inevitable red tidal wave. You need to back off, relax for several minutes and try again for the orange level, or let go and enjoy your genital explosion.

Let the erotic madness overwhelm you. Surrender to the excruciating ecstasy of being almost, almost, almost "there." It is an exquisite torture that is bound to bend your mind.

Taking breaks at least a few minutes in length is recommended. Just hold and feel each other, feel your breathing and blending together.

Use this time to taste and savor your union for what it is. Very often, lovemaking is used only as a means to an end like having orgasm, proving yourself or pleasing your partner. The hidden riches of the lovemaking opportunity remain hidden if you stay on the surface. Don't skim over it like a pelican gliding over the waves in search of fish. Become the deep-sea diver and discover buried treasure.

The Benefits

Women may find that with OTV practice they can bring on the orgasm or delay it to a much greater degree than they had believed. Judging from the large numbers of women who are concerned with not being orgasmic, who have difficulty having orgasm during intercourse or who are unable to initiate orgasm without primary clitoral stimulation, OTV may offer a unique skill building opportunity.

Too often women are trained to be so passive that they forget how to tap their own energy. Fully satisfying sexual activity requires an abundance or surplus of energy. OTV emphasizes the accumulation of energy, not its dispersion. You can't get off on what you don't have.

A man who is OTV may find that he actually can begin the ejaculation process and then stop it midstream. This may happen automatically. In this and other ways, a man can actually experiment with the sensation of "ejaculatory inevitability" and find out firsthand what brings it on. He may discover that this famous point of no return is not so inevitable after all. He may also discover that he can have pleasurable rushing sensations strongly resembling sexual orgasm without ejaculation, loss of erection or the usual PC muscle spasms. This we call the Non-Ejaculatory Male Orgasm (NEMO). The OTV style grew out of our experiments with Non-Ejaculatory Male Orgasm (NEMO) and voluntary female orgasm during intercourse.

The good news is, yes, NEMO can happen. The not so good news is we know of no way to reliably duplicate the experience at will.

Briefly, NEMO may be best achieved by relaxing as the ejaculation crisis is approached. Pleasurable orgasmic sensations are experienced without the usual ejaculation of semen taking place. Maximum PC muscle development seems to be a prerequisite. Male Multiple Orgasm (MMO) on one ejaculation or with no ejaculation seems to be developed the same way.

OTV places stress on a man's prostate gland. Therefore, male ejaculation orgasm is recommended at the conclusion of most sessions.

Both consorts may have extremely pleasurable experiences that are not the conventional sexual orgasm, simply cannot be described by words and must be experienced to be understood (see *Opening To Bliss*).

TAO OF SEX   According to traditional beliefs, the Yellow Emperor Huang Ti ruled China from 2697 B.C. to 2597 B.C. Many deeply respected ancient Chinese writings are attributed to him, including the single most important Chinese medical work, *The Yellow Emperor's Classic of Internal Medicine (Huang Ti Nei Ching Su Wen* or simply *Nei Ching*).

Among the ancient Chinese writings which bear the Yellow Emperor's name are several works on ancient Taoist (pronounced "*dow*-ist") sexology. One of these, the *Su Nui Ching (The White Madame's Classic),* disappeared in China about 1000 years ago. It reappeared 150 years ago in the possession of the Japanese royal family (in Japanese, of course). A Chinese version was finally found in China and the two were compared.

David attended a seminar based on the *Su Nui Ching* in San Francisco given by Dr. Stephen T. Chang, one of the foremost authorities on ancient Taoist medical practices and modern Chinese acupuncture (see *Appendix*). Dr. Chang wishes to make this vital information widely available and generously gave us permission to quote him at length here.

At The Table Of Love— Woman Dines As Man Waits

According to the wisdom of the *Su Nui Ching,* the woman should be, figuratively, served a nine course meal by her man. Ideally, the man plays the role of waiter and serves her course after delicious course until she enjoys the ninth and final delight, the Taoist total climax or blissful collapse.

But women nowadays are rarely taken all the way. The man usually ejaculates long before she has completed her meal. The result is, not surprisingly, indigestion. The ideal male Tao Of Sex consort, then, is a servant, a butler, a waiter.

Consistently harmonious sexual relations are possible only when the man makes loves with the attitude that serving female satisfaction is his first and foremost goal. The battle of the sexes would suddenly stop if men surrendered in this way. Nonetheless, by following the Tao male satisfaction is also greatly heightened.

Tao Of Sex is a completely cohesive, utterly logical systematic solution to the very real problem which is at the root of the sexual conflict. And what is that problem? Men and women have fundamentally different sexual goals.

Fire And Water

In the Taoist formulation, a man's inborn tendency is to rapidly heat up and explode. For this reason, he is symbolized as fire.

A woman's inborn tendency is to heat up slowly and cool down slowly. For this reason, she is symbolized by water.

But the differences are even more fundamental than this. During sexual intercourse not only does a man not know what a woman feels and a woman not know what a man feels during sexual intercourse, their destinations are completely different.

If a woman is taken to her ultimate destination, the ninth and final course of her erotic supper, she will experience a complete loss of sense of self. She will vanish, disappear,

THE JADE STEM AWAITS THE
FLOWER HEART *opposite*
After a painting on silk from
album of K'ang-hsi period,
C. T. Loo Collection, Paris.

melt into nothingness. She will not know where she is or who she is or what she is during this Tao Of Sex total climax.

This is the woman's Tao Of Sex climax of emptiness.

Paradoxically, this Tao Of Sex total climax of emptiness creates the feeling that she has returned to her deeper and truer self. She is stronger, more independent, more self-directed.

Her contribution to the celebration of sexual union is to lose herself. By acting in accord with the Tao, she also helps bring her man to a deeper sense of manhood, to a more confident, caring and easeful masculinity.

Her job is to let go completely. What is his job?

To use Dr. Chang's word, he is the "pilot."

She surrenders the she-boat of her body to the he-pilot who will, ideally, sail her beyond herself to bliss. Only a skilled navigator can fulfill his role as pilot. Most men must train their bodies, emotions and minds in order to fulfill this role.

Tao Of Sex couples enjoy the act of intercourse (apart from "foreplay") for half an hour, an hour or even longer. For ancient Tao Of Sex consorts, such prolonged lovemaking was standard fare.

In Tao Of Sex lovemaking, the woman may take 20 minutes or more to reach her ninth course, her total climax of emptiness. On the other hand, it is recorded in Taoist texts that some women have reached that stage in a few minutes.

There are many, many variables. For this reason, the Tao Of Sex draws upon ancient Chinese medical principles to describe in detail the nine stages (nine courses) of increasing female surrender and arousal ending in ecstatic emptiness.

- ○   *Lung:* she sighs and her breath is short
- ○   *Heart:* her heart speeds up
- ○   *Spleen/Pancreas:* her saliva increases so much she may have a cold tongue (a sure sign)
- ○   *Kidney:* she is very juicy from her vaginal secretions
- ○   *Bones:* she curls up and holds her man tight
- ○   *Liver/Nerves:* she starts to bite
- ○   *Blood:* she perspires heavily
- ○   *Muscles:* she is soft like silk, has no muscle tone and is completely relaxed
- ○   *Collapse:* total climax of emptiness

According to Dr. Chang, conventional orgasm is not the same thing as the Tao Of Sex complete climax of collapse and rejuvenating emptiness. The woman may or may not have regular orgasm with pubococcygeus (PC) muscle contractions. The two kinds of climax can occur at the same time, though.

Dr. Chang told the story of a wealthy woman who came to see him privately about her kidney problems and lack of energy. The solution was simple. When her husband began taking her to the ninth stage instead of the fourth (kidney) stage, her chronic kidney condition cleared up and her energy returned.

The Man's Pleasure Peaks

For the man, the routine of ejaculation orgasm with virtually every act of intercourse was viewed with horror by the Tao Of Sex experts. Though emptiness is definitely appropriate for and is to be sought by the female, the sensation of emptiness that may befall the ordinary man after he ejaculates is, according to the Tao Of Sex, a sure sign of significant loss.

However, the Taoists were not against ejaculation per se. The ordinary man was not advised to avoid ejaculation entirely but rather to regulate it according to his age and self-evident health and vitality. A man's semen was regarded

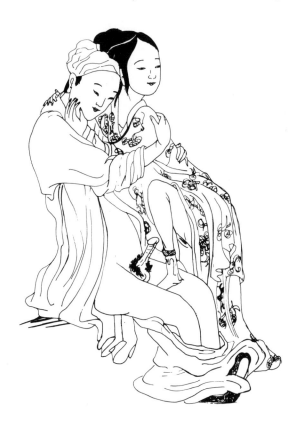

as life-giving and life-sustaining personally and merited a thoughtful and individualized conservation program.

The main obstacle to male–female harmony according to the Tao may well be the male addiction to ejaculation orgasm. As long as a man believes that his supreme pleasure can be found only in the ejaculation orgasm, the principle of the man as "pilot" will remain just another good theory.

Fortunately, however, no ascetic sacrifice of man's prime pleasure is implied or required by his taking on the Taoist pilot role. In fact, a significant gain in immediate pleasure and long-term sexual fulfillment (and long-term relationship fulfillment, perhaps) is waiting for him.

Some men do take their women to the ninth and final stage of Tao Of Sex and still ejaculate at the end. These men have discovered that as good as ejaculation orgasm feels, especially when delayed, there is something that feels even better.

What could possibly be even better than the ejaculation orgasm for a man? The answer is repeated almost ejaculation pleasure peaks. Just as a woman is capable of multiple orgasms, a man is capable of multiple almost ejaculation pleasure peaks.

The male pleasure peak in Tao Of Sex may be defined as approaching ejaculation orgasm inevitability, followed by retreat, relaxation, the male Deer exercise and, eventually, renewed thrusting.

The cycle is repeated to mutual satisfaction or as long as time or desire permit. Male satisfaction, by the way, is complete with this method without ejaculation. According to the Tao, this is the way of lovemaking for the man.

None other than the famed sex researcher Alfred C. Kinsey reported interviewing a number of men who practiced this kind of male climax. Kinsey made the point to his fellow sex researchers that they should not give the experience the coveted "orgasm" label. Still, he reported that these male sex adepts were themselves convinced that their dozen or so almost-ejaculation pleasure peaks during one lovemaking session were, in fact, actual orgasms, though admittedly of somewhat lesser intensity.

These "hold backs" (another of Dr. Chang's terms) are the main course for the man in Tao Of Sex. Male ejaculation orgasm becomes dessert and is enjoyed as an occasional delicacy of great sweetness.

For a man to commit to his pilot role it helps to keep in mind a supreme pleasure other than ejaculation orgasm. This new supreme pleasure is male multiple pleasure peaks.

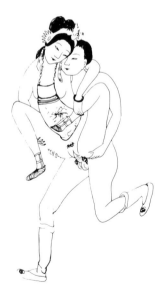

JADE STEM IN FLOWER
HEART RUNS *above*

Whether or not a man chooses ejaculation as a grand finale is a personal matter. Nonetheless, here is clear and sufficient motivation for him to last until his woman reaches the ninth stage of ecstatic total climax collapse.

One of the chief objections to this practice of parlaying for multiple pleasure peaks is the stress it can place upon the male prostate gland, particularly if relief is not provided at the end via ejaculation. Amazingly, the ancient Taoists had an answer for this one, too.

Male Deer— Inner Gland Massage

A woman's health is clearly benefited by being brought to the ninth stage. But where is the health benefit for the man in the Tao Of Sex male climax?

According to Tao Of Sex, his benefit is derived mainly from withholding the ejaculate and recycling the vital ingredients to the rest of his body. He may also receive benefit from her secretions and from excess vital energy released by her during orgasm.

However, some beneficial biochemistries are undoubtedly absorbed during extended lovemaking even if ejaculation does conclude the act.

There are men who for organic reasons, often as a result of surgery such as a prostatectomy, do not ejaculate when they orgasm (the ejaculate goes into the bladder). But there is no evidence that these men are any better off than men who emit semen from their bodies regularly.

Western men who avoid sexual activity altogether, such as Catholic monks, generally don't live as long as the average married man. If there is a health benefit gained from avoiding ejaculation, it certainly isn't just a matter of men avoiding seminal emission. One large, recent study of male health after vasectomy, though, does suggest that a slight health benefit may result.

Here the ever practical Tao Of Sex experts step in with a plausible modus operandi that makes perfect, though mind stretching, sense. During intercourse the man voluntarily contracts his anal and PC muscles firmly and frequently. This massages his slightly inflated prostate gland, encouraging it to release its hormonal treasures back into the bloodstream (see *Sexercises*).

Due to the prostate gland's mixing function, these secretions are a real pot pourri of male hormonal delicacies (see *Voluntary Orgasm For Men*). This semen "fertilizer" (to use Dr. Chang's term) is carried via blood to parts of the man's body needing the vital nutrients. Glands, nerves, bones and bone marrow, joints and the immune system are fertilized first by the rejuvenating hormones. This semen fertilizer also favors the hair and skin.

But there is another very practical reason for these voluntary PC–anal muscle contractions. As Dr. Chang put it, "the prostate must pump." Either you pump it or it pumps itself in ejaculation. If it doesn't pump, congestion of the prostate may result.

Dr. Chang suggested a variety of ways to pump. The man can stop completely, relax and pump for up to five minutes. The couple will need to lie still for this. He can also pump as he makes love, contracting the muscles as he pulls out. And he can pump as frequently during lovemaking as he likes and at any time he likes.

There are two main styles of pumping the prostate. With either approach, establish a pulsating rhythm.

The first way is to hold the contraction as long as possible, then totally let go and feel the relaxation. The second way is to do a set of them rapidly with complete relaxation of those muscles following. A set may be 50 repetitions.

Be aware of a tendency to slight the relaxation phase. Maximum contraction will result from maximum relaxation. Performance of this exercise during intercourse eventually enables the man to delay ejaculation indefinitely while intensifying his pleasure. This may or may not be followed by ejaculation.

The basic male Deer exercise is described elsewhere in this book (see *Sexercises*). A dedicated Tao Of Sex pilot practices on a daily basis separately from intercourse. However, even occasional practice should provide many valuable benefits. This exercise strengthens the muscles as well as intensifying the hormonal reabsorption process.

To summarize, the act of delaying final ejaculation and enjoying multiple pleasure peaks is, in fact, only half of the reality of the male Taoist climax. The other half is the conscious and voluntary act of pumping the prostate and recycling its hormonal cocktail throughout the male system.

Remember, Dr. Chang's pumping technique is an experimental method. It is not intended to replace the counsel of your physician. However, combined with very firm pressure on the Prostate Point (see *Voluntary Orgasm For Men*), pumping should aid in relieving prostate congestion and hormonal recycling. Please check with your physician now about the condition of your prostate and get regular prostate checkups. This annual evaluation should include a manual examination of your prostate via the rectum.

EROTIC ACUPRESSURE
opposite

When making love, the sequence of events is to pump

during intercourse and follow with manual pressure on the Prostate Point, which your consort may be willing to perform for you. Or pumping and manual prostate relief can be mixed during intercourse, which is the way we generally like to do it.

Acupressure And Sex Organs

The Taoist sexology of the *Su Nui Ching* teaches that sexual intercourse is actually a form of mutual, ecstatic acupressure. The end regions of the body, such as the hands and feet, and the open areas of the body, such as the ears and mouth, are rich with nerve endings and acupuncture energy points. The sexual organs are the richest of all such regions.

When male and female sex organs unite, a wonderful pressing together of acupuncture points takes place. In an acupuncture energy sense, the two bodies have literally become one. Among other things, this arrangement suggests a good match between male and female sex organs is required for whole body stimulation and release.

In the diagram below, Lung (L) includes the large intestine and skin, Heart (H) includes the small intestine and blood vessels, Spleen–Pancreas (SP) includes the stomach and muscles, Liver (LV) includes the nerves and gall bladder, and Kidney (K) includes urinary bladder and bones.

When a physically and emotionally compatible man and woman unite sexual organs, Kidney communes with Kidney, Liver communes with Liver and so on. According to this theory, there is simply no substitute for this all-points alignment. Even if the couple just lie still, abundant bio-energy is exchanged. They are both getting a free acupressure treatment.

Love Medicine

Tao Of Sex evolved in a more leisurely, more down-to-earth world that was very different from our own. People had not yet conceived of themselves as separate from nature, as we do today. In fact, we will probably never be able to fully understand how much and in what ways ancient Tao Of Sex couples appreciated lovemaking.

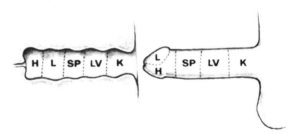

For one thing, they literally made it a part of their daily lives. Free of distractions like newspapers and television, many couples made love for hours on end daily.

When we get sick today, we receive a medical prescription, usually a drug. Although ancient Taoist physicians certainly did treat with medicinal herbs, they often advised frequent sexual intercourse utilizing very specific positions and thrusting protocols or pelvic movements.

So instead of taking pills one, two, three or four times a day, men and women were instructed to make love one, two, three or four times a day.

It was a very different world, indeed.

Enhanced Romance

A benefit of making love without male ejaculation that we have found is that romance is enhanced.

It is a common observation that the lightning of love strikes and then, just as swiftly, is gone. The mysterious magic quickly fades, leaving familiar struggles.

Being in love is a kind of creative tension. To get one's fill, to be sated, this is not the mood of a person in love. To be in love is to be ravenously hungry, to be ever unsatisfied, to be longing, to never get enough. Happy lovers enjoy a paradox of fulfilling non-fulfillment.

According to Tao Of Sex, some of this loss of magic is the result of one or both lovers losing rather than gaining via their lovemaking. Not only the man but the woman also can lose. The two who once felt so full with each other quickly exhaust the gift.

Karezza master J. William Lloyd echoes the Taoist sages. "Lovers glow, radiate, move in an enchanted world. This is attributed to love itself. But it is the wine of sex that gives love its enchantment and divine dreams. Lovers who express their transports via unrestricted orgasms waste the wine of sex by their reckless embraces. The irresistible attraction and radiance and magnetic thrills are gone. There is a strange drop into cool, critical intellection or indifference, or perhaps dislike. But as the wine of sex reaccumulates and lifts again in the glass, the old magic and charm reappear."

Wise lovers will never get enough of each other. Wise lovers will stay with the tension, the unknowing, the insecurity, the hunger of the beginning, the suspense of the fall into love. One way to sustain the magic is the Tao Of Sex.

In the words of the ancient Taoist sage Lao Tzu, "know the yang (the expressive energy) but dwell in the yin (the receptive attitude)." When intimacy and giving are the main focus, the ultimate in pleasure is enjoyed as well.

J. William Lloyd. *The Karezza Method or Magnetation.* Hollywood: Phoenix House, 1973, page 54.

RAGAMAYA TANTRA

The Ragamaya Tantra is a series of Tantric sexual instructions (or initiations). The modern Tantra Master who relayed it to us commented "Anyone who thinks they are or have a body is at a major disadvantage when it comes to doing Tantric sex."

Below we have excerpted some of his suggestions. As you will see, he has a rather bizarre sense of humor. However, there is a method to his madness: these playful games are bound to evoke some healthy self-observation.

Into The Light

At orgasm, switch attention to the third eye and look for the light. Do not think about how to do it. Just do it.

In The Gap

Attend to the gap in the breath after inhalation or exhalation.

Melt

Melt into your lover. Your skin is fluid like liquid butter.

Pop Top

Pretend that the top of your head is the most sensitive and erotic part of your body. Feel that you are open there in a sexual way. If you have a thought, it occurs in the perineum. Be aware of a connection but do not try to create it. Inverted yoga postions are excellent practice.

Open Eyes

Breathing slowly together and looking in each other's eyes, contemplate the other as love, energy or the void.

Alarm Game

Go to sleep together and set the alarm for the middle of the night. As soon as the alarm rings, reach for your lover and begin to make love to them.

Name Game

As you make love, invent spontaneous names to erotic parts of your lover's body—breasts, mouth, vagina, penis. Say them out loud. "I want to play with your bazongpa."

Sacred Consort

Imagine that you are making love to Jesus Christ, Mary Magdalene, Buddha, Tara, Kwan Yin, Radha, Krishna, Kali, Shiva or some other holy being, saint or enlightened one. How do you feel?

Time Clock

Make love at the same exact time of day or night for seven days in a row.

Dreaming

As you make love, imagine that this is a dream and you will soon be waking up.

Empty

Your bodies are completely empty, filled with space.

Heavy Think that your body is very heavy, made of stone, weighing at least two tons. You can move it but every gesture requires concentration and effort.

Balloon Think that your body is very light, like a balloon filled with helium. You feel yourself constantly starting to float up and away. To stay on the ground, on the bed, requires moment-to-moment concentration and effort.

True Colors Imagine that your lover's body keeps changing colors, going through all the colors of the rainbow and black and white.

My Ragamaya Before making love, stand before your lover and point to your body, saying "This is my Ragamaya. I have donned it like a suit of clothes in order to make love to you. When we are done, I will take it off."

I, Android You are an android. You have no soul.

Android Lover Your partner is an android. He or she has no soul.

No Souls You are both androids. Neither of you has a soul.

Earplugs Make love wearing earplugs.

Blindfold Make love wearing a blindfold.

Gloves Make love with gloves on.

My Bag Make love with a paper bag over your head. Make holes for breathing but keep the eyes covered. (Do *not* use a plastic bag as they are unsafe.)

Your Bag Make love with a paper bag over your lover's head.

Heart Dot With a felt-tip pen place a green dot on the center of your lover's chest. Concentrate there the whole time you make love.

Thought Dot Place a red, blue or black dot on your lover's forehead. Concentrate there the whole time.

Eyes Of Palm Paint eyes on the palms of your hands. Imagine that you can see through these eyes as you caress.

Strip Joker Play strip poker with a Tarot deck.

Bang A Drum   Buy a drum. Have a friend bang the drum from outside your bedroom at the rate of once every two or three seconds for at least twenty minutes. Or record this on tape, but live is much better.

Special Spot   Find the most sensitive spot on your lover's body other than the usual erotic locations.

Tied Down   Make love with one of you tied down spreadeagled. Be sure to switch roles.

Executive Dress   Begin lovemaking with the woman fully dressed in a formal or business outfit and the man naked except for his watch.

Male Stripper   Begin lovemaking by having the man do a striptease dance starting with his best business suit and tie. The man should do a serious job of dressing up as if he is going to a big meeting or a job interview.

Blank Face   Imagine that your lover's face is completely blank.

10,000 Faces   Imagine that your lover's face keeps changing, becoming the faces of lovers you have never known.

Animals   Imagine that you and your partner have suddenly become your favorite animal(s). Try to maintain this feeling.

Non-Verbal   Experience that neither of you speak English and that you have no language in common. Verbal communication is useless.

Food Or Love   At a time when you are very hungry, place a favorite food on a table and ask your lover to sit next to it. Which do you choose?

No Body Home   While making love, you discover that you cannot find your body anywhere.

Simple Sign   Create a simple sign out of white cardboard and loop it around your neck with a strong string. The sign reads "You love me."

Reflections   As you selflove, watch your face or genitalia in a mirror.

Art Appreciation   Take a picture of your favorite piece of art and concentrate on it in the same way.

Get Naked   Before making love, in separate rooms put on at least five layers of clothing, including gloves. Do this regardless of the temperature. Sit down and watch TV for half an hour. Then, without speaking, go to your bedroom. Still silent, slowly remove the layers of clothing until you are naked. Make love.

Smashing Time   Before making love, bring into the room where you will make love on a nice tray a small inexpensive object that you are not interested in keeping. Without saying a word, take it gently and reverently off the tray, and then smash it to pieces, yelling loudly as you do so.

No Image   Bring a recent photo of yourself and a pair of scissors. Exchange photos. Slowly cut up the photo of your partner into many pieces. Smile and enjoy this. When you are done, put the pieces in a sack and place it outside your bedroom door. Close the door. Later, throw the bag away. Even better, burn the bag outside over an open fire.

Mystery Memo   Type or write up a mystery memo that says something you want your lover to do that they have never done before. Fold it in half. On the outside, if it is to a man, write "Your Assignment." If it is to a woman, write "This is my dream." Repeat until stale.

Violet Vision   Paint your bedroom violet. Have violet sheets, pillows, etc. Use a violet filter on your lamp. You will automatically have fantastic experiences.

Holy Vision   Take a picture of your favorite deity or savior or guru and place it where you can see it while making love or selfloving, i.e., the ceiling or wall. Maintain eye contact the entire time. Wear glasses or contacts if you need to in order to see the image clearly.

Don't Know   As you make love, silently repeat "I don't know what this is."

Be Forehead   Take the holy or art picture and tape or paste a small xerox of it on your lover's forehead. Watch this picture and maintain eye contact with it.

Price Tag   Hand your partner a check (imaginary or real) in the amount that having sex with them is worth to you.

Do You Mind?   Lie down next to each other, eyes closed. Without physical contact, make love in your minds.

Morning After	If you are married, when you wake up the next morning imagine that you had sex with this person last night and do not know who they are. If you are single, imagine that you are married to them.
Condemned	You have been condemned to death. The local magistrate has an offer. Make love to him or her and you will be free.
Celibacy Or Me	You have been a celibate monk or nun since you were 13. This is your first time. You have no idea what to do and you admit that you are uneasy.
Eyes Only	Make love with your eyes only.
Slave Day	You are a slave. They are your owner. Switch roles.
$100	Go to the bank and get 100 crisp new $1 bills. Have your lover lie down on your bed. Pour the money over them. Lie on top of them briefly, not moving, the money sandwiched between you. Now gently sweep the money on to the bed. Make love on top of the money. If you are concerned about cleanliness ("dirty money"), you can wash the money and then dry it (but not in the oven!). Also, this softens the money so you avoid paper cuts.
Headache 108	Whether you are a man or woman, be irritated and bitchy. Complain of a headache. Make love anyway.
Lost My Head	Free to kiss, of course, make love as if your heads are totally, quite literally, gone.
Yes!	Instead of the usual sounds, remember to say only "Yes!"
Laughter	Make love for awhile. Then, in a flash, you are laughing. Laugh for five minutes at least.
I–I–I	Repeat "I-I-I" continuously, perhaps with the waves of your movement. Whenever you notice a part of your body more, put your attention there and repeat "I-I-I" continuously.
Who?	Repeat "Who is making love?"
I Love You	Before making love, spend 15 minutes in front of a mirror saying "I love you" over and over again.
You Love Me	Repeat but say "You love me."

Beautiful Repeat but say "You are so beautiful."

Last Time Decide that this is the last time you are having sex. You don't know what you will be doing afterwards, but you are sure that this is the very last time.

Burning House Imagine that your house is burning down around you while you are making love. You choose to continue your lovemaking and die in each other's arms, consumed by the flames.

Meditation Gong Buy a meditation gong (a round bowl) or equivalent. Place it next to the bed. Hit the gong and move until the sound dies away. When you get tired of this game, give the gong to a friend or fill it with earth and plant flowers in it. Do not meditate with it.

Bowls Of Fruit Take two large bowls and fill them with fruit. Sit across from each other and act as if you are making love to each other, but do so with the fruit. Do not touch each other during this.

Distant Love Sit naked facing each other from across the room. Decide that you will make fantastic love with each other from a distance. Do so.

Instant Love When acting on the impulse to make love, move to do so swiftly, instantly, without the slightest thought process. Be action only, without any anticipation or planning (except for contraception or AIDS issues).

Infant Love Have a hypnotist regress you to infancy. Make love in this state.

Angry Love Alone in another part of the house, act out being angry, yell, scream, jump around, hit a pillow. Then lie down for about 10 minutes. Go completely limp. Now make love.

Rock Love Pick up a small, nondescript rock and decide to establish a relationship with it. Stroke it, caress it, talk to it, hold it in your arms and rock it like it was your baby. When you feel close to the rock (this may take two weeks), bring it with you to your lover. Place it next to the bed. Remember what you did with the rock. Do the same with your lover.

Do, Don't Do Some time when you really want to make love, don't. Some time when you really don't want to make love, do. Compare notes.

Forbidden Food   Sit at your table, facing across from each other. Without leaving the table, drink or eat your favorite, forbidden food, i.e., chocolate cake, soda, ice cream, cookies. Eat or drink until you do not want anymore. Talk, tell stories and get drunk. No TV allowed. Then try to be sexual with each other in some way—if you can still move. Make love doggie style. Laugh about it the next morning.

Ra Ga Ma Ta   Repeat "Ra Ga Ma Ta" as you make love.

Ra Ga Ma Da Ta Ya   Repeat "Ra Ga Ma Da, Ra Ga Ma Ta, Ra Ga Ma Ya" coordinated with the breath. With Ra, breathe in through your third eye. With Ga, breathe out your solar plexus. With Ma, breathe in through your heart center. With Da, breathe out and straight down through the perineum.

Repeat "Ra Ga Ma" breathing as before but breathe out through the top of your head with Ta. Repeat "Ra Ga Ma" breathing as before but breathe out through the entire front surface of your body to your partner, releasing your whole being with the Ya sound. Or you can just repeat "Ra Ga Ma Ta" with the breathing to match.

Next Time   The next time you make love, don't do anything.

SLOW MOTION   Slow motion is exactly what its name implies. As you make love, move as slowly as possible. Whatever you think is slow, move even more slowly still. At times, you may become absolutely motionless. Allow this. The next impulse to move will originate from deep within you. You will discover a greater depth in your lovemaking, perhaps much greater than you had imagined, because you will be moving from a deeper part of yourself.

You may find that doing this is more difficult than you thought. It is a good idea to agree ahead of time to make love in slow motion for a specific time period. Do slow motion for at least five minutes. However, 20 to 40 minutes is ideal.

Slow motion can be smoothly incorporated into your regular lovemaking as a prelude to sensitize you or as an interlude to slow things down. Slow motion is both an exercise and a way to make love.

One of the great benefits of this technique is that it tends to increase awareness of detail. You may notice literally hundreds of new things about your partner—the pulsing of blood in their throat, the softness of their belly, a fleck of green in their otherwise blue iris—and about yourself. You may discover that the usual quiet current of non-verbal signals that flows between you when you make love has suddenly become a torrent of meanings.

Slow motion can begin even before you touch each other. Lie side by side on your bed. Only when you are moved from deep within to reach out to the other should you do so, and then with supreme slowness. You may feel awkward at first, but this won't last long.

Do several slow motion lovemaking sessions in a row so that the impact accumulates. Every now and then add this style to your repertoire. You will see the positive effects spill over into your love life, perhaps your personal life as well.

Slow motion is a way to bring the consciousness of meditation to the act of making love. Specifically, by going very slowly you are practicing mindfulness of body sensations, of tactile sensations especially. Just as there is slow walking meditation, so is there, for those who follow the way of Tantra, slow lovemaking meditation.

Some lovers report that this technique takes them to a place of silence and stillness that is exquisitely beautiful and wholly satisfying. This need not be an ascetic experience. Like a beautiful sunset, it is naked and rich as well as pure. Beauty is in the eye of the beholder, and doing it slowly is another way to see more clearly.

IMSAK   Imsak ("im-sak" or "im-shak") is an Arabic word that means, literally, "retention." In this respect, Imsak resembles *Karezza*. The man retains his semen by not ejaculating. However, it's difficult to tell from the sketchy records whether this meant ejaculation was delayed only until the woman was satisfied or that it was foregone entirely (probably either, depending on the occasion).

According to one tradition, Imsak was developed out of necessity: no ordinary man could satisfy an entire harem of passionate (and bored?) young women. A man who had mastered Imsak could satisfy 10 women or more a night. Such a man might still have had a favorite(s) and, when appropriate, shared the joys of mutual orgasm with her.

All of this sounds irredeemably sexist and it certainly is. Nevertheless, a woman stands to gain a great deal by enjoying this prolonged ecstasy with her consort.

Very little is known with certainty about the details of the Imsak method. The generic label of "retention" can be applied to several of the Sexual Energy Ecstasy styles. Fortunately, Robert Meister researched this method and has unearthed what are probably the essentials. The key to Imsak is found in its uniquely systematic way of combining *coitus interruptus* and *Pompoir* so that higher and higher levels of ecstasy and energy are attained and absorbed.

Since as far back as Roman times, man has pulled out before ejaculating to avoid (they hoped) impregnating the woman. In Imsak, the man pulls out well before he reaches his point of ejaculatory inevitability in order to achieve cumulative erotic and consciousness altering effects for the loving couple together.

Teasing is universally recognized as a way to build passion and desire to such a pitch that the final release is unforgettable. To a point, the greater the erotic tension and frustration, the better the release. Teasing, however, is too weak a word to convey the mind-boggling power of Imsak.

The Essence   In Imsak, the man enters and pulls out up to 10 times, allowing their mutual arousal to build with each successive penetration. Ejaculation is delayed until the final union or, perhaps, altogether.

Some lovers content themselves with two or three re-entries. The sensations that accompany even just this much erotic self-discipline can be far superior to the usual fare. These lovers may believe they have scaled the heights of erotic ecstasy when, in fact, they have only reached the foot of the mountain.

The acme of Imsak is reached after about 10 unions. The exaltation that permeates the lovers who go that far is, according to Meister, the pinnacle of erotic possibility.

All of this depends, of course, on male ejaculatory control as well as female cooperation. Fortunately, the essence of Imsak is also what makes it feasible for just about any man unless he is physically impaired.

Pulling out is a great way to delay ejaculation orgasm and is also a popular way to train a man to last longer. Ordinarily, a man feels awkward pulling out. Imsak enables him to pull out as needed, rest and then re-enter and be confident that he is adding to mutual bliss.

What do you do during these rest periods?

First, allow the man a few minutes of non-stimulation so that his erection and his need to ejaculate subside.

Stroke, caress and touch anything and everything except his genitals. Show affection while at the same time creating arousal as needed.

All is done very gently and with great sensitivity. The skin becomes sensitive due to the accumulated whole body arousal. Therefore, tender gestures are strongly preferred.

One thing leads to another. Soon you will be kissing and *El besiss,* "the impudent one," will rise once again. With great care and cooperation, re-entry is achieved once more.

Take enough time in the rest periods, though, that you actually do experience some rest and relaxation and cool down a bit. Also, these rest periods are your opportunity to recollect and focus your heart-felt feelings for each other and spread energy for health and rejuvenation. You may want to use some of this time to go within.

For Meister's Imsak, some *Pompoir* (kabbazah) ability is essential. Compared to *Kabbazah Sex,* though, the skill level required is not that demanding, and some women will have sufficient strength and control without any specific exercises. If Meister's formula is followed precisely, the first five unions (the man has pulled out and repenetrated four times) are mergers without male thrusting motion.

The woman is in control of their arousal through her kabbazah skill. This way the erotic fire builds and builds as an experience of the whole body and is not localized in the genitals.

Naturally, you are free to deviate from his formula according to your own needs and capacities. But you will know the precise and, perhaps, ideal Imsak formula.

On the first entry, Meister suggests that the man enter but not thrust, though he should push with his pelvis and penis against the woman as firmly yet comfortably as he can. The pressure he can exert in this way is a major stimulating factor and can be used during any unions without motion. Either partner can manually stimulate her clitoris.

If she is on top and facing him, this is the position known as *es sibfahheh,* "swimming." The position gets its name from the ease with which the clitoral bud is manually stimulated and intense arousal is achieved, especially when combined with voluntary contractions of the sexual muscles.

She also begins clenching and letting go, starting with delicate little flicks and building up to real manhandler grips and, if advanced in the art, rolling and milking motions.

He is encouraged to work his PC and anal muscles, too. She will probably need to stimulate her clitoris manually only during the first union. Even though he is not moving his penis, it won't be long before he has to pull out.

At this time begin the affectionate yet eventually arousing rest period. Avoid direct genital stimulation unless it is

ES SIBFAHHEH
opposite
Anyone for a swim?

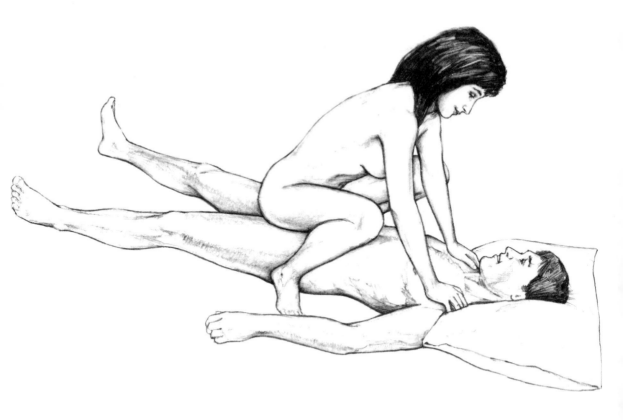

needed to achieve re-entry. Relax and cool down as needed. Literally take a break to drink or eat something light, if you wish, for this removes the mind from the heat of stimulation in addition to timely refueling.

After about the fifth such cycle the couple is now ready for the second half of the technique. During the next cycle the thrusting strategy outlined below is followed.

This cycle is followed by a motionless cycle as above. This cycle is followed by another thrusting cycle and so on up to about 10 completed cycles. The man pulls out between each cycle.

Advanced Imsak practicioners capable of completing all 10 cycles will follow a protocol consisting of five *Pompoir* cycles followed by thrusting, *Pompoir,* thrusting, *Pompoir* and thrusting cycles, in that order. The man voluntarily climaxes on the final thrusting cycle. However, she is not deprived.

In practice, the woman is orgasming by the third *Pompoir* cycle unless she is holding back intentionally. The male beginner will probably experience (very intense) ejaculation orgasm before reaching the second set of five cycles.

During the unions without motion, she determines their arousal through her *Pompoir.* During unions with motion, he determines their arousal with his thrusting.

This alternation of giving and taking, or sending and receiving, is one of the secrets to elevating your ecstasy. Each alternation is but one more breathtaking step up the *Stairway To Heaven.*

As mentioned earlier, out of 10 cycles total, only three involve male thrusting. Meister suggests that a systematic thrusting method in the midst of the madness of intercourse will bring the greatest fulfillment. Echoing the traditional recommendations of the *Tao Of Sex* masters, Meister advises the following thrusting strategy.

o   Thrust 10 times after entering, then pull out.
o   Stay near the entrance of the vagina on the first three thrusts. Don't go deep. This is to stimulate her.
o   Follow with two fast thrusts into the depths of her vagina to arouse her.
o   Follow with three more thrusts near the entrance of the vagina to tantalize her.
o   Conclude with two leisurely thrusts into the depths of her vagina to satisfy her.
o   Voluntary orgasm is ideally achieved with a long, leisurely, fully felt thrust that goes all the way to her "North Pole," to her very depths. This is to fulfill ("full-fill") her utterly.

As artificial as Meister's thrusting regimen may seem, it is a valuable aid to ejaculatory control as well as an intensifier of her pleasure. Through the magic of rhythm, the thrusting techniques add elegance and sophistication to the act of lovemaking.

Mastery of such a routine, particularly if it is performed as a team effort, is analogous to learning to dance with style instead of moving on impulse this way and that. Randomness can be great fun, but the joy of flowing together through a series of fluid position changes brings an exquisite delight.

This thrusting sequence works very well with any active lovemaking style. It is a concentrated recipe for ecstasy that takes into account both depth of penetration and speed of penetration. He may want to vary the angle of penetration, making straight, slanted, up and down, and circular thrusts.

Naturally, she is free to move and clench in concert with him. The caveat is this may bring him to climax long before the incomparable Imsak saturation effect can be tasted.

**In The Sack
With Imsak**

The words of wisdom to the male Imsak beginner are "Discretion is the better part of valor."

Success with this method, however, depends as much on female cooperation as it does on male discipline. Her sensitivity to his arousal—how close he is to genital climax—will determine whether to squeeze or not to squeeze. When a man is near the edge, one little compulsive twist of the waist or clench of the circumvaginal muscles can put him over.

Keep in mind your ultimate goal as you make love, that acme of erotic arousal in which each touch is like a miniature orgasm. Of course, your goal with this method may differ from time to time. This will motivate cooperation in delaying his ejaculation orgasm.

Keep in mind, too, that transcending ordinary pleasure may only be the beginning. You may find valuable personal insights, soak in an overwhelming sense of oneness or bathe in a peaceful calm of total contentment. These are just some of the possible benefits to you. It is likely that these experiences will occur to you when you are united but not moving.

Should you opt for the traditional orgasm as your grand finale, it will probably be an unforgettable tidal wave straight from paradise. The experience will prove to you that building up the erotic tension far beyond usual tolerance is the best way to guarantee a fabulous climax. Because you have built up such an abundance of energy, mutual orgasm will probably be easier to achieve.

Try to follow Meister's method to the letter, at least at first. There is something uniquely challenging and satisfying about following an effective erotic procedure precisely. This kind of training brings out the sexual artist in you. Any feelings of artificiality will melt away in the fire that engulfs you.

Once you are acquainted with the basics of Imsak, improvise. Simply use the Imsak secret of repeated *coitus interruptus* as an erotic elevator to new pinnacles of sexual ecstasy. Each re-entry takes you higher than you were before. Each rest period is yet another peace-filled realm to explore. Ride your Imsak elevator to the penthouse of paradise any way you like. As the first Tantra master, Shiva, said, "Do it. Then you will understand it. Not before."

FUSION BREATH SEX

We cannot emphasize enough the power of the breath in sex. Just as as people breathe differently when they are anxious or angry or excited or sad, so do different forms of lovemaking have their characteristic breath patterns.

Not only does each emotional state induce its own unique breath signature, the inverse is also true. Intentionally altering the breath to match a particular signature tends to induce the corresponding emotion.

Conventional hard, yang sex follows its well-known pattern largely because the breath patterns typically are the same. Though lovers tend not to think about it, they are actually using the breath to create this experience. Alter the breath and you will alter the experience.

Altering the breath is a radical act. It may be important to discuss this with your partner beforehand.

Many types of energy exercise and meditation are based on a deeper understanding of the power of the breath. Some meditators discover from just following the breath that as the breath becomes calm and peaceful, so does the mind. There is a direct link.

This method is based on David's experience of Tantric orgasm with a yogini in Mendocino, California (see *Co-Inspiration*). One key factor for attaining that mystical experience was the power of the breath. The other essential ingredient was surrender.

Wave Breathing

Wave Breathing is based on learning to perceive and extend your breath envelope. Practice stretching the breath out as far in front of you as possible. Pursing your lips, strive to prolong the exhalation as long as you can. Make an effort to literally feel the end of the breath, the furthest distance that it extends out in front of you.

You are not so much looking for the physical movement of the air, although that is a beginning. Look for, feel, sense the wave of energy, its solidity and radiance, where it ends. As a training tool, it may help to extend your hand in front of you as if it were marking the spot where the breath energy terminates.

Pay special attention to the moment when it ends. Stay in that gap for awhile. Explore the space in front of you during this gap, feeling for the energy that is there from your exhalation.

You may find it helpful to concentrate on your lips where the breath is going out. Concentrate either here or at the point in front of you where the breath seems to stop and turn around. It may also help to close your eyes.

Don't worry about the inhalation. It will take care of itself. If the exhalation is full, you will find that a deep inhalation is more or less automatic.

When you apply the Wave Breath to intercourse, approach it as a serene communion, as meditation. Bodily movement must be secondary to maintaining this long exhalation breath. With practice, you can move very slowly and rhythmically with this breath.

Always let the breath command, not your desires for direct stimulation. Then you will feel the touch of the subtle energy and taste a bliss that transcends conventional orgasm. There is a very delicate tone to this approach, but you will not be missing anything. As the erotic fire courses through you while doing the Wave Breath, inevitably you feel yourself merging with an ecstatic ocean of energy. A greater breath is breathing you.

You may have the experience that you are making love to the breath, and it is making love to you. You and your consort are expressions of the breath, not the other way around. It is best to have no preconceptions about this. Let go of mystical notions, too, for this is primal, before thought.

Circle Of Joy   The Circle Of Joy is an advanced co-breathing process with several variations. The basic skill was decribed in *Charge Up*. Here we elaborate, so that the breath is rotated around your bodies in a circle. This is perhaps best accomplished in the YabYum position.

In *Charge Up,* you alternated breathing and stopped at the top of the head. Now you will complete the circuit.

To begin, visualize a ring of light that connects your bodies in a perfect circle of wholeness. The gold wedding band symbolizes this living mandala of unity. Likewise, the well-known Yin-Yang or *T'ai Chi* circle expresses this as well as other philosophical truths. Know that this perfect circle already exists. You are just rediscovering it.

Let us say the woman starts. She does the breath a few times before he joins in, so that he knows her rhythm. Then he joins her on her inhalation, breathing out as he does so. If you have trouble following the total pattern, just concentrate on doing your part.

As she inhales, she pulls energy from both sex centers up, out and over the top of her head. As she exhales, she pushes the energy down through his crown and spine and through the genital juncture.

As he exhales, he pushes energy from both sex centers up, out and over the top of her head. As he inhales, he pulls energy down through his crown and spine and through the genital juncture.

You will notice that the energy is going in one direction only—up her spine, down his spine. This can be reversed so that you see energy going up his spine and down hers. You may find that it feels more natural for one partner to draw energy down through the crown and for the other to draw energy up through the root. Follow these inclinations. It will be good to exchange roles, though, in another session.

Whoever is drawing energy down should really concentrate on opening the top of the head and pulling the

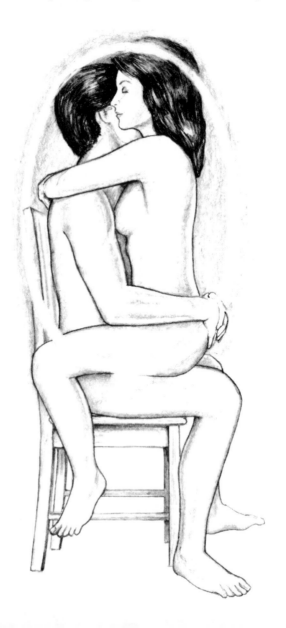

power down through there. Whoever is drawing energy up will deeply focus on opening the pelvis and pulling the power up through there.

Keep the pelvis loose. Rocking gently back and forth or swaying sinuously side to side may help get energy moving.

Strive to feel tangible contact with the breath, there at the crown or the genitals. Do not be surprised if you experience a distinctly erotic feeling in the crown or the sense that your whole body has become open up like a tube.

Remember, you are two halves of a unity. The balance that is found in nature is being celebrated by you now. What you are is beyond even the sum of your two parts. Play your part and do not be concerned about which body is which. Relax, float, be one with the ocean and the waves.

For some people, it is comfortable to take in the breath of the other. This can be shared to the point of sealing your loving exchange with a sustained kiss meditation, so that you do the entire technique in this pose.

As alternate co-breathing can be a bit confusing, here is an approach where you breathe together. If it seems more natural, you may want to try this first.

Breathe together three to six times. Once your breath rhythms are matched, begin the visualization. As you inhale, see energy rise up your own spine from the genital juncture through your head. As you exhale, send the energy in a curve down into your partner's crown and down their spine.

Draw up with your inhalation; pull down with your exhalation. The fact that your breath patterns seem to be going in opposite directions makes no difference at all.

A weather metaphor may be helpful here. Just as hot, moist air rises up into the sky to create clouds, which then bring the cooling and nourishing rains, so you are drawing the warm, earth-based passion fire up and then pulling down the cool, sky-based rain of contentment.

The ascending energy, symbolized by fire, may feel like a thrilling rush of intensity. The descending energy, symbolized by water, may feel like a soothing, saturating sweetness. To use religious terminology, the ascent is the aspiration of your souls, the descent the response to that aspiration in the form of a shower or mist of grace.

When you do this process alone within your own body, you draw the descending force down the front of your body. The connection is then made through the tongue, which is pressed to the roof of the mouth (the Tongue Press).

Esoterically, this is autosexual, as the tongue symbolizes the lingam, the mouth the yoni. You can certainly do this

CIRCLE OF JOY
(YABYUM ON CHAIR)
opposite

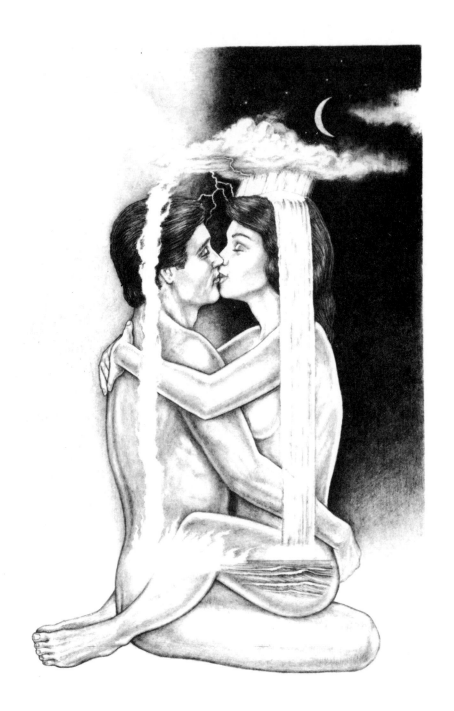

with these advanced breath styles if you wish. In general, do the Tongue Press when you want to contain energy. When you want to release energy, as with orgasm, let it go.

This breath is a good time to do *Elevate Energy*. When you draw the breath up, do the PC clench and hold it. Sniff in to send the energy up through and out the top of the head whenever you are ready. Your consort will take this as a cue and do the same. Remember, never force yourself beyond your comfort zone. The best results come from a relaxed, almost effortless attitude.

Brigitt's Ladder

Brigitt's Ladder is a fusion breathing technique for Tantric orgasm that David received from a *Dream Lover*. It has three steps: co-breathing up through the *chakras,* visualizing a God and Goddess in YabYum and a ball of light, and melting them into your bodies. Though this sounds elaborate, it is actually quite simple.

Sitting in a comfortable YabYum, begin breathing slowly and deeply together. After establishing an easy rhythm with each other, breathe three times at the root *chakra,* three times at the second *chakra* and so on up to the sixth *chakra,* the third eye center (see *Energy Centers*). Feel that you are exchanging and blending your energies with each breath, so that you are becoming one.

After breathing three times in the sixth *chakra,* perform an extra long exhalation and do One Eye Love, anointing your consort's forehead with saliva and touching foreheads (see *Pair Bonding And Tuning*).

After three more breaths, take a deep inhalation. On the exhalation, pop out through the crown of the head and emerge as God and Goddess. The God above his head quickly merges with the Goddess above her head.

Contemplate this sacred union of a God and Goddess taking place above you. Become them and feel what they feel. Share their exalted mood, their sense of immortality and greatness, their power to fuse as one. Visualize their bodies and ornaments in detail. There is no time limit for this segment. Simply keep your attention there as God and Goddess above your heads.

Eventually, you see a perfectly round ball of glowing light, the blissful quintessence of their union, appear above the heads of the God–Goddess. Now you switch your focus to this ball of light. Eventually, due to the heat of your attention, it begins to melt. The ball of the light and the God–Goddess in YabYum on top of your heads both begin to melt.

FIRE AND WATER
opposite
When your energies are perfectly balanced, you realize your oneness with nature and return to the Garden of Eden.

This precious liquid flows down into your body. You specifically taste its nectar-like sweetness on your tongue. You feel how this nectar seeps through every part of your body, saturating it with cool bliss and deep, lasting satisfaction. As the nectar empties into the ground beneath you, it takes with it impurities cleansed from your bodies. These impurities are quickly consumed by natural forces in the earth and turned into valuable minerals.

A playful yet thoughtful attitude is best. The God and Goddess and ball of light that you create need not conform to traditional images. Let them express how you feel about yourself and your consort. Enjoy their YabYum as an idealized expression of your love. There is no need to match images or compare notes. The feeling is more important.

Fire Flute   The Fire Flute is more forceful than the other fusion breath techniques. Ideally, it is performed in YabYum on a chair or in a modified Seesaw with plenty of pillows behind both of you for support. There are similarities to *Elevate Energy,* but the Fire Flute is done with a go for broke, all or nothing attitude.

The key here is that you want to be able to feel a clear route through the soles of your feet, your body and the top of your head. This is easier to experience when your feet are straightened out rather than bound up as in the classic Yab-Yum.

Unlike the other fusion breaths, which can be performed for a few minutes at a time, repeat the Fire Flute only five times. Breathing together, take five very strong, deep, rapid breaths. Breathe in through your nose, out through your mouth. These are very forceful breaths that will make your body shudder with effort.

As you breathe in, imagine that you are drawing energy up through the soles of your feet and out the top of your head. As you breathe out, imagine that you are drawing energy down through the top of your head and out the soles of your feet. While you do this visualization together and breathe together, see this happening within your own body only. Focus totally on the sensations you are feeling.

On the fifth inhalation, hold the breath at the top of your head as long as it is comfortable. Then, exhale slowly and gently through the mouth.

When you do the last exhalation, place your attention at a point about two feet above your heads between your bodies. You can roll your eyes up if you wish. From this point see and feel glowing, scintillating golden energy pour down on top of you and all around you, thoroughly soaking your bodies and the space around you with blissful light. You will now feel as if you are in a giant ball of light, that you are surrounded all around by a bright radiance. Feel that the top of this ball of light is above your heads and that a rain of blissful energy falls down upon you from there.

If you are inspired to do so, feel free to hang out at the apex point above your head. Come down only when you feel you are ready to do so.

Three or four cycles of the Fire Flute is usually enough. If you do it too forcefully, you may feel like you are going to pass out. Of course, you may like this feeling!

As with any other technique that alters your natural breathing pattern, be sure to do it in moderation. Also, do not do this breath or any other special breath pattern, especially ones that involve holding the breath, while on drugs. Drugs can definitely override the body's natural safeguards, creating a very serious health risk.

Since all these techniques tend to bring energy up to the head, grounding afterwards may be a good idea. Personal grounding also helps you to feel your own identity again after all this energy merging (see *Ground And Store Energy*).

Fusion breathing can be a style in itself or just a phase in your extended lovemaking session that takes you to another level while reducing the arousal of the man, essential for prolonging intercourse. Just as in *War And Peace* you took a break, perhaps to have iced tea and oranges, now you take a break to do ecstatic fusion breathing.

A nice way to transition back is to simply hold each other close for awhile, feeling the tenderness of the moment. Heart To Heart, One Eye Love and Trespasso from the *Pair Bonding And Tuning* sequence are also a good way to continue to share the delightful subtleties of your energy exchange before returning to a more vigorous style of lovemaking or transitioning into rest or sleep.

Fusion breathing techniques certainly will lead to an energy high in which a momentary sense of ego loss is experienced. However, our experience has been that integrating fusion breath and other sexual energy experiences into daily life requires a firm and lasting commitment to personal and spiritual growth. We especially recommend the practice of meditation or the equivalent (see *Deep Relaxation, Hara, Making Love Is A Touching Experience, Meditation And Tantra, Taoist Circle Of Gold, Wave Of Bliss*).

TANTRIC RITUAL SEX

Tantra does not approach sex as an indulgence. Instead, it seeks to elevate the sexual act to its highest possible level. The thrilling fusion that is briefly felt during conventional orgasm is experienced so consciously and completely that the individual unites with cosmic consciousness.

Sometimes called *samadhi,* this experience is attainable by a loving couple provided they are able to cultivate an attitude of serene surrender and stay with the sex yoga discipline. Hindu Tantra Yoga, from which this style is taken, is easily adapted to the needs of Western couples.

While the Buddhist Tantrics seem to advocate a sort of absolute yogic commitment that would exclude the average seeker, the Hindu Tantrics believe that a sincere, mindful ritual is a sufficient sacrifice for beginners. As long as the attitude of sacrifice is cultivated, the Tantric couple is encouraged to approach the rite at their level.

The mighty oak tree grows from a tiny acorn. Sooner or late, the sex yoga will be fulfilled and *samadhi* attained.

Sacred Chemistry

Since the Tantric ritual has been outlined in great detail in Bharati, Garrison, Mookerjee and Saraswati (see *Bibliography*), we will concentrate on the inner yoga, the alchemy of attitude that is the sacred intent of the ritual.

The Tantric vision is to embrace all life. Tantra teaches that you cannot transcend sex by denying it. Only the full, conscious experience of sex can lead to a higher awareness in which intrinsic bliss transcending even sexual pleasure is realized.

Mental and emotional stability, the ability to achieve a degree of meditative calm and an eagerness to experience the spiritual dimension of sex are the basic prerequisites. Beyond that, though, there must be a willingness to embrace the divine or infinite dimension of life.

The woman is worshiped as the perfect expression of divine energy *(Shakti).* The man is worshiped as the ideal expression of divine awareness *(Shiva).* Together, they represent the pure, primordial consciousness which has neither beginning nor end, one without a second, the perfect, eternal peace and bliss that is our ultimate nature.

The participants must have as their mutual goal a higher consciousness, even enlightenment, rather than reproduction or erotic pleasure. If they are unable to step beyond their usual view of themselves as man and woman and achieve a sense of reverence for each other as god and goddess, as holy beings, then the ritual should be aborted.

According to tradition, only if this sacred chemistry of

TANTRIC RITUAL
opposite
In a Tantric ritual, she is
worshipped as a Goddess.

mutual devotion to each other as an embodiment of higher consciousness is achieved will the ritual bear fruit. In fact, with practice, this state of mind does develop. Exotic as this method seems to those of us with Judeo-Christian backgrounds, the results are quite reliable.

Sacrificing The Elements

In the traditional ritual, called *panchatattva sadhana,* five types of objects—parched grain, fish, wine, meat and intercourse—are enjoyed as sacraments. These items offer many layers of symbolic meaning for those who have cultivated that knowledge. However, they can also be enjoyed simply as a mindful sacrifice that purifies the senses.

As with the Buddhist approach, the ideal is that the aspirants receive direct instructions from a guru and practice yogic disciplines for several years prior. Nonetheless, as the Hindu Tantra has great faith in the efficacy of ritual, some prominent gurus have waived even these requirements for sincere seekers.

Passionate cultivation of the "divine mood," unimpaired by false modesty, inhibiting doubts or emotional fragility, is thought to overcome technical limitations. Blind adherence to technique, in contrast, may lead to a dryness or rigidity that fails to please the impulsive Kundalini, sometimes symbolized as a ravishing, passionate young woman.

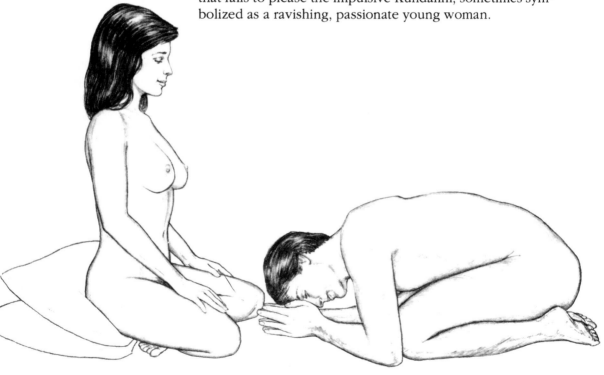

Here sexual union, or *maithuna,* is a ritual sacrifice of body, mind and self. Ancient belief is that we descended from light. Via this ritual of the five elements, the direction is reversed. We return into the light.

Maithuna, symbolizing space, is the culminating stage of the ancient sequence of earth, water, fire and air. While *Third Eye Sex* attempts to attain union with this light directly by leaping straight up to the third eye above the brows, this ritual method follows a gradual approach that progressively refines the senses and uses them to springboard into illumination (see *Energy Centers*).

The various ingredients of the ritual create a recipe that encourages this upward progress of energy. Incense and perfume appeal to the sense of smell, stimulating the root energy center in the cervix or perineum. Wine and other liquid refreshment arouse taste awareness at the sex center in the lower belly. The sight of the beloved and the dancing fire of the ritual candles awaken the solar plexus. The practice of *nyasa* as well as other forms of touching during the ceremony activate the heart in the chest region. Sounds, such as ritual music and the mantras that you repeat together, stimulate the throat center. At the top of this sensual ladder of ritual love lies the third eye, linked to the core of the brain. The kiss of your undivided attention will wake it up.

Ritual Reality   The basic setting is simple enough. After purifying the environment, decorate it in a beautiful manner with rich hues of red, purple and gold. The preferred incense is sandalwood. Rose, jasmine or musk can be added. Hibiscus or other red flowers, candlelight and an altar complete the ritual space.

To finalize the physical setting, on the floor (or other suitable surface) draw a large mandala, or geometrical mystic diagram, that shows two triangles interweaved within a circle. One is pointed up, the other down. You may recognize this ancient symbol of integration as the Star of David or the Seal of Solomon.

Other classic preparations include washing the body and perfuming it with oils such as rose, jasmine, patchouli and sandalwood. The purpose is to literally transform the body into a temple of cosmic consciousness, an appropriate vessel for the divine descent.

Physical purification is followed by mental purification. After meditating on a mantra such as "Om" or "God is love," contemplate the unity of cosmic male and female represented by the symbol of interlaced triangles within a circle.

The aspirants anoint each other on the palms, feet, third eye, eyelids, ear lobes, lips, breasts, navel and genitals. Known as *nyasa,* this can be performed in silent reverence. Or, with each anointing of a body part, repeat "Om" or affirm aloud "You are my god/goddess." Classic mantras for *nyasa* can be found in the published accounts of the sacred ritual.

Now the first four elements are enjoyed as sacraments.

Maithuna— The fifth and final element, *maithuna,* is enjoyed in a very
Joy Of Space specific way if the union is to follow the strict Hindu Tantric formula. Variations include *Extrasensory Sex* or *Kabbazah Sex* as consciousness raising strategies. The approach included here is a very traditional, very disciplined sex yoga method. Performed with dedication, it is one of the most powerful awareness techniques known.

The consorts sit in front of each other and breathe together so that the inbreath and the outbreath are of the same duration. Mindfulness of this balancing breath is maintained for the entire *maithuna.* They may chant "Om" together on the exhalation if they wish. The mind is concentrated on the *muladhara,* or root, *chakra* at the cervix, perineum or the base of the spine (see *Energy Centers*).

After awhile, the couple experiences an energy that starts to rise up the back. This energy is consciously drawn up the spine with the inhalation and then given to the consort with the exhalation.

When this energy is very strong, the male *Shiva* draws the female *Shakti* to him. Lingam and yoni are briefly worshipped. She sits in his lap in the classic YabYum position. Now she brings the lingam into the yoni. Completely motionless, the couple begins the sex meditation proper.

Dedicated To The The eyes and mental focus are placed at the third eye.
One Eye Love Continuing the breath awareness, the couple unites foreheads. They join their eyes into one (the One Eye Love). Awkward as this may seem, it quickly leads to a fusion of consciousness (see *Pair Bonding And Tuning*).

Staying with this merging of the eyes is important. Like psychic glue, the technique keeps the mind alert, preventing daydreaming, sleepiness and self-consciousness. Attention is kept firmly on the third eye, resulting in a definitive break from the usual pull towards genital stimulation.

Fixed in this spiritual embrace, awareness is purified as the energies and subtle bodies of the *Shiva* and *Shakti* interweave, unite, intensify and balance. When total polarization is achieved, which may take a few minutes or several hours, the regenerative Tantric orgasm results and a lasting experience of superconsciousness occurs.

While this kind of meditation for the attainment of higher consciousness is certainly not unique to India or the Hindu Tantra Yoga, this particular technique, also called *lata sadhana,* has been tried and tested over the centuries. Demanding as this practice is, when a couple does experience this total fusion, the relationship is forever elevated to a higher, more fulfilling plane.

There is perhaps no greater gift that we can give as a lover to another. Though obviously not for everyone, here is the total fulfillment implied by the primal gesture towards union that we call sex. Those interested in the yoga training behind this method may want to explore the Tantra Yoga system (see *Appendix*).

KABBAZAH SEX

In the old days in the Middle East, a woman who had mastered *Pompoir* (voluntary control of the circumvaginal muscles during sexual intercourse) was known as kabbazah or "holder." If you've ever had the experience, from either side, then you know just how appropriate the label is.

Back then this style was much more widely known and kabbazahs were more numerous. We are convinced that Kabbazah Sex was at one time a stock in trade of many of the more talented prostitutes in India, China, Japan, Persia and other countries in the East. This tradition is still alive today.

A man taking one of our workshops reported that while he was stationed in Japan during its occupation following World War II, he went to a Japanese prostitute. She bathed him and asked if he wanted to try something new. Without hesitation, he agreed. After he entered her, he was instructed to lie still and fully relax while she did all the work.

The sensations he experienced were incredible and truly exquisite, unlike anything he had ever felt before while inside a woman. Eager, innocent of expectation and starved for the feel of a woman's body, he was the ideal candidate. Because the nature of their relationship was that of leader and follower, or expert and novice, he was not hampered by the obstacle of male pride and followed her suggestions to the letter.

Within half an hour, he reported, they were sharing the ecstasies of the classic Tantric orgasm experience of energy oneness. It was, he said, to put it mildly, an unforgettable experience.

The ancient institution of sacred prostitution, which was active in Southern India as recently as the 1930s, must have made use of Kabbazah Sex in a similar way. If ever there was a way that a woman could offer a man the ecstasy of the gods, it is with Kabbazah Sex. Her kabbazah ability makes this experience possible, but she enjoys the same ecstasy.

It is difficult for us today to appreciate the training some of the prostitutes, sacred and otherwise, underwent in those days. Some, particularly those destined for temple service, were trained from an early age, much as apple-cheeked cherubs are sent off to their first ballet classes.

In some parts of Africa today, girls receive kabbazah training and may even be forbidden to marry unless they display mastery of it.

The practical point in this is that real mastery of *Pompoir* is usually needed to bring off the technique elegantly. If the female partner is struggling and straining to fulfill her part, to "do all the work," Kabbazah Sex can become quite cumbersome. She will not enjoy it and will suffer from performance stress in much the same way that men do when they "do all the work." She will experience fatigue and that will be the end of that lovemaking session, at least in Kabbazah Sex style.

Strategic abstinence is sometimes helpful. If a couple is willing to forego sexual release for three to seven days and yet encourage their sexual feelings for each other, the increased genital sensitivity and cumulative desire intensity may be sufficient to put them over the edge. A good time to try this is when you are reuniting after a physical separation. Still, the best guarantee of satisfactory results using this ancient technique is that she be kabbazah.

For communion this intimate, the quality of the feeling and the depth of the honesty between the man and woman can be decisive. Thoughts and emotions withheld from the consort, though invisible, act as solid barriers to merging the currents of your total selves. Well before trying this kind of lovemaking, confess any acts that have separated you from each other.

Role Reversal   The Kabbazah Sex style follows a very specific format. Like many of the styles already discussed, prolonged motionlessness may be necessary. The woman plays a precise and dynamic starring role. In *Imsak,* her *Pompoir* is encouraged. In Kabbazah Sex, it is the very heart of the method.

The concept of utter male passivity will strike some people as bizarre, perhaps even offensive. Actually, it is a wonderful experience. It can be a great relief for the man to be completely free of familiar performance demands during lovemaking.

He is also released to focus completely on the not un-challenging process of achieving total relaxation while being sexually stimulated. Finally, if he is a contemplative man, he will find the experience of going into contemplative reverie or some other form of meditation uniquely satisfying in this context.

Kabbazah Sex makes use of an authentic ancient secret, which is the power of kabbazah itself. Most men and women live, make love and die, never suspecting the awesome power of the virtuoso vagina. So great is this power that it could revolutionize current lovemaking if it became popular.

STANDARD SEX	KABBAZAH SEX
man is on top	woman is on top
man moves penis	woman moves vagina
woman is passive	man is passive
man is in control	woman is in control
man is aggressive	man is receptive
tension-relief orgasm	Tantric orgasm of total relaxation

Although the orgasm of total relaxation can be achieved in other ways, making use of the kabbazah power holder is one of the most logical and reliable methods. Kabbazah Sex successfully restructures the human sex act and achieves an ingenious total reversal of the stereotyped male-dominated sex act (see *Doing It Rite, Tantric Ritual Sex*).

Ancient Secret   We would like to emphasize staying in the sensory present. Kabbazah Sex is an ancient secret, but fulfillment will not be found by duplicating the past but rather in rediscovering the present.

What is the best way to prepare for Kabbazah Sex?

In the past, elaborate ritualistic procedures, designed to induce the requisite mood of total male surrender, often accompanied this Kabbazah Sex style. As the experience of the American serviceman with the Japanese prostitute il-lustrates, however, for Westerners a state of deep relaxation is probably even more fundamental. For some people, ob-viously, rituals do result in relaxation and, perhaps, a con-venient trance state that makes concentration much easier.

A suitable environment, physical and mental relaxation, setting aside plenty of time, a woman who is kabbazah and a man who is willing to be blissfully passive, these are the basic ingredients (see *Boudoir Basics*).

Repetitions of the Root Lock and the Thunderbolt Gesture prior to intercourse are considered helpful by sexual yogis. These, of course, are breath-intensified Kegel exercises, so you can do Kegel squeezes instead. There is something to be said for the impromptu union, too.

Now for the essence. Here is one of the most powerful techniques for experiencing a blissful, lasting alteration of consciousness discovered by humankind.

Here is the key to the Kabbazah Sex:

SHE ONLY MOVES—WITHIN.

Yes, it really is that simple.

The way she moves is internally. She does not even shuttle back and forth or circle around with her body. She does what no man can do—*Pompoir.*

Allow at least the minimum 30 to 40 minutes of genital union that is standard for all of the soft, yin styles.

Keep in mind that total relaxation is the secret.

Some positions are definitely better. The classic YabYum is difficult for most people to hold properly. Sitting on a fat pillow or meditation cushion, i.e., a Zen *zafu,* may help. Place giant pillows behind both of you to modify the Yab-Yum and provide the back with support. Or try a chair, a small pillow under her buttocks for comfort (see page 348).

Most positions in which the man is lying down on his back and the woman is on top will do just fine. *Es sibfahbeh* or *viparita maithuna* (see page 343) is specific for Kabbazah Sex, as this position brings lingam and yoni into forceful contact, intensifying sensation. Though the Scissors makes it harder for the yoni to grasp the lingam, its comfort can be sheer luxury (see *Peaceful Positions, Bio-Electric Sex*).

Step-By-Step To Tantric Orgasm

Here is the formula. Even if you don't stick to it, or you don't have the same experience, isn't it reassuring to know that there is a step-by-step way to achieve what may be the ultimate sexual experience?

○ Only she moves *(Pompoir).*
○ He does not move his hips or pelvis at all (never the entire time—not even once).
○ She does not move her hips or pelvis at all.

o Remember, all the action is internal via *Pompoir* only.

o The couple remains motionless except for the drama of the jewel in the lotus occuring in her womb. This is the classic recommendation. You may find, though, that you can caress and kiss and gaze in each other's eyes without accelerating into the usual arousal, resulting in thrusting and the standard orgasm. Basic motionlessness enables maximum focus on the genital sensations. Stillness, not stiffness, is what is being asked here.

o Remember, she, not he, is in control.

o Take your time. Easy does it. The tendency is to rush. Rush where? Ecstasy beyond convenient pleasure takes time.

o You want peace, serenity, calm. Your mood and every action, every response, is an affirmation of peace.

o At the same time, you deeply feel and encourage your desire and arousal. Your passions are slowly climbing to a white-hot temperature, hotter even than red-hot. You are experiencing genital arousal dialog. As she stimulates him, his penis throbs. As his penis throbs, she is further aroused, stimulating him more. As he gets more stimulated, so does she. And so it goes on and on in a seemingly never-ending upward spiral. Remember, she will have to ease up at certain times to avoid stimulating him into genital orgasm.

o After awhile, you reach what can be called the "too much" stage of throbbing and pulsating sex organs. You may feel like you are going out of your mind, the urge for relief will be so great. Or, you may not experience this stage so intensely. You may not experience it at all and move right through to the next one.

o After about 15 minutes of *Pompoir,* you will experience a bioelectrical force field effect. An aura of peace and benign energy is felt. The best word to describe the feeling is probably sacred. You may feel that you are on truly holy ground. You feel startlingly alive and clear-headed. You feel that the two of you are one.

o You are both now enjoying a wonderful out of this world (meditative) state. You feel inspired, aglow, rejuvenated. She stimulates the man as needed.

o Tantric orgasm takes place for both about 30 minutes from the beginning of the union. This is 15 minutes after the force field effect was first felt.

By all means, do not take this outline as gospel. We are all individuals and each couple is a unique combination.

There is one action the man can take which we haven't mentioned. He can contract his PC and anal muscles to join in. It is also possible, at the outer limits of sexercise practice, to develop the muscles that move the penis up and down and side to side to such an extent that the penis can be moved around within the vagina without moving the rest of the body. Then two can tango in quiet body sex meditation.

We have said nothing about visualizations, affirmations and the like. If you like them, use them.

THIRD EYE SEX What you've got to understand—this is the whole point—is that Tantra isn't about techniques. It's about changing, rearranging, sacrificing your usual mood. Attaining to a holy mood, a mood of worship, reverence, awe, devotion, wonder, glory, innocence, veneration, adoration, no mind.

The techniques, the ritual, the lovecraft are all about how to achieve this alchemy of mood, which is a very great thing, a magic. Then, when the mood is right, pure, refined, true, sacred, holy, authentic, then whatever you do will be right.

Spend most of your time on creating the mood. The sex union will take care of itself. But as long as you are still thinking self-limiting, socially conditioned thoughts, "We are a man and a woman making love," then it is not yet Tantra.

Go For The Glow When you start to see or feel or sense the soft, lush luminescence that is around all the edges of everything and the glow seeps through and you are suddenly wondering and not knowing and not in control but somehow surprised and happy—then it is right. Then it's not fucking. Then it's God. Goddess. Lover. Beloved. You're home. You're in the light.

If your mind is already totally sexed, if you are in its lavishly lustful grip, then Tantra could be for you. Take your fascination with sex and use it. Relax and go into that warm, sweet honey place, into the magnetic center of it, yield to it, open to it, explore it, be pulled down to your root by it.

Relax and melt wide awake into the soft, flowing, glowing, golden pit. Let the life force rise up in rushing, roaring, singing, soaring waves that melt your mind and spread all through you and lift you up in a fountain of love to the top in bliss explosion beyond death.

Sex is not what you think. Sex is natural LSD.

Samadhi Flash During lovemaking there can be continuous unity perception, *samadhi*. There is that flash of lightning, yes, but we can grab it, hold onto it, cultivate it. It sizzles for a second, almost an hallucination, but it is real.

It flashes there in the middle of intercourse and then vanishes. Know it, love it, become a friend of that light. In those moments when you become one with it, you are, paradoxically, beyond the body, beyond all the bodyness of anybody and everybody, weightless, flying, beyond, gone.

Then, having glimpsed it, having seen the glory of your being, of your brightness, you fall deeply in love with yourself. You passionately seek to fully uncover who you are.

Long, Slow, Deep

Notice three things: that the longer intercourse lasts the more opportunity there is for seeing the light, that it is important that your breathing be calm and slow, and that the place to put the mind is at the third eye.

Arousal can be none, some, overwhelming. It is challenging to play with the edge of fire but ambition has no place in the bedroom. The early embers are easier to handle. Know your limitations. You are already One—no amount of effort can make it so. This is just a way to taste it.

If the breathing is fast, intercourse will be short. If you want to use sex to reach superconsciousness, to go beyond ego, beyond time, breathe slowly. When the breath is slow, slow, slow, you go deeper, deeper, deeper into your root, into sex, into source, into essence, into life, into death, into *samadhi*. The other thing is this: keep the attention between the eyes at the *ajna chakra,* the third eye, the psychic center in the center of the brain. Then an ineffable Tantric climax of many hours is possible.

Just keep the attention between the eyebrows or in the center of the head, where the inner light of the mind is seen. Right away making love will be much deeper, will move closer to the core, will become sublime, will invoke the blissful light of wholeness.

Prayer Mat Of The Flesh

The body is the temple. The heart is the door. Yoni and lingam are the holy of holies. Lips are the sacrament, tongues the wafer, juices the wine, moans the liturgy, our waves of ecstasy, my beloved, the baptism.

Now you realize that your attraction to sex was not just to fuck, not just to come, not just to feel good just to feel good, but to soak in *samadhi,* to sweat with light, to swim in endless, timeless seas of joy, to dance in the heart of space.

This pull is magnetic, it is total, it is ultimately pure. It is ourselves. We are making love to ourselves. We seek our selves, our real selves, our authentic selves.

Through love, we seek the self, the One True Self. There is no other choice. We will not rest until we find it.

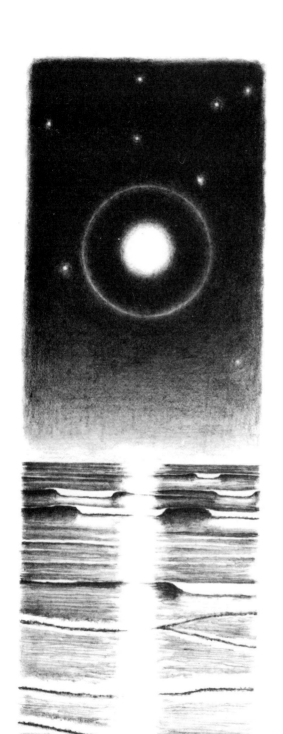

Wave
Of
Bliss

HAPPINESS IS KNOWING YOU ARE SINGLE

happiness is knowing you are single

alone forever
are you

whether your consorts are none, one, few or many
they have but one face

a reflection in the mirror

those who are joined
will eventually part

those who are a part
will eventually be whole

all is a process of
uniting and separating

do not be fooled by appearances

how can relationships be permanent
when life itself is not?

no one can love you
unless you love you

the greatest love, the sweetest love, the best love
stands on ground sanctified
by a love of freedom

without fresh air
even the finest fire
dies

ENDLESS ORGASM

We are advocates of the endless orgasm (climax). We are advocates of the endlessly orgasmic relationship.

Orgasm is a state of mindbody. In the sexualove play between man and woman, male and female polarities, the potential exists for endless orgasm.

When people speak of endless love, of ultimate romantic love, what they are actually referring to is this dynamic condition of endless orgasm.

Once it is understood how to maintain that subtle ongoing sense of orgasm, of thrilling dynamic circulating aliveness, it need never end but only expand and go higher and higher and deeper and deeper.

What is non-stop orgasm?

Endless orgasm is a kind of recycling.

Not that you're always in a state of physical orgasmic spasming. But that your lovemaking never really ends. You make the transition from bed to head and heart and retain the ecstatic glow in daily life. Life is foreplay, arousal, orgasm and afterglow all rolled into one resonant bursting forth, for so much of the time that the fundamental tone or quality of your relationship is, somehow, orgasmic.

Endless orgasm is for those who can be responsible for staying in love, for stepping out of the mental trivia trap, out of everyday thinking mind.

Thoughts can kill endless orgasm, just as they can kill ordinary orgasm during ordinary sex.

Desire, left to itself, will try to end the interaction. Desire wants to achieve the goal, the orgasm, the relief. Desire is not concerned with what will be after.

Love, on the other hand, wants never to end. Lovers long for immortality together. The heart is at home in heaven. Endless orgasm is endless giving to and receiving from love.

But love, by itself, cannot be enough for lovers. Otherwise, lovers are just friends, mutual benefactors. Desire, an undefinable yet irrefutable magnetic attraction, is needed. Steady desire, stable desire, desire to make love, desire to be with your lover, desire to share joy, desire fostered by Sexual Energy Ecstasy lovemaking.

Desire is the fuel and the fire. Love is the oven and the temperature control. Life energy is the bread upon which you feast as you exchange essences via your union.

The love, the respect, the esteem between love partners provides the special space in which this one act play of polar opposites may playfully yet intensely go on and on in endless cycles of expansion and contraction, of rising and falling, of in and out, of for and against, of yes and no, of pain and pleasure, of birth and death of self.

This is possible because the man holds the essence of woman in him, and the woman holds the essence of man in her. What is outside male is inside female. What is outside female is inside male.

The ideal of growth is nurtured by a relationship that recognizes the value of the twenty-four hour day after day orgasm, of lovemaking that never ends.

The differences are only in what is on the outside and what is in the inside, not in what is. The differences provide the track, the circuit, the two poles of positive and negative polarity needed for energy flow to begin and continue, for energy and ecstasy. The same polarity is demonstrated at the level of the universe and the atom and man-woman.

Enjoy this polarity. It is a form of balance. In the game of balance lost, sought and regained three needs are at work: the need to reach for the other, the need to commune and the need to release that union and return to the integrity of self alone.

Authentic action is the key, and it is based on having a deep practical understanding of life's everyday dramas.

What must be understood is the natural cycle, the fundamental reality of rhythm as it applies to a relationship. The ocean tides flow in and out. The sun and the moon share the sky in a rhythm of day and night. Man and woman, as phenomena of nature, are part of this rhythmic process.

The feeling of closeness will appear and disappear. The feeling of distance will appear and disappear. The feeling of neutralness, of being neither attracted nor repelled by the other, will appear and disappear.

This cannot be changed. You might as well try to grab the sun out of the sky and carry it in your pocket.

What can be changed is your relationship to it.

It is an impersonal process. In and out, back and forth, together and apart, up and down, like the breath which never ends as long as you are alive. It is quite uncontrollable.

Since you cannot defeat it, join it.

Your feelings of anger and alienation are blessings in disguise. Your feelings of indifference and neutrality are a hidden delight. It is the natural time to take a break, to renew the primary relationship, the relationship with yourself. At such times be relieved of the need for others.

Glory in your self-sufficiency. Revel in your self-reliance.

Taste the sweetness of your supreme aloneness. Be the eagle, free to soar confidently through an empty sky of shimmering blue, above and beyond the lonely confusion below.

The key to fulfilling your possibility for endless orgasm in a relationship is to become harmless. Harmlessness is the absence of ill will. It is objective compassion, neutral caring, unqualified good will, high indifference.

Harmlessness is self-esteem in action.

To become even a little harmless brings great freedom.

Become harmless.

There comes a time when it is seen that everything in our world around us, and in our relationships in particular, is a reflection of our relationship with ourselves.

On the outside opposites may attract, but inside it is sameness, agreement, that attracts.

Endless orgasm is a celebration of the exciting friction created by the differences between two polarized persons who can remain in emotional agreement with one another. It is not a new standard, a new goal, a new measure of love.

It is a form of fire walking.

It is an invitation to dance, and, in the dancing, to remember why you came to this party in the first place.

WAVE OF BLISS

my beloved
you are the gate
you are the way
you are the answer

every pore a portal
every breath a blessing
you are the secret joy body
that will never end

your halo
precious one
a sparkling rainbow of desires
glistening in the burning kisses
of a self-consuming sun

love's hot pursuit
undying fuel for
this endless dream
will outlive
even that golden witness

Shankaracharya, a complex mystic, called you
Anandalahari—Wave Of Bliss

oh, you are a crazy lover
your wave of bliss
is so strong
you swept me away
and dissolved me
in your endless seas
of delirious vibration

WAVE OF BLISS *below*
After *View Of Mount Fuji*
by Kurosawa.

you showed me the way:
honor the Goddess
honor the act of making love
honor oneness at every level
honor my Self

find the peaceful place
beyond time and space
future faceless
past erased

yes, you burn in my body
loving you is loving me

still
to believe in you
as you appear—separate from me
is the bittersweet trap

the search is endless
once I take that sleepy step

ecstatic yet serene
the ultimate lover
I sing the song of Myself
and celebrate You

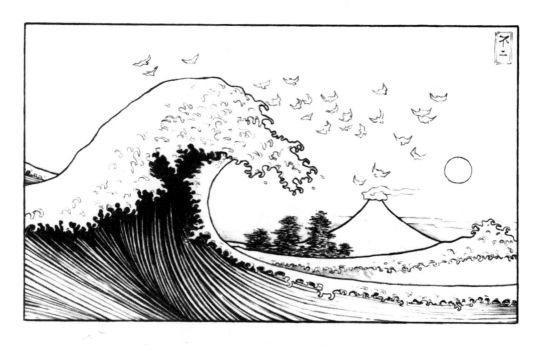

APPENDIX

Acupressure:
The G-Jo Institute, Box 8060, Hollywood, FL 33024.

Essential Perfume Oils And Incense:
Attar Bazaar, Ltd., Box 99, Sidney, NY 13838.
Garuda, Box 1162, Fairfax, CA 94930. Tibetan products.

Foot Reflexology:
Reflexology, Box 12642, St. Petersburg, FL 33733.
Laura Norman Reflexology Center, 117 E. 24th St., Suite 4B, NY, NY 10010.

Health Organizations:
Academy of Orthomolecular Psychiatry, 1691 Northern Blvd., Manhasset, NY 11030.
American Holistic Medical Association, 6932 Little River Turnpike, Annandale, VA 22003.
Huxley Institute, 1114 First Avenue, NY, NY 10021.
Int'l Acad. of Preventive Medicine, 10409 Town & Country Way, # 200, Houston, TX 77024.
National Association of Naturopathic Physicians, 2613 N. Stevens, Tacoma, WA 98407.
National Health Federation, 211 W. Foothill Blvd., Monrovia, CA 91016.
National Women's Health Network, 224 7th St. S.E., Washington, DC 20003.
Society for Clinical Ecology, 109 W. Olive St., Fort Collins, CO 80524. Allergy help.

Health Technology:
Biocircuit™ can be ordered from Peak Skill Publishing, Box 5489, Playa Del Rey, CA 90296.
Duro-Test Corp., 2321 Kennedy Blvd., N. Bergen, NJ 07047. Full spectrum lighting.
Floatation Tank Association c/o Alma Daniel, 300 Central Park N., NY, NY 10024.
Special Fx Lighting, 3665 W. Diablo, No. 6, Las Vegas, NV 89118. Natural spectrum lighting.

Herbs:
Herbalist & Alchemist, Box 458, Bloomsbury, NJ 08804.
Herb Products Co., Box 898, North Hollywood, CA 91603.
House Of Hezekiah, 4305 Main St., Kansas City, MO 64111.
Herb-Pharm, P.O. Box 116, Williams, OR 97544. Source for pygeum bark in liquid form.
St. Jude Herb Center, Box 563, Huntington Station, NY 11746.

Kundalini Assistance:
Dhyanyoga Centers, Box 3194, Antioch, CA 94531. Asha Ma/Dhyanyogi Madhusudandasji.
Guruji Thapasyogi, C.K.S., Thapas Yoga Ashram, 5 Rathas Road, Mahabalipuram, India.
Stuart Sovatsky, Ph.D., The Kundalini Clinic, Oakland, CA.
Spiritual Emergence Network (SEN) c/o I.T.P., 1010 Doyle, Suite 10, Menlo Park, CA 94025.

Meditation:
Advaita Fellowship, Box 911, Redondo Beach, CA 90277. Ramesh Balsekar, successor to
    Sri Nisargadatta Maharaj of *I Am That* fame. Advaita Vedanta at its very best.
Anandashram P.O., 670531, Kanhangad, Kerala, South India. Sri Swami "Papa" Ramdas.
Center for Sacred Sciences, 1430 Willamette, #164, Eugene, OR 97401-4049. Joel Morwood.
Community Meditation Center, 1041 S. Elden Ave., Los Angeles, CA 90006. Shinzen Young.
Hanuman Tape Library, Box 61498, Santa Cruz, CA 95061.
Inner Light Foundation, Box 761, Novato, CA 94948. Betty Bethards.
Insight Meditation Society, Pleasant St., Barre, MA 01005. Vipassana.
Insight Meditation West, Box 9658, Berkeley, CA 94709. Vipassana.
Jean Klein Foundation, Box 940, Larkspur, CA 94939. Contemporary Advaita Vedanta.
Justin Stone, Box 397, Santa Barbara, CA 93102. T'ai Chi Chih master.
Nityananda Institute, Box 1973, Cambridge, MA 02238. Kashmir Shaivism.
Self-Studies Foundation, Box 93, Ojai, CA. Ligia Dantes.
Sri Lakshmana Ashram, Chillakur, Gudur, Nellore Dist., 524412, Andhra Pradesh, India.
Sri Ramanasramam P.O., Tiruvannamalai-606 603, South India.
Vipassana Meditation Center, Box 24, Shelburne Falls, MA 01370.

Music:
Backroads Distributors, 417 Tamal Plaza, Corte Madera, CA 94925, 1-800-825-4848.
Bindu, 1 Penn Plaza, Suite 100, NY, NY 10119. Tantra yoga resources.
Chidvilas, Box 17550, Boulder, CO 80308. Osho (Rajneesh) meditation music.
Kahua Institute, Box 1747, Makawao, Maui, HI 96768. *Tantric Wave* and Raphael's music.
Sound Rx Productions, Box 2644, San Anselmo, CA 94960. Steven Halpern tapes.

Relationship Astrology:
David A. Ramsdale, M.A., Peak Skill, Box 5489, Playa Del Rey, CA 90296.

Ritual Skills:
Al G. Manning, E.S.P. Laboratory, Box 216, Edgewood, TX 75117.

Sacred Sexuality Seminars:
Dr. Stephen Chang, Tao Academy, 2700 Ocean Ave., San Francisco, CA 94132.
Deer Tribe, Box 1519, Temple City, CA 91780. Cherokee Quodoshka sacred sexuality path.
Joseph Kramer, "The Dear Love of Comrades" unique training for gay and bisexual men in
    Tantric/Taoist and Reichian approaches, 6527A Telegraph Ave., Oakland, CA 94609.
Kahua Institute, Box 1747, Makawao, Maui, HI 96768. Oceanic Tantra. Kutira & Moonjay.
Sexual Energy Ecstasy® Seminars, Box 5489, Playa Del Rey, CA 90296.
Source Retreats, Charles & Carolyn Muir, Box 69, Paia, Maui, HI 96779.
Stephanie Wadel, M.A., Box 60971, Palo Alto, CA 94306. Cherokee Quodoushka path.

Safer Sex:
AIDS Hotline of US Public Health Service: 1-800-922-AIDS. Tape: 1-800-342-AIDS. Voice:
    1-800-342-7514 (Information).
AmFAR, Suite 406, 40 W. 57 St., NY, NY 10019.
Nat'l AIDS Network, 1012 14th St., NW, Suite 601, Washington, DC 20005, 202-347-0390.
For additional information, contact your local county health care service, local AIDS
    hotline, local chapter of the American Red Cross or check your Yellow Pages.

Sensuality Training:
Kenneth Ray Stubbs, Ph.D., Secret Garden, 1352 Yukon Way, #20, Novato, CA 94947.

Sex Accessories:
Eve's Garden, 119 W. 57th St., #420, NY, NY 10010. Created by women for women & their
    partners. Sensual accessories and books to enhance selflove & shared love. $3/catalog.
Good Vibrations, 1210 Valencia St., San Francisco, CA 94110. $3/catalog. Popular vibrator
    & sex toy source. Also home to extensive The Sexuality Library mail order $3/catalog.
Xandria Collection, Box 31039, San Francisco, CA 94131.

Sex Therapists:
AASECT, 11 Dupont Circle, N. W., Suite 220, Washington, DC 20036.
James Benson, Ph.D., 1400 S. Sunkist St #199, Anaheim, CA 92806, creator of "Hypnosex."
Bryce Britton, M.S., Certified Sex Therapist, 4111 Lincoln Blvd., #631, MDR, CA 90292.
J. Giovannoni, M.A., Certified Sex Therapist, 1481 S. King St., #402, Honolulu, HI 96814.
Jonathan Robinson, M.A., M.F.C.C., Box 1045, Santa Barbara, CA 93102.
Society for the Scientific Study of Sex, Box 208, Mount Vernon, IA 52314.

Sexual Enrichment Seminars:
National Sex Forum, 1523 Franklin St., San Francisco, CA 94109. Advanced sex education.

Tantra Yoga:
Swami Satyananda, Bihar School of Yoga, Monghyr 811201, Bihar, India.
Swami Janakananda, Scandinavian Yoga & Meditation, S-340 13 Hamneda, Sweden.

Videos:
Tantra Love, Peak Skill Publishing, Box 5489, Playa Del Rey, CA 90296.
Intimacy And Sexual Ecstasy, Love Alive Productions, Box 1045, Santa Barbara, CA 93102.

BIBLIOGRAPHY

Allen, Gina and Clement Martin. *Intimacy*. Chicago: Cowles, 1971.

Ayres, Alex. "Running and sexuality." Running Times. April, 1984, 12-22.

Anderiesz, Godfrey. "Where the bee sucks—oriental techniques of oral love." Forum. February, 1972, 22-27.

Beck, Renee and Sydney Metrick. *The Art of Ritual*. Berkeley: Celestial Arts, 1990.

Benton, Holly and Elliot Tanzer. *Celebrate Your Love*. Tantrix: Malibu, 1989.

Berkeley Holistic Health Center Staff. *Holistic Health Lifebook*. New York: Greene, 1984.

Bethards, Betty. *Sex and Psychic Energy: Beyond the Sexual Revolution*. Novato: Inner Light Foundation, 1977.

Bharati, Agehananda. *The Tantric Tradition*. New York: Samuel Weiser, 1975.

Bieler, Henry and Sarah Nichols. *Dr. Bieler's Natural Way To Sexual Health*. Los Angeles: Charles, 1972.

Bindrim, Paul and Helaine Harris. "The Ultimate Sexual Experience." Los Angeles: On-Site Taping, 1982.

Brauer, Alan and Donna. *ESO*. New York: Warner, 1983.

Breaux, Charles. *Journey Into Consciousness*. York Beach: Nicolas-Hays, 1989.

Britton, Bryce. *The Love Muscle*. New York: New American Library, 1982.

Burton, Sir Richard, trans. *The Kama Sutra of Vatsyayana*. New York: E.P. Dutton, 1964.

——, trans. *The Perfumed Garden of the Shaykh Nefzawi*. New York: G.P. Putnam's Sons, 1964.

—— and F.F. Arbuthnot, trans. *The Ananga Ranga of Kalyana Malla*. New York: G.P. Putnam's Sons, 1964.

Bush, Patricia. *Drugs, Alcohol & Sex*. New York: Richard Marek, 1980.

Calhoun, Marcy. *Are You Really Too Sensitive?* Nevada City: Blue Dolphin, 1988.

Carter, Mildred. *Helping Yourself With Foot Reflexology*. West Nyack: Parker, 1969.

Castleman, Michael. *Sexual Solutions*. New York: Simon & Schuster, 1980.

Cerney, J.V. *Acupuncture Without Needles*. West Nyack: Parker, 1974.

Chang, Jolan. *The Tao of Love and Sex*. New York: E.P. Dutton, 1977.

——. *The Tao of the Loving Couple*. New York: E.P. Dutton, 1983.

Chang, Stephen with Richard Miller. *The Book of Internal Exercises*. San Francisco: Strawberry Hill Press, 1978.

Comfort, Alex, ed. *The Joy of Sex*. New York: Crown, 1972.

——, trans. *The Koka Shastra*. New York: Stein and Day, 1965.

Cook, Keven. "The Brawning of America." Playboy, July, 1982, 146-150, 184-190.

Corey, Douglas and Jeannette Maas. *The Energy Couple*. Springfield: Charles C. Thomas, 1980.

Culling, Louis T. *A Manual of Sex Magic*. St. Paul: Llewellyn Publications, 1971.

Cutler, Winnifred. "Q&A interview: Researcher leads men and women through the menopause myths." Michael Fink, ed., L. A. Herald Examiner, October 18, 1983, B7.

Da Free John. *Love of the Two-Armed Form*. Middletown: Dawn Horse Press, 1978.

Dass, Ravi and Aparna. *The Marriage & Family Book: A Spiritual Guide*. New York: Schocken, 1978.

Dean, Carole. "Bach Remedies." Whole Life Times, L. A., January/February, 1982, 49.

Denning, Melita and Osborne Phillips. *The Llewellyn Practical Guide to The Magick of Sex*. St. Paul: Llewellyn, 1982.

Diamond, John. *Your Body Doesn't Lie*. New York: Warner Books, 1979.

Dodson, Betty. *Sex For One: The Joy of Selfloving*. New York: Harmony/Crown, 1987.

Dong, Paul and Aristide Esser. *Chi Gong: the ancient Chinese way to health*. New York: Paragon House, 1990.

Douglas, Nik and Penny Slinger. *Sexual Secrets*. Rochester: Destiny Books, 1979.

Dowman, Keith. *Sky Dancer*. Boston: Routledge & Kegan Paul, 1984.

Downing, George. *The Massage Book*. N. Y./Berkeley: Random House/ Bookworks, 1972.

Dunkell, Samuel. *Lovelives*. New York: New American Library, 1980.

Dunn, Jean, ed. *Seeds of Consciousness: The Wisdom of Sri Nisargadatta Maharaj*. New York: Grove, 1982.

Eliade, Mircea. *Yoga: Immortality and Freedom*. Bollingen Series LVI: Princeton University Press, 1969.

Feuerstein, Georg, ed. *Enlightened Sexuality*. Freedom, CA: The Crossing Press, 1989.

Ferguson, Marilyn, ed. "Endorphins trigger isolation tank euphoria." Brain/Mind Bulletin, January 23, 1984, 1.

Flatto, Edwin. *Warning: Sex May Be Hazardous to Your Health*. New York: Arco, 1976.

Garrison, Omar. *Tantra: the Yoga of Sex*. New York: Avon Books, 1973.

Gillies, Jerry. *Transcendental Sex*. New York: Holt, Rinehart and Winston, 1978.

G-Jo Institute. *The G-Jo Institute Sexual Pleasure Enhancement Program*. 1980.

Gold, E.J. "Alchemical Sex." Canada: Fourth Way Research Associates, no date. Audio cassettes.

—— and Cybele. *Tantric Sex*. Playa Del Rey: Peak Skill Publishing, 1988.

Godman, David. *No Mind—I Am The Self*. Sri Lakshmana Ashram: Gudur, India, 1988.

Gottlieb, Adam. *Sex Drugs and Aphrodisiacs*. Manhattan Beach: 20th Century Alchemist, 1974.

Gunther, Bernard. *Energy Ecstasy and Your Seven Vital Chakras*. Los Angeles: The Guild of Tutors/IC Books, 1978.

Haimes, Leonard and Richard Tyson. *How To Triple Your Energy*. New York: New American Library, 1977.

Halpern, Steven. *Sound Health*. New York: Harper & Row, 1988.

Harris, A. *Sexual Exercises For Women*. New York: Carroll & Graf, 1985.

Hewitt, James. *The Complete Yoga Book*. New York: Schocken, 1978.

Hirsch, Edwin. *The Power to Love*. New York: Garden City Publishing, 1938.

Hollander, Xaviera. *Xaviera's Supersex*. New York: New American Library, 1978.

Holzer, Hans. *Psycho-Ecstasy*. New York: Lancer, 1971.

Ishihara, Akira and Howard Levy. *The Tao of Sex*. Lower Lake: Integral Publishing, 1989.

Iyengar, B.K.S. *Light On Yoga*. New York: Schocken, 1979.

"J". *The Sensuous Woman*. New York: Lyle Stuart, 1969.

Kassorla, Irene. *Nice Girls Do*. Rockville Centre: Playboy, 1982.

Keyes, Laurel Elizabeth. *The Mystery of Sex: A Book About Love*. Denver: Gentle Living Publications, 1975.

Kilham, Christopher. *Stalking The Wild Orgasm*. San Diego: ACS, 1984.

King, Serge. *The Secret Science & Sex*. Malibu: Huna International, 1982.

Kingsland, Kevin and Venika Kingsland. *Complete Hatha Yoga*. New York: Arco, 1983.

—— and Venika Kingsland. *Hathapradipika*. Devon, England: Grael, 1977.

Kinsley, David. *Hindu Goddesses*. Berkeley: University of California Press, 1988.

Kline-Graber Georgia and Benjamin Graber. *Woman's Orgasm*. NY: Popular Library, 1976.

Koestenbaum, Peter. *Existential Sexuality*. Englewood Cliffs: Prentice-Hall, 1974.

Kuhn, Franz. *Jou Pu Tuan*. Franz Kuhn's interpretation in German of Li Yu's masterpiece translated by Richard Martin. New York: Grove Press, 1963.

Leeson, Francis. *Kama Shilpa*. Bombay: D.B. Taraporevala Sons & Co., 1962.

Ladas, Alice, Whipple, Beverly and John Perry. *The G Spot and Other Recent Discoveries About Human Sexuality*. New York: Holt, Rinehart and Winston, 1982.

Leboyer, Frederick. *Inner Beauty, Inner Light*. New York: Knopf, 1978.

Leonard, George. *The End of Sex*. Los Angeles: J.P. Tarcher, 1983.

Levine, Stephen. *A Gradual Awakening*. Garden City: Anchor, 1979.

Lloyd, J. William. *The Karezza Method or Magnetation*. Hollywood: Phoenix House, 1973.

Lynn, Alice. "Female Orgasm Clinics." Penthouse Forum, November, 1975, 53.

"M". *The Sensuous Man*. New York: Lyle Stuart, 1971.

McCary, James. *Human Sexuality*. New York: Van Nostrand Reinhold, 1978.

MacLaine, Shirley. *Going Within*. New York: Bantam, 1989.

Maltz, Maxwell. *Psycho-Cybernetics*. New York: Pocket, 1969.

Masters, William and Virginia Johnson. *Human Sexual Response*. Boston: Little, Brown & Co., 1966.

Meister, Robert. "Prolonging Pleasure—An Exotic Technique." Forum, Nov., 1975, 16-18.

Miller, Richard. *The Magical and Ritual Use of Herbs*. Seattle: Organization for Advancement of Knowledge, 1982.

Moffett, Robert. *Tantric Sex*. New York: Berkley Medallion, 1974.

Mookerjee, Ajit. *Kali: The Feminine Force*. New York: Destiny, 1988.

— and Madhu Khanna. *The Tantric Way*. Boston: New York Graphic Society, 1977.

Moore, Marcia & Mark Douglas. *Diet, Sex & Yoga*. York: Arcane, 1970.

Morgenstern, Michael with S. Naifeh and G. Smith. *How To Make Love To A Woman*. New York: Ballantine, 1983.

Morin, Jack. *Anal Pleasure & Health*. Burlingame: Down There Press, 1986.

Motoyama, Hiroshi. *Theories of the Chakras*. Wheaton: The Theosophical Publishing House, 1981.

Muir, Charles and Caroline. *Tantra: The Art of Conscious Loving*. San Francisco: Mercury House, 1989.

Mumford, Jonn. *Ecstasy Through Tantra*. St. Paul: Llewellyn, 1990.

—. *Psychosomatic Yoga*. London: Thorsons, 1962.

—. *Tantra Sexual Yoga Course*. Audio cassette tapes. St. Paul: Llewellyn, no date.

Namikoshi, Tokujiro. *Shiatsu: Japanese Finger-Pressure Therapy*. Tokyo: Japan, 1972.

Neff, Dio Urmilla. "Tantra: A Tradition Unveiled." Yoga Journal, February, 1983.

—. "Tantra: A Tradition Unveiled Part II." Yoga Journal, April, 1983.

Nelson, Dee Jay and David Coville. *Life Force in the Great Pyramids*. Marina del Rey: DeVorss & Co., 1977.

Nobile, Phillip, ed. "Mysteries of Male Multiple Orgasm: Can A Man Learn To Double His Pleasure?" Forum, August, 1983.

—, ed. "The Forum Interview: Germaine Greer." Forum, April, 1984, 15-17, 70-72.

Omega, Kane. *Cosmic Sex*. New York: Lyle Stuart, 1973.

O'Relly, Edward. *Sexercises*. New York: Crown, 1967.

Osbourne, Arthur. *The Collected Works of Sri Ramana Maharshi*. York Beach: Samuel Weiser, 1968.

Otto, Herbert and Roberta. *Total Sex*. New York: New American Library, 1972.

Patten, Leslie and Terry. *Biocircuits*. Tiburon: H.J. Kramer, 1988.

Pearson, Durk and Sandy Shaw. *Life Extension: A Practical Scientific Approach*. New York: Warner Books, 1982.

Penney, Alexandra. *How To Make Love To A Man*. New York: Dell, 1982.

—. *How To Make Love To Each Other*. New York: G.P. Putnam's Sons, 1982.

Powell, James. *Energy And Eros*. New York: Morrow, 1985.

Rajneesh, Bhagwan Shree (Osho): *The Book of Secrets-I. Discourses on "Vigyana Bhairava Tantra."* New York: Harper Colophon, 1977.

—. *The Book of Secrets-III. Discourses on "Vigyana Bhairava Tantra."* New York: Harper Colophon, 1980.

—. *From Sex To Superconsciousness*. New Delhi: Orient, 1976.

—. *Tantra: The Supreme Understanding*. Rajneeshpuram: Rajneesh Fnd. Internat'l, 1984.

Rama-Andre. *Sexual Yoga*. New York: Quantum, 1974.

Ramsdale, David. "Tantra, the Ecstatic Discipline of Love." L.A. Resources, Fall, 1982, 7.

Rawson, Philip. *Tantra*. London: Thames and Hudson, 1973.

Reagan, Harley Swiftdeer. *The Whirlwind-Serpent Fire*. Deer Tribe, 1983.

Reid, Daniel. *The Tao of Health, Sex, & Longevity*. New York: Fireside, 1989.

Reuben, Carolyn. "Sex and Your Health." L.A. Weekly, Oct. 1, 1982, 34-35.

Reuben, David. *Everything You Always Wanted To Know About Sex But Were Afraid To Ask*. New York: Bantam, 1971.

Rosenberg, Jack. *Total Orgasm*. New York/Berkeley: Random House/Bookworks, 1973.

Sannella, Lee. *Kundalini—Psychosis or Transcendence?* Lower Lake: Integral Publishing, 1988.

SAR. *SAR Guide for a Better Sex Life*. San Francisco: National Sex Forum, 1975.

Saraswati, Swami Janakananda. *Yoga, Tantra and Meditation in daily life*. New York: Bindu, 1991.

Saraswati, Swami Satyananda. *Meditations from the Tantras*. Monghyr, India: Bihar School of Yoga, 1981.

—. *Sure Ways To Self Realization*. Monghyr, India: Bihar School of Yoga, 1983.

Schultz, William. *Shiatsu Japanese Finger Pressure Therapy*. New York: Bell, 1976.

Shankaranarayanan, S. *Glory Of The Divine Mother (Devi Mahatmyam)*. Dipti Publications, Sri Aurobindo Ashram, Pondicherry-2, 1973.

Shapescope. "Lean, healthy, but not pregnant." Shape, October, 1982, 115.

Shih, Tzu Kuo. *The Swimming Dragon*. Barrytown: Station Hill, 1989.

Shivanandan, Mary. *Natural Sex*. New York: Berkley Books, 1981.

Siegel, Ronald. "Herbal Intoxication: Psychoactive effects from herbal cigarettes, tea, and capsules." Journal of the American Medical Association, August 2, 1976, 473-476.

Silburn, Lilian. *Kundalini: The Energy of the Depths*. Tr. by Jacques Gontier. New York: State University of New York Press.

Smith, Bob and Linda. *Yoga For A New Age*. Seattle: Smith, 1986.

Smith, David. *The East/West Exercise Book*. New York: McGraw-Hill, 1976.

Smith, Howard. *The Sensual Explorer*. New York: G.P. Putnam's Sons, 1977.

Smith, Manuel. *Kicking The Fear Habit*. New York: Dial Press, 1977.

Stockham, Alice B. *Karezza: Ethics of Marriage*. Mokelumne Hill: Health Research.

Stone, Justin. The Joys of Meditation. Albuquerque: Sun Books, 1973.

Strange de Jim. *How To Be The World's Second Greatest Lover*. San Francisco: Ash-Kar, 1987.

Stubbs, Kenneth Ray with Louise-Andrée Saulnier. *Erotic Massage: The Touch of Love*. Larkspur: Secret Garden, 1989.

—— with Louise-Andrée Saulnier. *Romantic Interludes: A Sensuous Lovers Guide*. Larkspur: Secret Garden, 1988.

Sui, Choa Kok. *Pranic Healing*. New York: York Beach, 1990.

Svoboda, Robert. *Aghora: At the Left Hand of God*. Albuquerque: Brotherhood of Life, 1986.

Tannahill, Reay. *Sex In History*. New York: Stein and Day, 1980.

Teeguarden, Ron. *Chinese Tonic Herbs*. New York: Japan, 1985.

Thapasyogi, Guruji. *Yoga and Bhoga*. Mahabalipuram: Thapas Yoga Ashram, 1989.

Thirleby, Ashley. *Tantra: The Key to Sexual Power and Pleasure*. New York: Dell, 1978.

Thomas, P. *Kama Kalpa*. Bombay: D.B. Taraporevala Sons & Co., 1963.

Tierra, Michael. *The Way of Herbs*. Santa Cruz: Unity Press, 1980.

——. *Planetary Herbology*. Santa Fe: Lotus Press, 1988.

Van Lysebeth, Andre. *Pranayama: The Yoga of Breathing*. London: Unwin, 1979.

von Urban, Rudolf. *Sex Perfection & Marital Happiness*. New York: Dial Press, 1949.

Waldemar, Charles. *The Mystery Of Sex*. Laura and Andrew Tilburg, tr. New York: Lyle Stuart, 1960.

Walker, Morton and Joan. *Sexual Nutrition*. New York: Kensington, 1983.

Wander, Zev and David Radell. *How Big is Big?* New York: Warner Books, 1982.

Watts, Alan. *Nature, Man and Woman*. New York: Vintage, 1970.

White, John, ed. *Kundalini, Evolution and Enlightenment*. Garden City: Anchor Books, 1979.

Woods, Margo. *Masturbation, Tantra & Self Love*. San Diego: Mho and Mho Works, 1981.

Wright, Gridley Lorimer. *The Tantric Transmission of the Shivalila Kinship Society*. New Delhi: Children's Liberation Front/Allied, 1979.

Young, Lawrence and Linda, Klein, Marjorie and Donald and Beyer, Dorianne. *Recreational Drugs*. New York: Berkley Books/Macmillan, 1979.

Zilbergeld, Bernie. *Male Sexuality*. New York: Bantam, 1978.

Zitko, Howard. *New Age Tantra Yoga*. Tucson: World University Press, 1975.

INDEX

A

abstinence benefit, 296, 359
acupressure, 135-142, 169-171, 203, 204, 226, 279, 331
affirmations, 95, 96, 104, 114, 209, 228, 229, 233, 258, 266, 316
afterglow, 246-248
AIDS (*see also* sex, safer), 90, 94, 177, 184, 248, 372
allergy effect, 55, 56
Ananga Ranga, 93, 104, 190, 228
Anderiesz, Godfrey, 184
anger (*see also* fighting), 25, 88, 134, 256, 257, 277, 338, 368
anticipation effect, 166
aphrodisiacs, 56, 57
    herbal, 70-74, 149
    toxic, 74
art, 156
astrology, 168
attitude effect, 83, 118-121, 127, 128, 354, 364

B

Bach flower remedies, 259
Barbach, Lonnie, *For Yourself*, 282
bathing, sensual, 96, 136, 160
bearing down maneuver, 104, 224
Bethards, Betty, 150, 177, 221
big toe fellatio, 137, 138
Bindrim, Paul, 322
biocircuit™, 126, 127
bio-electric sex, 304-307
Blate, Michael, 136
blood flow, 107, 283, 284
boudoir, (*see also* lighting, pillow), 146-149, 153, 154, 355, 357
brain, 45, 47, 65, 82, 112, 118, 131, 165, 204, 227, 234
Brauer, Alan and Donna, 178, 189
breasts, 55, 106, 149, 169, 186
    nipples of, 165, 170, 186, 231, 240
breath, 88, 109, 113, 150, 174, 175, 200-203, 206, 207, 221-227, 244, 277, 287, 301, 346-353, 357, 364
    alternate nostril, 45, 46
    and pelvis, 85, 86
    complete, 42-46
    hara, 68-70
    holding of, 42, 43, 194
    PC clench, 78, 91, 184, 200, 207-209, 223, 224
    spoon, 201
    through nose, 48, 51, 275
    together, 145, 200-203, 215, 243
Breaux, Charles, *Journey Into Consciousness*, 76
Britton, Bryce, *The Love Muscle*, 91, 92
butterfly stretch, 87, 88

C

Castleman, Michael, 268
cat pose, 86, 87
celibacy, 94, 298, 301
cervix, 114, 278, 287, 356, 357
chakras (*see* energy centers),
Chang, Stephen, 78, 106, 107, 325-330
charge up technique, 150, 151, 302-304
Christianity, sexual tradition of, 216, 296, 300, 314,
Chuluaqui Quodoushka, Cherokee, 191, 223
circle of gold, Taoist, 122-126, 206
circle of joy, 347-351
circuits, complete, 109, 131, 203-207
clitoris, 72, 89, 98, 106, 107, 113, 169, 187-193, 196, 222, 223, 236, 237, 241, 249, 281, 287, 290, 311, 323, 342
clove oil, 100, 275
co-inspiration, 174, 200-203, 215, 333, 347-353, 357
coitus, interruptus, 95, 341, 345
    reservatus, 300, 314
    saxonus, 274
concentration, and lovemaking, 62, 92, 172, 213, 234, 277, 283, 284, 289
    during sexercises, 104, 105, 107, 108, 112-114
condoms, 94, 182, 183, 248, 275, 305
confession of affection, 22, 153, 159, 359
conservation chant, 242
consort, 21
    attracting, 41
    chemistry, 80, 132, 201, 296
contraception, barrier, 305
Cook, Keven, 67
crown, 64-66, 207-212, 244, 297
    sealing the, 205, 206, 263
crystal, use of, 94
cuddling, 300, 301
Culling, Louis, *A Manual of Sex Magic*, 73
cunnilingus, 72, 143, 184-193, 282
Cutler, Winnifred, *Menopause: A Guide for Women and the Men Who Love Them*, 82

D

damiana, 73
dancing, 84, 118, 153, 156, 166,
    belly, 287
death, 200, 266
deer exercise (*see* sexercises, Tao),
Denckla, W. Donner, 120
desire, role of, 199, 296, 332, 341, 359, 362, 367

detachment, 214, 275
Diamond, John, 227
diet, and lovemaking, 40, 54-62, 283
    and menstruation, 55, 56, 60, 61
    and prostate, 56, 58-60
    and vagina, 60-62
    vegetarian, 55, 59, 61, 71, 181
dildo, training with, 89, 93, 191, 192
Dodson, Betty, *Sex For One*, 61, 95, 96, 222
donnoi relationship, 300, 301
Dowman, Keith, *Skydancer*, 76
dream lover, 97, 156-159
drugs, 109, 140, 332, 363
    side effects of, 62, 63, 353

E

earth, 168
    and grounding, 212, 220, 221
    caring for, 35, 49, 71, 292
eduction, 159-162
Ehrlich, George, 120
ejaculation, 80-83, 99, 183, 242, 248, 332, 340-345
    and emptiness feeling, 82, 327
    multiple almost, 328-331
    voluntary, 90, 99, 103, 108, 138, 216, 228, 268-281
el besiss, 342
emotion, extremes of, 167, 168
    ritual use of, 152, 156, 355
energy, elevate, 207-213, 216, 227, 249
    level of female, 62, 289
    life, 28, 105, 122, 312, 313
energy centers, 63-66, 145, 146, 150, 157, 185, 194, 232, 264, 265, 278, 356, 357
energy field, 80, 167, 194, 221, 307, 312, 313, 351, 363
energy tools, 126, 127
erotic zones, 80, 88, 164, 165, 169-170, 185, 186
es sibfahheh, 289, 290, 292, 342, 343
exercise, 67, 68
    and ejaculation, 67, 277, 278
    and orgasm, 62, 67, 283
extrasensory sex, 144, 150, 155, 176, 302-304
eyes, contact of, 175, 200, 207
    movement of, 187, 207-209, 281

F

face, fierce, 276
fantasy (*see* visualization),
fasting, effect of, 261
fear, 25, 88, 134, 156, 259
fellatio, 72, 143, 178-182, 276
Feuerstein, Georg, *Enlightened Sexuality*, 201

fighting (*see also* anger), 198, 256, 283, 294, 307, 333, 368
fingertip Om, 175, 176
flotation tank, 47
flowers, 147, 153, 184, 356
food (*see* diet, herbs)
foot washing, 138, 153
full stop, 200, 214-216, 227, 243
fusion breath sex, 158, 346-353

G

Gandhi, Mahatma, 299
Garrison, Omar,
    Tantra: The Yoga of Sex, 304
genitals (*see* penis, vagina)
ginseng, 73, 74
god, and goddess, 21, 22, 97, 153, 155-157, 216-218, 351, 352, 354-357, 363
goddess, 185, 289, 290, 292, 307, 355, 370
    in Tantra, 216, 292, 295
    mother, 35, 212, 238
Gold, E. J. and Cybele, *Tantric Sex,* 177, 217
Gottlieb, Adam, 72
grounding, 68, 211, 212, 219-221, 244
G spot, 81, 98, 99, 182, 189-192, 238, 248, 249, 289, 290
Gunther, Bernard, 163
gypsy potency formula, 58

H

Halpern, Steven, 143-146
hara, 45, 68-70, 123, 206, 277, 297
Harris, A., *Sexual Exercises For Women,* 242
harmony signs, 130-132
health improvement, and sex, 105-109, 119-121, 327, 331, 332
heart, and feeling center, 36, 37, 155, 199, 218, 259, 270, 342
    and sex energy, 100, 186, 208, 230, 315, 321
    and thymus gland, 36, 140, 227
    opening, 25, 172-174, 232, 238, 244, 259, 356
    physical, 89, 117, 140, 212, 221
heart to heart exercise, 172-174
heart to pulse exercise, 174
Heider, John, 311
helicopter stroke, 195
herbs, aphrodisiac, 70-74, 149
Hill, Napoleon, *Think And Grow Rich,* 82
Hollander, Xaviera, *Xaviera's Supersex,* 181, 314
hormones, 107, 108, 329
horse gesture (*see* sexercise),
hypnosis, 126, 159

I

imagination (*see* visualization),
impotence, 108, 116
imsak, 280, 340-346, 359
incense, 96, 147, 148, 356
intimacy (*see also* heart), 27, 127

K

kabbazah, 91, 239, 358-363
kama salila, 190
Kama Sutra, 185, 187, 191, 224, 228, 289
karezza, 207, 313-320
kava kava, 71-73
kechari mudra (*see* tongue press),
Kegel, Arnold, 101
kegel exercise (*see* sexercises),
Kingsland, Kevin, 116
Kinsey, Alfred, 328
kissing, 130, 169, 170, 187, 188, 206, 280, 281, 296, 349
Kline-Graber and Graber, *Woman's Orgasm,* 241, 282
Koka Shastra, 186, 190
Kramer, Don, 296
Kulvinskas, Viktoras, 61
Kundalini, 65, 77, 99, 102, 104, 114, 118, 185, 191, 205, 355
    and cervix, 114
    kegel, 114-116, 200

L

Ladas, Whipple and Perry, *The G Spot,* 98
lata sadhana, 358
Leonard, George, *The End Of Sex,* 270
lighting, effect of, 66, 148, 149, 152, 153, 217, 356
lingam (*see also* penis), pleasuring of, 177-184, 236-240
    sacredness of, 177
Lloyd, J. William, *The Karezza Method,* 314, 317, 318, 332
love (*see also* heart), 127, 128, 140, 153, 160, 161, 172, 173, 176, 199, 207, 213, 227, 295, 300, 363-370
lover, archetypal, 97, 217, 218
    dream, 156-159
    inner, 97, 126
love spot, 19, 36-38, 83, 227, 228, 243, 244, 257, 261
lubricants, use and selection of, 94, 103, 178, 188, 267, 276, 287, 303

M

magnetic sex, 311-313
maithuna, 17, 356, 357
    viparita, 289

mandala, 18, 97, 234, 347, 356
mantras (*see also* sounds), 65, 66, 104, 242-245, 356, 357
marriage, renewal of, 296
massage, 135-142, 153, 160-165, 185, 193-196, 264, 280, 313
Master of the Cave Profound, 81
Masters and Johnson, 135, 282
    squeeze technique of, 279
masturbation (see *selfloving*),
McCandless, Jacquelyn, 227
meditation, 69, 124, 199, 200, 207-213, 227, 297, 304, 308, 311, 319, 347, 353, 363, 364, 367-370
    and energy centers, 65, 66, 82, 351, 356
    and orgasm, 82, 252, 253, 257-263
    and pleasure, 97, 114-116, 205
    and ritual, 65, 156, 357, 358
    and Tantra, 74-77, 114-116, 218
    and thoughts, 132-134, 228-234
    basics of, 47-54,
    Taoist, 122-126
    touch mindfulness, 77, 132-134, 213, 315, 339, 340
    with partner, 171-177, 193-196
Meister, Robert, 341
menstruation, 55, 56, 60, 61, 78, 88, 106, 107, 111, 116, 168, 290
Merrell-Wolff, Franklin, 214
mirror, use of, 61, 96, 186
Moffett, Robert, *Tantric Sex,* 6, 66
moon, 53, 168, 190, 306
motionlessness, benefit of, 234, 235, 303, 304, 359, 362
muscles, anal, 88-90, 105, 108-113, 169, 183, 184, 242, 329, 330, 363
    circumvaginal, 91-94, 283, 284, 291, 345, 358-362
    pubococcygeus (PC), 78, 101-116, 109, 154, 184, 223, 227, 239, 244, 284, 329
    smooth, 269, 270, 284
music, 66, 84, 104, 142-146, 153, 156, 172, 228, 300

N

nauli, 117, 118, 287
negative ions, 146, 147, 153
Nelson, Dee Jay, 147
nonoxynol-9, 94
nose tip, 170, 185, 186
Noyes, John, 314-317
nupercainal®, 275
nyasa, 206, 356, 357

O

oils, essential, 100, 136, 147, 149, 153, 356, 357

ojas, 83
one eye love, 172-174, 351, 357
Oneida community, 314
oneness, degrees of, 75, 353
on the verge (OTV), 183, 314,
    320-324
orgasm 100, 102, 144, 168, 204, 205,
    221-224, 228, 230, 241, 245,
    252-292
    achievement of, 90, 91, 97, 102,
    105, 111, 138, 162, 211, 259
    attitude towards, 83, 118-122,
    214
    and drugs, 62, 63, 72
    and energy level, 284, 289, 324
    and energy loss, 78-83, 126
    and nervous system, 282-284,
    311, 315, 320
    and nutrition, 56, 57, 290
    conservation of the, 78-83, 100,
    101, 119, 126, 166, 242, 264, 265,
    275, 297, 327, 332
    endless, 366-369
    extending, 183, 184, 191,
    257-263
    female, 78-80, 91, 92, 184-193,
    282-292
    fire, 191
    internal, 78, 79, 114-116, 281
    male, 182-184, 268-274
    metasexual, 264, 265
    multipe female, 79, 80, 286
    multiple male, 324, 327-329
    non-ejaculatory male, 324
    Tantric, 31-33, 65, 66, 94,
    201-203, 207, 211, 223, 227, 236,
    311-313, 346, 354, 358, 362-364
    total, 266, 267
    total relaxation, 33, 360
Otto, Herbert and Roberta, *Total Sex,*
    91

P
pair bonding and tuning, 171-177,
    353
peak experience program, 265, 266
Pearson and Shaw, *Life Extension,*
    56, 57
pelvic expression, 84-88
penis (*see also* lingam), 72, 89, 108,
    111, 113, 170, 177-184, 231-233,
    236-240, 243, 281, 303, 311, 344,
    363
perfume, 143, 147, 356
Perls, Fritz, 77
Physician's Desk Reference, 63
pills, birth control, 62, 63
pillow, big, 65, 154, 361
    crescent, 147, 288
pineal gland, 79, 83, 106, 107, 118-
    120, 137, 138, 148, 212, 226

pituitary gland, 65, 79, 83, 106, 107,
    112, 118-120, 137, 204, 212, 226
Playboy, 67
pleasure, and pain, 294, 295
poetry, use of, 153, 228, 316
pompoir (*see also* muscles), 91-93,
    239, 289, 291, 342, 344, 358-363
positions (*see also* yoga), and G spot
    stimulation, 81, 248
    carriage, 239
    cobra, 246
    cry of the eagle, 215
    es sibfahheh, 289, 292, 343
    missionary, 84, 279
    peaceful, 234-236
    prayer mat of the flesh, 254
    psychology of, 234, 235, 289,
    292
    rear entry, 249
    scissors, 236, 305, 306, 361
    seesaw, 214, 236, 247, 248
    sequence, 248, 249, 310
    sixty-nine, 131, 177, 206
    statues, 262
    surrender, 245, 247
    tension, 248-250
    viparita, 289, 292
    woman on top, 288, 289, 292
    yabyum, 65, 158, 214, 227, 248,
    263, 350, 361
    yabyum on chair, 348
pregnancy, 87, 88, 106, 117, 140, 303
prostate gland, 55-60, 73, 83, 90, 99,
    108, 111, 116, 183, 184, 269, 270,
    272-274, 329-331
    point, 99, 216, 273-275, 291
prostitute, sacred, 135, 136, 289, 290,
    292, 358, 359
psychic attunement, 167, 174, 175
pubococcygeus (PC) muscle
    (*see* muscles),
pull out, 278, 279, 341, 342
push out, 104, 224, 269, 279

R
Rajneesh (Osho), 277
Ramana Maharshi, 66
Reagan, Harley Swiftdeer, 191
Reid, Daniel, *The Tao of Health, Sex,
    and Longevity,* 60
relaxation (*see also* meditation,
    tension, yoga), 268, 307
    and release, 29, 261
    and sexercises, 103
    before making love, 144, 153,
    160-165, 280, 321
    deep, 46-50, 195
reverie state, 159, 220, 304, 321, 360
ring of calm, 17, 203, 204
ritual, 63, 65, 149, 152-156, 168, 206,
    354-358

Robinson, Jonathan, 195
roles, exchange of, 161, 162, 245, 246
romance, enhanced, 21, 22, 75, 76,
    79, 153, 160, 292, 296, 300, 304,
    313, 332, 358, 366-370
root lock (*see* sexercise),
Rosenberg, Jack, *Total Orgasm,* 84,
    266

S
sacred sexuality (*see* meditation,
    ritual, sex, Tantra, Tao, touch,
    ultra-intimacy, visualization)
safe sex (*see* AIDS, sex, safer),
samadhi, 74, 363, 364
Secrets of the Jade Bedroom, 81
selfloving, 61, 80, 95-101, 114, 218,
    271, 290, 297
    mutual, 99, 193
semen, content of, 82, 83
    recycling of, 82, 83, 242, 281,
    328
    stopping, 274
    swallowing, 181
    taste of, 55, 181
sensuality, creative, 53, 77, 134, 153,
    158-167, 290
sex (*see also* breath, heart, lingam,
    orgasm, positions, Tantra, Tao,
    yoni), and making love, 33-35,
    169, 171-177, 315, 328
    and media, 156
    and mysticism, 21-25, 38, 63-66,
    74-79, 83, 354-370
    arousal, 196, 199, 287, 308
    energy recycling, 77, 78,
    105-127
    freedom, 35, 36, 41, 128
    games, 162, 182, 196, 207, 214,
    215, 217, 264, 265, 277, 333-339
    levels of, 75, 135, 362
    natural, 296
    safer, 94, 182-184, 248, 267, 300,
    301
    therapy, 282
    timing of, 167-168, 296, 306
sexercises (*see also* breath, muscles,
    pompoir, visualization), 93-118
    and health, 59, 60, 62, 78, 83, 92,
    105-109, 117, 289
    and personal growth, 105-107
    deer, female, 105-107
    deer, male, 107-109, 328-331
    during intercourse, 93, 269, 330
    horse gesture 110, 111,
    Kegel, 60, 92, 96, 101-105, 269,
    283
    root lock, 111, 112, 361
    stomach lift, 116-118
    thunderbolt gesture, 112-113,
    269, 361

sexual energy ecstasy, 15-17, 76, 296
styles of, 127, 298, 299
workshop, 84, 102, 104, 195, 268, 302, 358
Shakespeare, 142
Shakti, 125, 289, 292, 295, 354-358
shambhavi mudra (see also third eye), 114
Shankaracharya, 369
Shiva, 66, 177, 289, 295, 354-358
Shivanandan, Mary, 296
slow motion, 339, 340
smell, sense of, 64, 130, 131, 356
Smith, Jr., Howard, 149
snapping pussy, 91
soaking, 236-240
Society for Clinical Ecology, 55
soft entry, 276, 303
solar plexus, 64, 100, 196, 208, 222, 223, 245, 339
peace exercise, 171-174
sounds, making of (see also mantra), 65, 66, 97, 224, 225, 240-245, 277, 278
spine, 71, 86, 116, 208
and sex energy, 77-79, 108, 112, 212, 226, 227, 347, 357
heating of, 170, 174
spreading technique, 127, 182, 193-196, 297, 321
Sri Da Kalki (Heart Master Da Loveananda), 66
Stockham, Alice, 313-317
Stone, Justin, The Joys Of Meditation, 122
Strange de Jim, 264
stress effect, 40, 82
stuffing, 302
Sufi tradition, 177
Sun, Master, 320
Sun, Patricia, 61
Sundar, 236
Su Nui Ching, 325, 331
symbol, mystical, 18, 97, 310, 356

T

t'ai chi, 18-20, 310, 347
Tantra, 63-66, 134, 137, 145, 156, 158, 206, 289, 292, 361-365, 369, 370
and orgasm, 31-33, 79-83, 94, 99-101, 176, 201-203, 236, 242, 267, 361, 364
Buddhist, 74, 76, 155, 218, 243, 354
contemporary, 157, 201-203, 236-240, 307, 333-339, 346-353
global practice of, 295
Hindu, 66, 74-77, 147, 149, 169, 177, 185, 216, 244, 354, 358
tenets of, 23-25, 122, 128, 289, 290, 292, 295, 354, 363

yoga, 45-47, 83, 109-118, 121, 144, 205, 249, 250, 269, 357
Tao, way of the, (see also T'ai chi), 18-20, 121, 122, 135, 219, 310, 347
and female, 78, 79, 95, 184, 185, 188, 275, 276, 281, 325-327
and orgasm, 78-82, 274, 325-332
sexology of, 105-109, 167-171, 184, 185, 275-281, 324-332, 344
yoga of, 67, 105-109, 120-126, 206, 213, 219, 220, 281
teasing, 166, 191, 192, 287, 341
techniques (see breath, muscles, orgasm, penis, sounds, Tantra, Tao, vagina, visualization)
tension, voluntary, 261, 263, 264, 345
testicle tug, 280
testosterone, 67, 120
third eye, 64, 65, 157, 158, 194, 196, 210, 217, 231, 234, 244, 265, 333, 339, 354, 356, 357, 364
and orgasm, 83, 100, 297
and psychic rapport, 174, 357
and sex energy meditation, 114-116, 155, 209
thought, management of, 132-134, 165-167, 228, 229, 244, 258, 316, 356, 357, 359
thrusting sequence, 281, 332, 344
thunderbolt gesture (see sexercise),
thymus gland, 36, 106, 227, 228, 243, 257, 281
tide of yin, 189, 282
Tierra, Michael, Planetary Herbology, 60
tiger tonic, Ellen's, 57, 58
Tolstoi, Leo, 313
tongue press, 114, 203-206, 208, 209, 224, 227, 242, 281, 349, 351
touch, 77, 160, 165, 166, 194, 206, 207, 296, 297, 312, 315, 316, 345
and sensory present, 134, 213, 214, 221, 228, 340
inner sense of, 15, 21, 77, 210-213, 312
just, 77, 134, 213-216
penetrating, 233, 234, 320, 323
toy, sex, (see dildo,vibrator)
trespasso exercise, 175
triple tuner exercise series, 172-174
turtle stretch, 281
Tzu, Lao, 332

U

ultra-intimacy, 20, 127, 128, 229, 256, 313, 319, 358, 359, 363,
unity, experience of, (see also meditation, orgasm) 32, 75, 172, 239, 256, 313, 314, 347, 349, 353, 354, 358, 364

V

vagina (see also muscles, yoni), 229-231, 236-240, 243, 284, 303
healing of, 56, 60-62, 92
nectar from, 185, 281
pleasuring, 184-193, 281
secretions of, 55, 242
sensitizing, 92, 289
vampirism, sexual, 79
vibrator, use of, 89, 90, 96, 99, 182, 188, 191, 284
visualization (see also meditation), 54, 155-159, 220, 225, 232-234, 253, 254, 269, 304, 305, 346-353
and fantasy, 97, 126, 157-159, 216-218, 229-232
and Kundalini, 114-116
and sexercises, 92, 104, 105, 284
before making love, 150-152, 165-167, 234, 287, 312
lingam and yoni, 231, 236-240
of light, 147, 209-213, 220, 232, 233, 320-322, 351, 352, 364
Tantric, 24, 65, 66, 155, 201-203, 216-218, 333-339, 354-358, 363, 364
Taoist, 122-126, 219
vitamins, 56, 57
von Urban, Rudolf, Sex Perfection & Marital Happiness, 304-307

W

Walker and Walker, Sexual Nutrition, 56
war and peace, 307-310
West, Mae, 291
woman, wild, 292
womb gesture, 205
Woods, Margo, Masturbation, Tantra, and Self Love, 99

Y

Yellow Emperor's Classic, 324
yoga (see also Tantra), 45, 46, 75-77, 86-88, 106, 108, 109-118, 283
positions, 86-88, 116, 118, 153, 195, 208, 249, 250
sexercises, 109-118, 153
yogini, 202, 346
yohimbine, 74
yoni (see also vagina), 184-194, 232, 236-240, 357, 364
yoni mudra, 205

Z

Zen, 69, 264
Zilbergeld, Bernie, 268
zinc, 56, 57
Zitko, Howard John, 206

AFTER YOU READ THIS BOOK

Sacred sexuality is an intuitive experience, not a technique. You may find it very helpful to participate in a group with like-minded people who, like yourself, are eager to open to the higher possibilities of their erotic potential. We offer trainings at several levels, ranging from the introductory SEXUAL ENERGY ECSTASY® and LOVE FIRE ORGASM courses to advanced week-long retreats once a year. The introductory courses are regularly offered at several locations around the country.

While our trainings emphasize rich, liberating experiences, not dry theory, we feel it is very important to honor the sacredness of the individual. Our seminars do not involve nudity, orgies, bizarre rituals or other activities that might offend you. We simply share how the pleasure of union with a beloved can expand into the ecstasy of oneness.

Practical courses on sexual healing, erotic massage, loving relationships, goddess wisdom, men's liberation and many other contemporary issues are offered at our centers or by an instructor in our national network. We also offer a wide variety of educational books, audio and video tapes and sensual products to enhance your sacred lovemaking.

We offer our personal insights about sacred sexuality in the following instructional tapes. On audio: *Zen Sex I & II, The Secret of Sexual Satisfaction, Working with Sex Energy, Your Relationship—Your Mirror* and *Tantra—Bliss of Reality*. On video: *Tantra Love—Eastern Secrets of Intimacy and Ecstasy for Western Lovers* (with Kevin Kreisler, M.D.).

If you would like to receive information about our seminars and courses and/or our sacred sexuality products, write us at the address below. Please enclose a self-addressed stamped envelope with your request.

Attn: David Ramsdale
c/o Bantam Books
1540 Broadway
New York, NY 10036

ABOUT THE AUTHORS

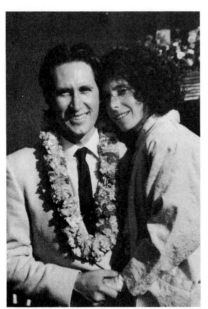

Photo credit: Lee Perry

David A. Ramsdale, M.A., has a gift for taking people beyond their ordinary expectations and experiences of sexuality. In his private practice he educates and counsels individuals and couples in the sacred sexual rituals of the East, including ancient Tantric and Taoist methods. A member of the Society for the Scientific Study of Sex, he has a B.A. in Psychology and an M.A. in Humanities/Philosophy.

Ellen Ramsdale is a talented ceramic sculptor, artist, massage therapist, and vegetarian cook. She received her B.A. in Studio Art from the University of California, Santa Barbara. She is especially interested in helping to heal and empower women through sacred sexuality and goddess wisdom practices.

Inspired by their sexual experiences of a higher consciousness, they meditate regularly and do T'ai Chi and hatha yoga. They believe that meditation or an equivalent practice helps lovers to remain relaxed while aroused and to reach higher levels of sexual rapture together.

Married in 1987, David and Ellen Ramsdale have appeared on numerous radio and TV shows, incuding "People Are Talking" and "A Current Affair." Articles featuring their work have appeared in *The San Francisco Examiner, The Wall Street Journal,* and the book *Enlightened Sexuality.*

In addition to *Sexual Energy Ecstasy,* the Ramsdales are the authors, with Kevin Kreisler, M.D., of the video "Tantra Love: Eastern Secrets of Intimacy and Ecstasy for Western Lovers" and of the audiotapes "Tantra—Bliss of Reality," "Zen Sex," "Your Relationship—Your Mirror," "The Secret of Sexual Satisfaction," and "Working with Sex Energy."